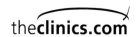

CLINICS IN
CHEST MEDICINE

Contemporary Chest Imaging
GUEST EDITOR
David A. Lynch, MD

March 2008 • Volume 29 • Number 1

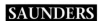

An Imprint of Elsevier, Inc.
PHILADELPHIA   LONDON   TORONTO   MONTREAL   SYDNEY   TOKYO

W.B. SAUNDERS COMPANY

A Division of Elsevier Inc.

Elsevier Inc. • 1600 John F. Kennedy Boulevard • Suite 1800 • Philadelphia, Pennsylvania 19103-2899

http://www.chestmed.theclinics.com

CLINICS IN CHEST MEDICINE
March 2008
Editor: Sarah E. Barth

Volume 29, Number 1
ISSN 0272-5231
ISBN-13: 978-1-4160-5866-3
ISBN-10: 1-4160-5866-4

Reprints: For copies of 100 or more, of articles in this publication, please contact the Commercial Reprints Department, Elsevier Inc., 360 Park Avenue South, New York, New York 10010-1710. Tel. (212) 633-3813; Fax: (212) 462-1935; e-mail: reprints@elsevier.com.

The ideas and opinions expressed in *Clinics in Chest Medicine* do not necessarily reflect those of the Publisher. The Publisher does not assume any responsibility for any injury and/or damage to persons or property arising out of or related to any use of the material contained in this periodical. The reader is advised to check the appropriate medial literature and the product information currently provided by the manufacturer of each drug to be administered to verify the dosage, the method and duration of administration, or contraindications. It is the responsibility of the treating physician or other health care professional, relying on independent experience and knowledge of the patient, to determine drug dosages and the best treatment for the patient. Mention of any product in this issue should not be construed as endorsement by the contributors, editors, or the Publisher of the product or manufacturers' claims.

Clinics in Chest Medicine (ISSN 0272-5231) is published quarterly by Elsevier Inc., 360 Park Avenue South, New York, NY 10010-1710. Months of issue are March, June, September, and December. Business and Editorial Offices: 1600 John F. Kennedy Blvd., Suite 1800, Philadelphia, PA 19103-2899. Customer Service Office: 6277 Sea Harbor Drive, Orlando, FL 32887-4800. Periodicals postage paid at New York, NY and additional mailing offices. Subscription prices are $232.00 per year (US individuals), $370.00 per year (US institutions), $113.00 per year (US students), $255.00 per year (Canadian individuals), $444.00 per year (Canadian institutions), $149.00 per year (Canadian students), $297.00 per year (international individuals) $444.00 per year (international institutions), and $149.00 per year (international students). International air speed delivery is included in all *Clinics* subscription prices. All prices are subject to change without notice. **POSTMASTER:** Send address changes to *Clinics in Chest Medicine,* Elsevier Periodicals Customer Service, 6277 Sea Harbor Drive, Orlando, FL 32887-4800. Customer Service: 1-800-654-2452 (US). From outside the United States, call 1-407-563-6020. Fax: 1-407-363-9661. E-mail: JournalsCustomerService-usa@elsevier.com.

Clinics in Chest Medicine is covered in *Index Medicus, Current Contents/Clinical Medicine, EMBASE/Excerpta Medica, Science Citation Index,* and *ISI/BIOMED.*

Printed in the United States of America.

GUEST EDITOR

DAVID A. LYNCH, MD, Professor, Division of Radiology, National Jewish Medical and Research Center, Denver, Colorado

CONTRIBUTORS

DENISE R. ABERLE, MD, Professor of Radiology and Bioengineering; and Vice Chair of Research, Department of Radiological Sciences, David Geffen School of Medicine, University of California, Los Angeles, Los Angeles, California

MASANORI AKIRA, MD, PhD, Chief, Department of Radiology, Kinki Cuo Chest Medical Center, Sakai City, Osaka, Japan

PHILLIP M. BOISELLE, MD, Director, Thoracic Imaging; and Associate Chief of Administrative Affairs; and Associate Professor of Radiology, Department of Radiology, Beth Israel Deaconess Medical Center, Harvard Medical School, Boston Massachusetts

SAMUEL BRAFF, MD, Clinical Instructor in Surgery, Fletcher Allen Health Care; University of Vermont College of Medicine, Burlington, Vermont

KATHLEEN BROWN, MD, Professor of Radiology, Department of Radiological Sciences, David Geffen School of Medicine, University of California, Los Angeles, Los Angeles, California

SUJAL R. DESAI, MD, FRCP, FRCR, Consultant Radiologist, Department of Radiology, King's College Hospital, London, United Kingdom

JEREMY J. ERASMUS, MBBCh, Professor of Radiology, Division of Diagnostic Imaging, University of Texas, MD Anderson Cancer Center, Houston, Texas

LAWRENCE R. GOODMAN, MD, FACR, Professor of Radiology, Department of Radiology, Medical College of Wisconsin, Milwaukee, Wisconsin

MELTEM GULSUN AKPINAR, MD, Visiting Associate Professor of Radiology, Department of Radiology, Medical College of Wisconsin, Milwaukee, Wisconsin; Associate Professor of Radiology, Department of Radiology, Hacettepe University Faculty of Medicine, Sihhiye, Ankara, Turkey

JOSHUA R. HILL, MD, Resident Physician, Department of Radiology, Oregon Health and Science University, Portland, Oregon

ERIC A. HOFFMAN, PhD, Professor of Radiology, Medicine and Biomedical Engineering, Department of Radiology, Carver College of Medicine, University of Iowa, Iowa City, Iowa

PEDER E. HORNER, MD, Fellow, Vascular and Interventional Radiology, Dotter Interventional Institute, Oregon Health and Science University, Portland, Oregon

TAKESHI JOHKOH, MD, PhD, Department of Radiology, Kinki Central Hospital of Mutual Aid Association of Public School Teachers, Itami, Hyogo, Japan

KIRK JORDAN, MD, Assistant Professor, Department of Radiology, University of Texas Southwestern Medical Center at Dallas, Dallas, Texas

LOREN KETAI, MD, Professor, Department of Radiology, University of New Mexico Health Science Center, Albuquerque, New Mexico

JEFFREY S. KLEIN, MD, A. Bradley Soule and John P. Tampas Green and Gold Professor of Radiology; and Associate Dean for Continuing Medical Education, University of Vermont College of Medicine; Chief of Thoracic Radiology, Fletcher Allen Health Care, Burlington, Vermont

DAVID A. LYNCH, MD, Professor, Division of Radiology, National Jewish Medical and Research Center, Denver, Colorado

EDITH M. MAROM, MD, Associate Professor, Department of Diagnostic Imaging, University of Texas, MD Andersen Cancer Center, Houston, Texas

STEVEN L. PRIMACK, MD, Professor of Radiology; and Vice Chairman, Department of Radiology; and Professor of Medicine, Division of Pulmonary Medicine, Oregon Health and Science University, Portland, Oregon

BRADLEY S. SABLOFF, MD, Associate Professor of Radiology, Division of Diagnostic Imaging, University of Texas, MD Anderson Cancer Center, Houston, Texas

ATHOL U. WELLS, MD, FRACP, FRCR, Professor and Head of Department, Royal Brompton Hospital, London, United Kingdom

FELIX WOODHEAD, MBBChir, MRCP, Specialist Registrar, Royal Brompton Hospital, Sydney Street, London, United Kingdom

EDWIN J.R. VAN BEEK, MD, PhD, FRCR, Professor of Radiology, Medicine and Biomedical Engineering, Department of Radiology, Carver College of Medicine, University of Iowa, Iowa City, Iowa

CONTENTS

FORTHCOMING ISSUES

RECENT ISSUES

CLINICS
IN CHEST
MEDICINE

Clin Chest Med 29 (2008) ix–x

Preface

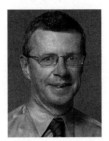

David A. Lynch, MD
Guest Editor

Since the last issue of *Clinics in Chest Medicine* dedicated to chest imaging, published in 1999, the field has expanded at an extraordinary pace. For example, CT angiography is accepted now as the primary tool for evaluation of pulmonary embolism, CT-positron emission tomography is established as an excellent technique for the diagnosis and staging of lung cancer, and high resolution CT plays a pivotal role in the diagnosis and classification of diffuse lung diseases. In this issue, our readers are fortunate that international leaders in thoracic radiology have agreed to provide up-to-date authoritative reviews of important topics for the pulmonologist.

This issue begins with three articles discussing lung cancer. Drs. Aberle and Brown deliver a scientific assessment of the role of CT and other techniques in screening for lung cancer. Drs. Klein and Braff provide a rational approach to the use of imaging in the evaluation of the solitary pulmonary nodule identified on chest radiograph or CT. Drs. Erasmus and Sabloff share their rich experience in the use of imaging to stage lung cancer.

Critical care imaging, pneumonia, and pulmonary embolism remain primary concerns for the hospital based physician. Drs. Hill, Horner, and Primack provide a practical and well-illustrated guide to the imaging evaluation of the critically ill patient. Drs. Ketai, Jordan, and Marom provide a comprehensive discussion of the imaging features of infection in normal and immunocompromised hosts. Drs. Akpinar and Goodman discuss the imaging diagnosis of pulmonary thromboembolism in the light of the recent Prospective Investigation of Pulmonary Embolism Diagnosis II trial.

Imaging often is pivotal in the diagnosis of diffuse lung diseases. Dr. Akira provides a unique perspective on the radiographic and CT features of common and uncommon occupational and environmental lung diseases. Dr. Johkoh illustrates and discusses the radiologic and pathologic features of idiopathic interstitial pneumonias. Drs. Woodhead, Wells, and Desai provide a clinically focused discussion of the pulmonary complications of connective tissue diseases. My article discusses the value of CT in diagnosis and differential diagnosis of small airways diseases. This is complemented by Dr. Boiselle's elegant demonstration of the use of multi-dimensional imaging in diagnosis of large airways disease. Drs. VanBeek and Hoffman conclude the issue by describing the state of the art evaluation of regional and global pulmonary function by CT and MRI.

doi:10.1016/j.ccm.2007.12.004

chestmed.theclinics.com

It has been an honor to participate with this outstanding group of authors, and I have been educated by reading their contributions. I am very excited about the quality of their articles, and my sincere thanks are due to them. Thanks also to Sarah Barth and Patrick Manley at Elsevier, who were very helpful in ensuring compliance with deadlines and production of this high-quality book. I hope that this snapshot of contemporary chest imaging will be of value to pulmonologists, radiologists, and others dedicated to the daily care of patients who have pulmonary disease.

David A. Lynch, MD
Division of Radiology
National Jewish Medical and Research Center
1400 Jackson Street
Denver, CO 80206, USA

E-mail address: lynchd@njc.org

ELSEVIER SAUNDERS

Clin Chest Med 29 (2008) 1–14

CLINICS IN CHEST MEDICINE

Lung Cancer Screening with CT

Denise R. Aberle, MD*, Kathleen Brown, MD

Department of Radiological Sciences, David Geffen School of Medicine, University of California, Los Angeles, 924 Westwood Boulevard, Suite 420, Los Angeles, CA 90024, USA

Lung cancer is the leading cause of cancer death in the United States. In 2007, it is estimated that 160,390 lung cancer deaths will occur in the United States, representing 29% of all cancer deaths [1]. Roughly 87% of lung cancers are attributed to cigarette smoking [2]. Although cancer risk is attenuated by smoking cessation, the risk is not eliminated, and lung cancer now occurs with equal frequency in current and former smokers [3]. Moreover, other factors clearly influence risk, including age; family history; chronic obstructive pulmonary disease; pulmonary fibrosis; and exposures to environmental radon, asbestos, and certain other occupational agents [4]. Realistically, lung cancer will likely remain at epidemic proportions for decades to come.

Non–small cell lung cancer (NSCLC), which accounts for 75% to 80% of all lung cancers, is typically diagnosed when disease is locally advanced or there are systemic metastases [5], explaining the dismal overall 5-year survival of 15% [6]. In contrast, the 5-year survival of individuals with surgically resected, early stage NSCLC approaches 75% [6,7]. These differences have fueled the impetus to find a screening test that can detect NSCLC in its early preclinical stages, when surgical resection is most likely to prolong life and potentially reduce lung cancer mortality. Although earlier randomized controlled trials (RCTs) of lung cancer screening using chest radiography and sputum cytology failed to show reduced lung cancer mortality, CT is a much more sensitive test for detecting small lung nodules, and has generated considerable enthusiasm as a potential contemporary screening tool for lung cancer.

Results of observational trials with low-dose helical CT

There are now published results of several cohort studies [8–18] investigating CT screening in groups at varying risk of lung cancer. The first published American study was the Early Lung Cancer Action Program (ELCAP) [8,9]. In this observational study, 1000 individuals aged 60 years or greater with a minimum 10 pack-year smoking history underwent prevalence screening; 841 underwent at least one incidence (annual repeat) screen. At the prevalence screen, 233 nodules and 31 lung cancers were detected (27 lung cancers based on the detection of a nodule and 4, which were excluded from analysis, based on the detection of mediastinal or airway lesions). Twenty-three (85%) of the 27 nodular lung cancers were stage I. On annual follow-up, there were seven incidence cancers and two interval cancers not detected by screening; of these nine cancers, five (56%) were stage I NSCLC. In this study, both CT and chest radiographs (CXR) were obtained on participants; three times more nodules and four times more lung cancers were detected by CT than by CXR [8].

Swensen and colleagues [10] recently reported their 5-year results on combined CT and sputum screening in 1520 high-risk individuals aged 50 years or older with a smoking history of greater than 20 pack-years. This cohort underwent four incidence (annual repeat) screenings; compliance rates were 95% or greater through the first three incidence screens and 80% for the final incidence screen at year 5. They observed 68 primary lung cancers in 66 participants (4% of participants

* Corresponding author.

E-mail address: daberle@mednet.ucla.edu (D.R. Aberle).

doi:10.1016/j.ccm.2007.12.001

and 2% of 3356 nodules), consisting of 31 prevalence, 34 incidence, and 3 interval cancers. Two
cancers were detected only by sputum cytology.
Of prevalence cancers, 71% were stage I; 49%
of combined incidence and interval cancers were
stage I. There was one postsurgical mortality in
a lung cancer patient. Thirteen participants underwent 15 surgeries for ultimately benign disease.
Although no surgical deaths were reported in individuals with ultimately benign disease, the rates of
unnecessary thoracotomies has raised concerns
about the potential for screening-related harms.

Three major cohort studies using different
clinical protocols have investigated low-dose helical CT screening in Japan [11–13]. Sobue and colleagues [13] performed both CT and combined
CXR with sputum cytology on 1611 participants.
In this study, CT detected fourfold more lung cancers than CXR across all screenings. Two studies
performed unselected population screening in
smokers and nonsmokers aged 40 years and older
[11,12]. In these two studies, lung cancer prevalence rates were low (averaging 0.4%); however,
roughly equal numbers of lung cancers were seen
in smokers and nonsmokers. The prevalence rates
of lung cancer in nonsmoking women averaged
0.44% and most were indolent bronchioloalveolar
cell carcinomas or well-differentiated adenocarcinomas; these detection rates represent a 10- to
15-fold increase over annual mortality rates in
Japanese women. Detection rates of lung cancer
in smoking men using CT screening were also increased by 2- to 15-fold [11].

Diederich and colleagues [14,15] reported their
findings with low-dose screening CT in a cohort
study of 817 smokers aged 40 and older in Europe. Of the original cohort, 668 participants
(81.8%) underwent at least one of five annual incidence (follow-up) screens. At prevalence screen,
they observed 858 indeterminate nodules in 408
participants (50%), of which more than 98%
were deemed benign based on follow-up or biopsy. There were 12 prevalence lung cancers in
11 participants (1.3% prevalence), of which 7
were stage I. At incidence screens, 174 new nodules were observed; over 93% were deemed benign. A total of 21 suspicious incidence nodules
(11 growing nodules and 10 new nodules) underwent additional diagnostic evaluation. Incidence
lung cancers were diagnosed in 11 (incidence of
0.86%), benign disease in 8, and in 2 nodules histology was indeterminate because biopsy was
refused (one patient with bladder cancer, one patient with growth of a nodule from 4–6 mm over

36 months). Five interval cancers were diagnosed
between annual screens, only one of which had
abnormalities visible on retrospective review of
screening CT, in the form of a hilar mass. Overall,
they reported that 26.7% of invasive procedures
were for benign disease, including one thoraco-
scopy and one thoracotomy.

The findings of Diederich and colleagues [14,15]
were consonant with prior observational studies in
that (1) a large number of nodules are seen at prevalence (baseline) and incidence screens using low-
dose CT, of which less than 10% represents lung
cancer; (2) using standardized diagnostic algorithms, the number of invasive procedures can be
minimized; and (3) nodules with documented
growth should undergo additional diagnostic testing, although benign disease is ultimately found
even in growing nodules. The conclusions of Diederich and colleagues [14,15] differed from the
American and Japanese trials in that they observed
that one third of lung cancers diagnosed after the
baseline examination were interval cancers (between screenings) because of symptoms; and their
lung cancers were not disproportionately adenocarcinomas, as reported elsewhere (rather, their
patients had relatively greater numbers of both
squamous cell and small cell carcinomas). From
these data, the number of early stage lung cancers
is higher with CT screening; however, the impact
of screening on lowering the number of late-stage
cancers is not clear.

Findings from preliminary randomized controlled trials

Preliminary data from four RCTs using CT
screening in the intervention arm have been
published [16–19]. Three of these trials were conducted in advance of large multicenter national trials to determine the feasibility of enrollment into
a randomized trial by generalists [16–18]. The Depiscan, conducted in France, involved 765 subjects
randomized to receive either low-dose CT or CXR
at baseline and annually for 2 years. Complete clinical and imaging baseline data were obtained in
81% of patients. One or more nodules were seen
in 336 participants (45.2%) in the CT arm versus
21 participants (7.4%) in the CXR arm. Eight
lung cancers were detected in the low-dose CT
arm versus one in the CXR arm. Trial limitations
included a 19% rate of noncompliance by participants who withdrew consent and only modest par-
ticipation of the enrolling generalists (only 41% of
232 investigators enrolled participants).

In 2003, the NELSON trial was launched, a Dutch-Belgian trial that randomized roughly 16,000 high-risk participants to receive either annual CT screening (at years 1, 2, and 4) versus a control arm receiving no screening [19]. The NELSON is the only trial in which the control arm receives no screening intervention, and has 80% power to show a lung cancer mortality reduction of at least 25% by 10 years after randomization. The data from the NELSON will be pooled with the Danish RCT; preliminary data are pending.

Gohagan and colleagues [18], representing the Lung Screening Study Research Group, reported the final results of the Lung Screening Study, in which 3318 individuals at high risk of lung cancer were equally randomized to receive either low-dose CT or CXR for two annual screenings. The study was not powered to address differential lung cancer mortality between the two arms, but rather, whether a large-scale multicenter randomized trial was feasible in the United States. Compliance rates at baseline and year 1 screenings were 96% and 86% for CT and 93% and 80% for CXR, indicating that a RCT was possible in the United States. Positive screens were seen in 20% and 10% of baseline CT and CXR screened participants, respectively, and in 18% and 7% of incidence screens. Over the study period, there were 40 CT-detected lung cancers and 20 CXR-detected lung cancers; stage I cancers comprised 48% of all CT-detected cancers and 40% of CXR-detected cancers.

Newest data from cohort studies

Two recent studies have further confounded the subject of the benefit of CT screening. The first was the report of the International-ELCAP (I-ELCAP), a multinational, observational study undertaken in the United States, Europe, Japan, and Israel in which 31,567 participants underwent prevalence screens and 27,456 incidence screens [20]. Each site determined its own eligibility criteria, which included smokers, never smokers, and individuals with exposures to various environmental and occupational carcinogens. Lung cancer was diagnosed in 484 participants: 405 at prevalence screen, 74 at incidence screen, and 5 interval cancers (eg, symptom-detected). Of these, 412 were clinical stage I; pathologic stage was not reported. Participants were followed for a median of 3.3 years; two participants were followed for 10 years. Using Kaplan-Meyer estimates, the 10-year

lung cancer–specific survival for all participants was 80% (95% confidence interval [CI], 74%–85%); among the 302 participants who underwent resection within 1 month of diagnosis, the estimated lung cancer–specific 10-year survival was 92% (95% CI, 88%–95%). Eight untreated lung cancer patients died within 5 years of diagnosis. Based on these survival statistics, the investigators concluded that such screening could "prevent some 80% of deaths" from lung cancer.

Subsequent to the I-ELCAP report, Bach and colleagues [21] described their findings in 3246 asymptomatic, high-risk individuals who underwent at least three annual CT screenings after a median follow-up of 3.9 years. They compared observed lung cancer rates, stages, surgical resections, and deaths with what would have occurred absent screening based on a set of validated prediction models [22,23]. They observed 144 individuals with lung cancer compared with 44.5 predicted cases (relative risk, 3.2), among whom 42 had advanced-stage disease versus 33.4 predicted. There were 109 individuals who underwent lung resection, representing a 10-fold increase over the expected number of surgeries. Lung cancer mortality was unchanged: 38 lung cancer deaths were observed, 38.8 were predicted. They concluded that CT screening might increase the rate of lung cancer detection and treatment without reducing the number of advanced lung cancers or lung cancer mortality, calling into question the benefit of CT screening in face of possible risk. The authors rightfully acknowledged that their data were preliminary, predicated on a small sample and on the validity of their risk model and assumptions. Nonetheless, their findings contrast with those of the I-ELCAP and underscore a quintessential concern in the discussion of lung cancer screening: the I-ELCAP reported increased survival; Bach and colleagues [21] reported no difference in mortality. At the heart of screening debate is the question of which end point provides adequate validation of the efficacy of CT screening for lung cancer.

Survival versus mortality end points in screening

At face value, increased lung cancer survival seems to be synonymous with decreased lung cancer mortality. Yet, such is not the case. Lung cancer survival is appropriately an end point in controlled trials that compare different treatment interventions. Under these conditions, the diagnosis of the disease precedes the intervention and all patients have the disease. In the case of screening, the individuals undergoing the screening intervention are asymptomatic, relatively few actually have the disease, and the screening intervention precedes the diagnosis. These differences place screening interventions in a profoundly different paradigm than treatment interventions because some healthy individuals become patients because of a positive screen, resulting in collective psychologic, economic, and medical jeopardy. Moreover, this paradigm introduces confounding variables that make disease-specific survival misrepresentative of screening efficacy: the biases of lead time, length, and overdiagnosis. Each of these can prolong survival without actually enhancing longevity, to produce an artificial semblance of benefit where none may exist [24–26].

Lead time bias refers to the fact that with screening, earlier detection increases survival time even if death is not delayed (Fig. 1A). Survival is measured from the time of lung cancer diagnosis or the initiation of treatment, events that are usually temporally proximate. To the extent that the time of diagnosis is advanced (lead time) by screening relative to symptom-diagnosed lung cancer, and assuming that early treatment intervention is not lethal, survival will increase even if death is not delayed. In point of fact, the early detection of lung cancer may favorably alter the natural course of disease by delaying death (eg, increase longevity). However, the phenomena of lead time and increased longevity are indistinguishable by survival statistics, particularly in a cancer with so heterogeneous a biology as lung cancer, because the rate of disease progression is not known.

The second bias that confounds the use of survival as a measure of efficacy is length bias. The purpose of lung cancer screening is to detect malignancy when it is preclinical, before the development of overt symptoms, providing the opportunity for treatment intervention that prevents or delays death. There is clear evidence that lung cancer is not the product of one single molecular construct: there is considerable variation in lung cancer growth rates, as has been amply demonstrated by several observed phenomena: by calculations of tumor doubling time using CT [27,28], by the propensity of a subset of pathologic stage IA lung cancers to recur following presumed curative surgery [29,30], and by the indolent growth characteristics of certain subtypes of adenocarcinoma [31,32]. Effectively, some lung cancers are biologically indolent and grow slowly; some lung cancers are biologically aggressive and grow and metastasize rapidly. Length bias refers to the tendency of

screening tests preferentially to select for more indolent lung cancers because of their longer preclinical phase (Fig. 1B). Aggressive cancers are less likely to be screen-detected because they have a shorter preclinical phase. As such, the survival of individuals with screen-detected lung cancers predictably is longer than that of individuals with symptom-detected lung cancers of the same stage. Similarly, if two screening tests are compared, the more sensitive screening test should detect more favorable (indolent) cancers than the less sensitive screening test.

The third bias peculiar to screening interventions is overdiagnosis bias, which can be considered an extreme form of length bias (Fig. 1C). Overdiagnosis bias refers to the screening detection of cancers that would not have contributed to the death of an individual (pseudodisease) [24–26]. Overdiagnosis can occur when screening detects a potentially lethal lung cancer, the course of which is superseded by competing comorbidities, such as chronic obstructive pulmonary disease and cardiovascular disease, conditions that are prevalent in lung cancer patients and may result in death before demise from lung cancer. Overdiagnosis also occurs when screening detects a lung cancer that satisfies histologic criteria of malignancy, but that is so biologically indolent that it never contributes to death. This concept is well established as a consideration in prostate carcinoma screening [33–35], but has been relatively ignored in lung cancer because of the high lethality of most symptom-detected cancers.

It is rarely possible to document pseudodisease in a living individual; once detected by screening, treatment is initiated, and longevity with later death from unrelated causes is ascribed to the successful treatment. In the I-ELCAP study, eight participants with clinical stage I cancers who did not receive treatment died within 5 years of diagnosis [36]. Although it is tempting to infer from this that pseudodisease is not a significant factor in lung cancer, it is not possible to draw meaningful conclusions, both because the numbers are so small and because the factors that prevented primary treatment intervention (access to health care, comorbidity, emotional state) also will influence survival.

The documentation of pseudodisease in lung cancer derives from necropsy studies in which unsuspected (surprise) lung cancers were observed in individuals who died of other causes. In a review of necropsies performed at Yale New Haven Hospital over a 30-year period, surprise lung cancers represented 13% of all lung cancers observed [37].

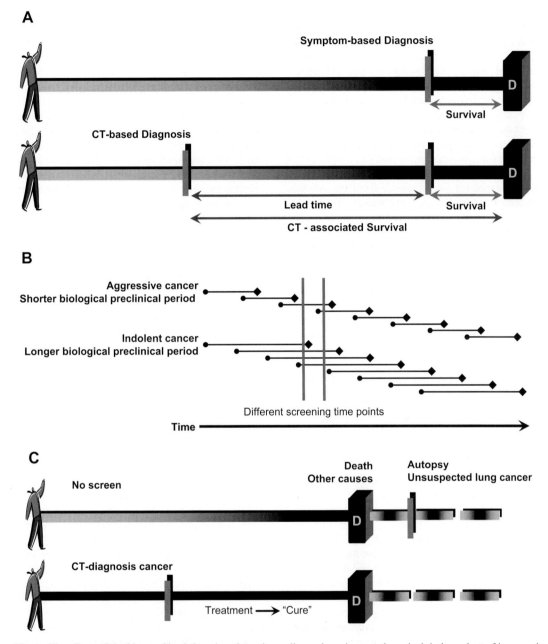

Fig. 1. The effects of the biases of lead time, length, and overdiagnosis on increased survival, independent of improved longevity or mortality reduction. (*A*) Lead time from the early detection of a lung cancer by screening prolongs survival independent of any delay in death. (*B*) Screen-detected lung cancers tend to be more indolent than symptom-detected or intervals cancers diagnosed between screenings. The survival benefit associated with these favorable cancers is ascribed to the screening test, even if screening does nothing to reduce the number of advanced-stage cancers or lung cancer deaths. (*C*) The pseudodisease detected because of overdiagnosis bias markedly increases survival, regardless of whether screening or associated treatments are effective.

Over the 30 years, the total number of surprise lung cancers increased; moreover, the proportion of resectable lung cancers in the surprise cases rose from 35% in the first decade to 70% in the third and final decade. The investigators postulated that necropsy documents a large reservoir of undetected lung cancers in the general population and that future advances in diagnostic technology would most certainly result in increased numbers of detected early stage lung cancers during life and would improve survival rates, particularly in women [37].

As if to confirm this premise, the most compelling evidence for overdiagnosis from the current screening studies is the observation of roughly equivalent rates of lung cancer among smokers and nonsmokers in Japanese population CT screening, where lung cancer detection rates with CT in nonsmoking women exceed annual mortality rates by several fold [11]. Some proportion of these excess screen-detected cancers is tumors that would never contribute to the death of the individual.

When analyzing statistical trends in lung cancer, and especially in screening trials, it is important to distinguish lung cancer mortality from case fatality rates.

Lung cancer–specific mortality is defined as:

$$\frac{\text{the number of lung cancer deaths}}{\text{the total number of individuals screened}}$$

Lung cancer–specific case fatality, often called "lung cancer death rate," is defined as:

$$\frac{\text{the number alive with lung cancer}}{\text{the total number with lung cancer}}$$

Lung cancer–specific mortality rates consider the number of lung cancer deaths among all individuals under surveillance and address the impact of the screening intervention across the entire population to which screening is applied. In contrast, case fatality rates consider lung cancer deaths exclusively in individuals with lung cancer. Because case fatality rates consider only individuals with lung cancer, these rates are subject to the same biases as survival statistics. Mortality rates address the essential question of screening impact across the entire population that undergoes screening. Mortality rates are meaningful in the context of a contemporaneous control arm, a population that has not undergone the intervention of interest.

Finally, CT screening for lung cancer is a special case of screening. Unlike screening mammography that images only breast tissue, cervical Papanicolaou smears in which cervical epithelial cells are analyzed, or colonoscopy in which the colonic epithelium is directly visualized, chest CT scans span a wide anatomic range from the lower cervical region to the upper abdomen–retroperitoneum. Imagers are obliged to report any potentially significant findings observed, whether related or not to potential lung cancer. These additional observations may themselves incur downstream diagnostic tests that involve additional risk and potential death [38]. Studies that follow and report medical outcomes on only the small percentage of individuals with suspected or diagnosed lung cancer cannot inform the benefits or risks of CT screening across the entire population being screened.

Summarizing the present knowledge base

There is much to be learned from the multiple single-arm observational studies and the preliminary experience of the RCTs of CT screening for lung cancer. Low-dose helical CT is a sensitive imaging tool and detects many more lung nodules than CXR, on the order of twofold to sixfold. Variations in the rates of nodule detection on screening CT are caused by primarily the lower size threshold used by various investigators to define a "lung nodule" and the spatial quality of the CT scan, determined primarily by slice thickness. Most CT-detected nodules, typically over 90%, are benign, even in a targeted, high-risk population.

CT screening detects roughly two to four times more lung cancers than CXR. The increase in lung cancer detection is associated with a higher proportion of stage I disease and a relative oversampling of adenocarcinoma. The impact of CT screening, however, on the absolute number of late-stage cancers is not known. A true stage shift requires that the increase in screen-detected early stage cancers occur in parallel with a decrease in the number (not percentage) of advanced lung cancers. Absent this, it is unlikely that CT screening confers benefit. In the study by Diederich and colleagues [15], one third of lung cancers were interval cancers not detected by screening, the implication being that aggressive cancers may escape screen detection.

CT detects smaller lung cancers than are normally visible on CXR. The average size of CT-detected prevalence cancers has ranged from 9 to 16.5 mm [10,15,28]. Some investigators have reported that CT-detected incidence cancers are smaller than prevalence nodules [36], albeit biologically more aggressive. A key premise by CT screening proponents is that the smaller tumors detected by CT have a different prognosis than larger lesions. In support of this, Wisnivesky and colleagues [39] analyzed 7620 patients with stage I NSCLC who had undergone resection from the Surveillance, Epidemiology, and End Results registry 2003 to determine survival statistics. They found that smaller tumor size at diagnosis was associated with improved survival within stage I NSCLC. Specifically, the 12-year survival rate for patients with tumors 5 to 15 mm in diameter was 69% (95% CI, 64%–74%) and 63% for tumors 16 to 25 mm in diameter (95% CI, 60%–67%). Similarly, Flieder and colleagues [40] retrospectively reviewed data on 503 patients with completely resected invasive NSCLC with invasive primary tumors less than or equal to 3 cm. They observed that primary NSCLC greater than 2 cm in diameter is twice as likely to have nodal metastases as tumors less than or equal to 2 cm, lending support for the notion that small lesions represent early stage disease.

Although other investigators have not observed a significant relationship between T1 lesion size and stage distribution [41], the preponderance of data suggest small, but significant, survival benefits for tumors within the T1 category less than or equal to 2 cm. This has provided the impetus for staging revisions in the seventh edition of the TNM Classification of Malignant Tumors, due in 2009, which will propose that T1 lesions be subclassified as lesions less than or equal to 2 cm and greater than 2 cm [30]. What is not known from these data is the efficacy of CT screening in reducing "underdiagnosis," meaning the detection of small primary lesions before metastases (advanced disease). Surveillance, Epidemiology, and End Results data suggest that up to 40% of lung cancers measuring less than or equal to 15 mm in diameter present with mediastinal or distant metastases at diagnosis [42]. Experimental studies have shown that a 1-cm tumor sheds 3 to 6 million tumor cells into the blood every 24 hours [43]. Tumor genetics, epigenetic phenomena, and tumor angiogenesis may be more influential than lesion size in determining cancer biology and metastatic potential.

It is to be expected that survival increases in individuals with CT screen–detected lung cancers. The increased survival may be caused by any of the biases inherent to screening: lead time, length, and overdiagnosis; or may be a consequence of a true increase in longevity (delay in the time of death). The essential concerns about the current data on CT screening are that (1) CT screening may be detecting biologically favorable lesions, some of which would remain subclinical during life, promoting unnecessary diagnostic and treatment interventions that themselves incur morbidity and mortality; (2) CT screening may not result in true stage shift (eg, reduce the number of advanced-stage lung cancers) and do nothing to significantly reduce mortality in small cancers destined to become advanced; and (3) the balance of benefit and risk have yet to be determined across the entire population subjected to screening.

Despite the lack of evidence of a mortality benefit from CT screening, the observational studies have informed several of concepts of best practices. One notable example is the evaluation of the positive screen. Screening is beneficial to the extent that it detects disease sufficiently early that intervention can increase survivability or prevent death. Diagnostic pathways to further evaluate CT-detected indeterminate nodules have been largely empiric. These algorithms have been refined through the experience of several different groups of investigators, however, with the goals of achieving the most efficient discrimination between malignant and benign disease while minimizing risks. With minor variation, different investigators have converged on very similar diagnostic pathways [36,44–46]. This is itself encouraging, and suggests that should CT be found to confer a legitimate mortality benefit, its implementation for public policy can be accomplished in concert with rationale diagnostic algorithms to manage indeterminate nodules detected by screening.

The current studies have also shown the considerations important to implementing standardized protocols across multiple sites for low-dose helical CT. The earliest screening studies were done using thick-section (10 mm) CT scans [8]. With CT screening, the detection task is to be able to reliably detect and follow the morphology of small, subcentimeter lung nodules, which mandate high spatial resolution on the order of 2-mm contiguous slice thicknesses. Moreover, the whole chest should be imaged at suspended full inspiration in a single breath-hold with minimal cardiorespiratory motion and using low radiation exposures [47]. Over time, the acquisition protocols for helical CT across different groups of investigators have converged on common techniques. Moreover, with the increasing potential of software designed for computer-aided nodule detection and volumetric analysis, helical CT technology lends itself to such image analysis in that additional high-resolution image datasets can be reconstructed from a single acquisition. The optimal datasets for computational analysis must be of high spatial quality, on the order of 1-mm contiguous intervals or better. These datasets serve automated image analysis purposes well, but are cumbersome for human interpretation needs. The standardization of acquisition parameters across different scanner platforms and the adoption of standardized image interpretation guidelines are critical to the validity and quality of CT screening data and its analysis across different cohorts.

The National Lung Screening Trial

Blueprints for a randomized trial that could validate the efficacy of CT screening for lung cancer were initially drafted in the late 1990s, partially in response to a series of workshops hosted by the National Cancer Institute (NCI). What ultimately became the National Lung Screening Trial (NLST) was the product of considerable collaboration and input by several researchers in both the extramural research community and the NCI. The NLST is a lung cancer screening trial sponsored by the NCI [48]. Now in its fifth year, this RCT compares the efficacy between two different screening tests: low-dose helical CT and CXR. The trial has randomized 53,476 individuals at high risk of lung cancer in a 1:1 ratio to receive either annual CT or CXR for three screens (Fig. 2). By the end of the trial, medical outcomes will have been collected for 4 to 6 years from randomization, depending on the time of enrollment. All trial-related data are reviewed at least twice annually by an independent data and safety monitoring board; interim analyses are also performed annually to determine potential

trends that might reflect differential benefits or risks between the two arms. The final analysis of the NLST is expected some time in 2009.

The primary end point of the NLST is lung cancer–specific mortality, for which the trial has 90% power to detect a 20% difference between the two screening arms. Secondary end points include all-cause mortality; differences in stage distribution of lung cancers at diagnosis; medical resource use (including complications of downstream diagnostic testing) in participants with positive screening tests; and the overall performance of the two screening tests. Additional secondary aims are being studied in a subset of the NLST participants who were enrolled at sites sponsored by the American College of Radiology Imaging Network (ACRIN) and include (1) quality of life issues in screenees and anxiety in participants with positive screening tests, (2) medical resource use in participants across all categories of screening result, and (3) the impact of lung cancer screening on smoking behaviors and beliefs. Specimens of blood, urine, and sputum have also been collected at each of the three screening time points in over 10,000 (ACRIN) participants; these specimens will be used to validate biomarkers or panels of biomarkers of early lung cancer that seem promising based on preliminary tests [49].

The eligibility criteria for the NLST were designed to investigate individuals at highest risk of lung cancer and include asymptomatic male and female cigarette smokers between the ages of 55 and 74 years with a minimum cigarette smoking history of 30 pack-years (total years smoked × packs per day). Current and former smokers were eligible, although the latter must have quit within 15 years before enrollment. Participants could not

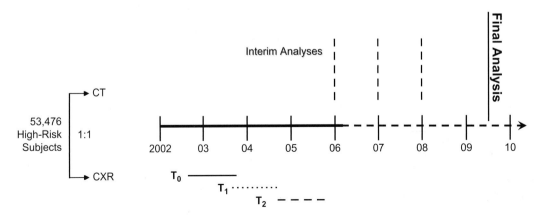

Fig. 2. NLST trial schema. T_0 is the baseline screen; T_1 is Year 1 incidence screen; and T_2 is Year 2 incidence screen.

have been previously diagnosed with primary lung cancer, and could not have been treated for, or have evidence of, another cancer within the preceding 5 years (excluding nonmelanoma skin cancers). Exclusion criteria were intended to ensure that participants can tolerate potentially curative lung resection.

National Lung Screening Trial screening interpretations

For both CT and CXR arms, there are three types of screening results as follows: (1) positive screen, based on the presence of one or more nodules greater than or equal to 4 mm diameter or other abnormality potentially related to lung cancer; (2) negative screen with no, or minor, abnormalities not requiring follow-up; and (3) negative screen with significant findings unrelated to potential lung cancer. For all positive screening results, radiologists are obliged to provide some form of diagnostic recommendation. Recommendations for the follow-up of positive CT screening examinations are based on guidelines that take

into consideration the size and attenuation characteristics of CT-detected nodules (Fig. 3).

The interpretation task with CXR screening is often twofold: to determine whether there is an abnormality and to evaluate further a visualized abnormality (Fig. 4). The NLST protocol provided diagnostic recommendations as guidelines; in all instances, the decision regarding the diagnostic recommendation for a given screening result was left to the discretion of the radiologist based on their best judgment and local institutional practices. Screening examinations in which significant findings unrelated to potential lung cancer also mandate some form of recommendation, although no guidelines were provided, given the diverse range of possible findings and variations in practices across institutions.

National Lung Screening Trial outcomes assessment

The intention of longitudinal assessment in the NLST is to determine the consequences, both positive and negative, that result from screening the population at risk. Participants are contacted at

Guidelines for CT-Detected Nodules at Screening

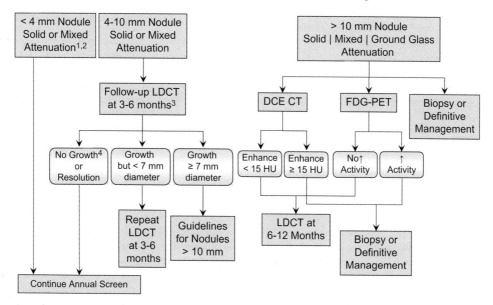

Fig. 3. Guidelines for diagnostic follow-up of CT-detected nodules in the NLST. **1** Pure ground glass nodules <10 mm can be followed-up with LDCT at 6–12 months. **2** At T2 (final year screen) new nodules <4 mm can be followed-up with repeat LDCT at 3–4 months. **3** The timing of repeat LDCT varies according to nodule size. Larger nodules should be followed-up sooner than smaller nodules. **4** No growth is defined as <15% increase in overall diameter or no increase in solid component. DCE-CT, dynamic contrast-enhanced CT; FDG-PET, 18-fluorodeoxyglucose positron emission tomography; LDCT, low-dose helical CT.

Diagnostic Guidelines for Positive CXR Screens in NLST

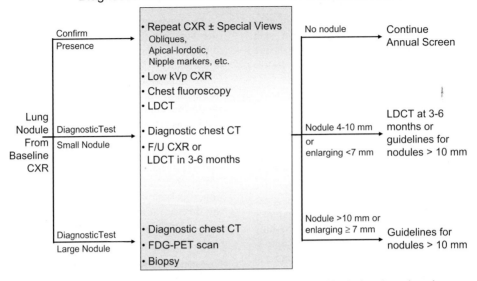

Fig. 4. Diagnostic guidelines for positive chest radiograph screening tests. Specific choices depend on the nature of the detected abnormality and institutional preferences. CXR, chest radiograph; FDG-PET, 18-fluorodeoxyglucose positron emission tomography; LDCT, low-dose CT.

least annually to determine their health status. In participants with positive screens, all diagnostic tests, complications of tests, and test results are obtained. In participants with the diagnosis of lung cancer, the histology, grade, and stage of cancer are documented, as are the diagnostic tests used to establish the diagnosis, complications of diagnostic evaluation, treatments, treatment complications, and cancer progression or recurrence. Subsets of participants with negative screens, both with and without significant other findings, are also followed to tabulate all health encounters so that differential medical resource use between the two screening arms can be determined.

Deaths are documented through annual follow-up with participants or their contacts, or by querying the National Health Index data linked to death certificates. In all trial decedents, death certificates are obtained and coded using the International Classification of Diseases-10 Revision. These codes, combined with screening results and the timing of death relative to screening or downstream diagnostic tests, factor into an algorithm to determine those trial decedents whose deaths should be independently evaluated by experts. An end point verification committee then reviews medical records and available documentation to establish cause of death independent of the death certificate. The intent of the end point verification committee is to minimize biases that may overestimate or underestimate the benefit of screening.

Beyond CT screening: molecular biomarkers

The potential of CT lies in its capacity to detect small lung cancers in the parenchyma. A total of 15% to 20% of lung cancers in previous screening trials, however, have been detected only by sputum cytology [50,51]. In particular, early squamous cell carcinomas in the large central airways escape CT detection, as do premalignant lesions like severe dysplasia and carcinoma in situ. These precursor lesions have been shown to progress to invasive squamous cell carcinoma in over 50% of cases in some studies [52]. Indeed, absent severe dysplasia, the progression of low-grade dysplasia to carcinoma in situ and invasive squamous cell carcinoma is not negligible, suggesting that each of these preneoplastic lesions must be independently considered to have malignant clones [53]. Although atypical adenomatous hyperplasia (now classified as a precursor lesion of lung adenocarcinoma) is detectable on CT and is known to have many of the same molecular alterations as adenocarcinoma [54,55], the progression of atypical adenomatous hyperplasia to adenocarcinoma has not been directly demonstrated, and it is not known with what frequency atypical adenomatous hyperplasia transforms into invasive cancer. Helical CT is only now providing the means by which to study this lesion; before CT, most investigations of atypical adenomatous hyperplasia involved specimens discovered incidentally in tissue resected by patients with adenocarcinoma [56].

Molecular studies show that lung cancers have multiple genetic and epigenetic alterations, numbering greater than 20 per cancer [57]. Many of the alterations in gene expression and chromosome structure seen in lung cancer have also been demonstrated in preneoplastic lesions, including hyperproliferation and loss of cell cycle control; abnormalities in the p53 pathway, the *ras* genes, and genes in the genomic regions of 3p14.2; aberrant gene promoter hypermethylation; angiogenesis; and altered expression of multiple proteins [58]. These observations support the concept of lung carcinogenesis as a multistep process developing from normal epithelium and involving successive genetic and epigenetic abnormalities, typically through exposure to tobacco-related carcinogens.

Although sputum cytology itself has not satisfied the criteria necessary for an effective screening tool, sputum, blood, and urine are attractive for screening strategies because they are readily attainable without invasive procedures and lend themselves to the exploration of potential molecular biomarkers. If reproducibly detected, biomarkers from these biospecimens could identify individuals destined to develop lung cancer and

could be applied to lung cancer prevention strategies rather than treatment strategies.

A number of molecular analyses have been applied to sputum. Among these are DNA evaluation techniques, such as fluorescence in situ hybridization, using probes for several genes known to be associated with lung cancer, including c-*myc*, EGFR, 5p15, and CEP6 [59]. These molecular biomarkers are relatively insensitive for the detection of lung cancer when considered alone (sensitivity 41%, specificity 94%), but become more sensitive when combined with sputum cytology (sensitivity 83%, specificity 80%).

The *RAS* family of proto-oncogenes (*HRAS*, *KRAS*) encode proteins that regulate key signal-transduction pathways involved in normal cellular differentiation, proliferation, and survival. Activating mutations in the *KRAS* genes are common in lung cancer of both adenocarcinoma and squamous cell histologies. A significant number of individuals with squamous cell carcinoma have *KRAS* mutations in sputum. These mutations are also found in individuals without subsequent lung cancer, however, and their significance as biomarkers of early disease has not been validated [60].

Among the more promising sputum biomarkers is the detection of aberrant methylation of DNA promoter genes, which occurs early in the development of lung cancer, and is associated with silencing of the transcription of genes involved in several aspects of normal cell function (Fig. 5). Belinsky and colleagues [61] recently

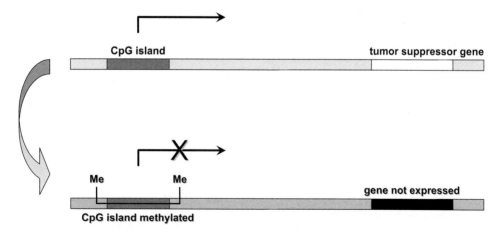

Fig. 5. The effect of hypermethylation of tumor-suppressor gene promoters. CpG islands are regions of the gene rich in cytosine-guanine dinucleotides. Most CpG islands are found in the proximal promoter region of nearly half of all genes in the mammalian genome and are normally unmethylated. In the human genome, methylation (Me) occurs only at CpG islands. Hypermethylation of the promoter regions of tumor suppressor genes occurs early in the development of lung cancer and silences the transcription of the gene. Silencing by hypermethylation affects genes involved in all aspects of normal cell function and is a critical trigger for malignant transformation and cancer progression.

reported that promoter hypermethylation in sputum is associated with lung cancer and may precede its clinical diagnosis.

Similarly, promoter DNA hypermethylation changes have been observed in blood samples from patients with lung cancer [62]. The levels of circulating cell-free DNA in blood are generally higher in patients with cancer than in healthy controls. The source of the increased DNA is assumed to be apoptotic or necrotic tumor cells that release DNA into the circulation. The circulating DNA in lung cancer patients exhibits many of the genetic and epigenetic changes typical of the primary tumor. For example, K-*ras* and p53 gene mutations have been found in between 20% and 30% of lung cancer patients [63]. These mutations in blood are identical to those in the primary tumor, and provide solid evidence that nucleic acids are released into the circulation by lung cancers.

Proteomic studies in lung cancer have taken two forms: protein profiling, in which patterns of protein expression are used to identify malignancy without knowledge of the specific proteins; and techniques to identify individual proteins that may serve as biomarkers. Many of the molecular markers for NSCLC are growth factors and their receptors, such as the epidermal growth factor receptor and c-ErB-2 (Her-2/neu), and serum cytokines, such as vascular endothelial growth factor, stem cell factor, and hepatocyte growth factor–scatter factor [64]. The field of proteomic biomarker discovery is rapidly accelerating, enabled by recent advances in high-throughput technologies and bioinformatics platforms. Substantial challenges, including instrument standardization, sample handling, reproducibility, and validation of preliminary results in larger prospective studies need to be met to see the translation of these molecular approaches to the clinical practice of lung cancer screening.

Summary

CT screening is highly sensitive for the detection of lung nodules. Among individuals at high risk of lung cancer, up to 10% of CT-detected nodules detected at prevalence screening ultimately prove to be lung cancer. CT detects more lung cancers than does CXR; a high percentage of these cancers are early stage when diagnosed. The survival of CT screen–detected lung cancers is increased relative to historical controls, which are typically symptom-detected.

Although these observations are provocative, the demonstration of prolonged survival is itself insufficient evidence of screening benefit. When applied to screening, survival statistics are subject to the biases of lead time, length, and overdiagnosis. Moreover, there is no evidence to date that CT screening reduces the number of aggressive, advanced-stage lung cancers. Because of these biases, prolonged survival can occur absent a meaningful decrease in lung cancer–specific mortality. The results of the ongoing large-scale RCTs, such as the NLST and NELSON trial, are essential to determine whether lung cancer–specific and all-cause mortality differs between those who do and do not undergo CT screening.

Beyond benefit, these trials must show that screening benefit outweighs risk, across all individuals screened, not only those with lung cancer. Chest CT provides a window to the evaluation of multiple organs and conditions. The collective consequences of all screening observations, the diagnostic follow-up associated with these imaging findings, the complications of downstream tests, and the potential to treat patients who neither require nor benefit from treatments must be weighed against the unbiased measure of mortality benefit [65].

Concurrently, molecular research is accelerating at extraordinary pace. Although there has yet to be found a single biomarker, or panel of biomarkers, that predicts lung cancer, it is reasonable to anticipate that this may occur in the foreseeable future. How molecular medicine and contemporary imaging will converge to subdue the scourge of lung cancer remains to be written. Certainly, both the prospects and the stakes are high; the hope for a screening test that will reduce lung cancer mortality must be balanced with the necessary scientific skepticism to keep the journey honest.

References

[1] American Cancer Society. Cancer facts and figures 2007. Atlanta (GA): American Cancer Society; 2007. p. 1–51.
[2] Strauss GM. Bronchogenic carcinoma. Textbook of pulmonary diseases. 6th edition. Philadelphia: Lippincott-Raven Publishers; 1998.
[3] Ebbert JO, Yang P, Vachon CM, et al. Lung cancer risk reduction after smoking cessation: observations from a prospective cohort of women. J Clin Oncol 2003;21:921–6 Artinian #12.
[4] Smith RA, Glynn TG. Epidemiology of lung cancer. Radiol Clin North Am 2000;38:453–70.

[5] Jemal A, Tiwari RC, Murray T, et al. Cancer statistics, 2004. CA Cancer J Clin 2004;54:8–29.

[6] Fry WA, Phillips JL, Merick HR. Ten-year survey of lung cancer treatment and survival in hospitals in the United States: a national cancer data base report. Cancer 1999;86:1867–76.

[7] Mountain CF. Revisions in the International system for staging lung cancer. Chest 1997;111:1710–7.

[8] Henschke CI, McCauley DI, Yankelevitz DF, et al. Early lung cancer action project: overall design and findings from baseline screening. Lancet 1999;354: 99–105.

[9] Henschke CI, Naidich DP, Yankelevitz DF, et al. Early lung cancer action project: initial findings on repeat screening. Cancer 2001;92:153–9.

[10] Swensen SJ, Jett JR, Hartman TE, et al. CT screening for lung cancer: five year prospective experience. Radiology 2005;235:259–65.

[11] Sone S, Li F, Yang Z-G, et al. Results of three-year mass screening programme for lung cancer using mobile low-dose spiral computed tomography scanner. Br J Cancer 2001;84:25–32.

[12] Nawa T, Nakagawa T, Kusano S, et al. Lung cancer screening using low-dose spiral CT. Chest 2002; 2 122:15–22.

[13] Sobue T, Moriyama N, Kaneko M, et al. Screening for lung cancer with low-dose helical computed tomography: anti-lung cancer association project. J Clin Oncol 2002;20:911–20.

[14] Diederich S, Wormanns D, Semik M, et al. Screening for early lung cancer with low-dose spiral CT: prevalence in 817 asymptomatic smokers. Radiology 2002;222:773–81.

[15] Diederich S, Thomas M, Semik M, et al. Screening for early lung cancer with low-dose spiral computed tomography: results of annual follow-up examinations in asymptomatic smokers. Eur Radiol 2004; 14:691–702.

[16] Garg K, Keith RL, Byers T, et al. Randomized controlled trial with low-dose spiral CT for lung cancer screening: feasibility study and preliminary results. Radiology 2002;225(2):506–10.

[17] Blanchon T, Bréchot JM, Grenier PA, et al, for the "Dépiscan" Group. Baseline results of the Depiscan study: a French randomized pilot trial of lung cancer screening comparing low dose CT scan (LDCT) and chest X-ray (CXR). Lung Cancer 2007;58(1):50–8 Epub 2007 Jul 12.

[18] Gohagan JK, Marcus PM, Fagerstrom RM, et al, The Lung Screening Study Research Group. Final results of the Lung Screening Study, a randomized feasibility study of spiral CT versus chest X-ray screening for lung cancer. Lung Cancer 2005;47:9–15.

[19] van Iersel CA, de Koning HJ, Draisma G, et al. Risk-based selection from the general population in a screening trial: selection criteria, recruitment and power for the Dutch-Belgian randomised lung cancer multi-slice CT screening trial (NELSON). Int J Cancer 2007;120(4):868–74.

[20] The International Early Lung Cancer Action Program Investigators. Survival of patients with stage I lung cancer detected on CT screening. N Engl J Med 2006;355:1763–71.

[21] Bach PB, Jett JR, Pastorino U, et al. Computed tomography screening and lung cancer outcomes. JAMA 2007;297:953–61.

[22] Bach PB, Elkin EB, Pastorino U, et al. Benchmarking lung cancer mortality rates in current and former smokers. Chest 2004;126:1742–9.

[23] Cronin K, Gail MH, Zou Z, et al. Validation of a model of lung cancer risk prediction among smokers. J Natl Cancer Inst 2006;98:637–40.

[24] Black WC, Welch HG. Screening for disease. AJR Am J Roentgenol 1997;168:3–11.

[25] Patz EF, Goodman PC, Bepler G. Screening for lung cancer. N Engl J Med 2000;343:1627–33.

[26] Reich JM. Assessing the efficacy of lung cancer screening. Radiology 2006;238:398–401.

[27] Hasagawa M, Sone S, Takashima S, et al. Growth rate of small lung cancers detected on mass CT screening. Br J Radiol 2000;73:1252–9.

[28] Lindell RM, Hartman TE, Swensen SJ, et al. Five-year lung cancer screening experience: CT appearance, growth rate, location, and histologic features of 61 lung cancers. Radiology 2007;242:555–62.

[29] Gu C-D, Osaki T, Oyama T, et al. Detection of micrometastatic tumor cells in pN0 lymph nodes of patients with completely resected nonsmall cell lung cancer: impact on recurrence and survival. Ann Surg 2002;1:133–9.

[30] Goldstraw P, Crowley J, Chansky K, et al. The IASLC Lung Cancer Staging Project: proposals for the revision of the TNM stage grouping in the forthcoming (seventh) edition of the TNM classification of malignant tumors. J Thorac Oncol 2007;2: 706–14.

[31] Noguchi M, Morikawa A, Kawasaki M, et al. Small adenocarcinoma of the lung: histologic characteristics and prognosis. Cancer 1995;75:2844–52.

[32] Suzuki K, Kusumoto M, Watanabe S, et al. Radiologic classification of small adenocarcinoma of the lung: radiologic-pathologic correlation and its prognostic impact. Ann Thorac Surg 2006;81:413–20.

[33] Stenman UH, Abrahamsson PA, Aus G, et al. Prognostic value of serum markers for prostate cancer. Scand J Urol Nephrol Suppl 2005;216:64–81.

[34] Telesca D, Etzioni R, Gulati R. Estimating lead time and overdiagnosis associated with PSA screening from prostate cancer incidence trends. Biometrics 2007 May 14 [Epub ahead of print]. DOI:10.1111/j. 1541-0420.2007.00825.x.

[35] Bangma CH, Roemeling S, Schroder FH. Overdiagnosis and overtreatment of early detected prostate cancer. World J Urol 2007;25:3–9.

[36] Henschke CI. New York Early Lung Cancer Action Project investigators. CT screening for lung cancer: diagnoses resulting from the New York Early Lung Cancer Action Project. Radiology 2007;243:239–49.

[37] Chan CK, Wells CK, McFarlane MJ, et al. More lung cancer but better survival: implications of secular trends in necropsy surprise rates. Chest 1989;96:291–6.

[38] Casarella WJ. A patient's viewpoint on a current controversy. Radiology 2002;224:927.

[39] Wisnivesky JP, Yankelevitz D, Henschke CI. The effect of tumor size on curability of stage I non-small cell lung cancers. Chest 2004;126:761–5.

[40] Flieder DB, Port JL, Korst RJ, et al. Tumor size is a determinant of stage distribution in T1 non-small cell lung cancer. Chest 2005;128:2304–8.

[41] Heyneman LE, Herndon JE, Goodman PC, et al. Stage distribution in patients with a small ($\leq$ 3 cm) primary nonsmall cell lung cancer. Cancer 2001;92:3051–5.

[42] Pastorino U. Early detection of lung cancer. Respiration 2006;73:5–13.

[43] Swartz MA, Kristensen CA, Melder RJ, et al. Cell shed from tumours show reduced clonogenicity, resistance to apoptosis, and in vivo tumorigenicity. Br J Cancer 1999;81:756–9.

[44] Xu DM, Gietema H, de Koning H, et al. Nodule management protocol of the NELSON randomized lung cancer screening trial. Lung Cancer 2006;54: 177–84.

[45] MacMahon H, Austin JH, Gamsu G, et al. Guidelines for management of small pulmonary nodules detected on CT scans: a statement from the Fleischner Society. Radiology 2005;237(2):395–400.

[46] Aberle DR, Black WC, Goldin JG, et al. ACRIN Protocol 6654 (NLST): contemporary screening for the detection of lung cancer. Available at: http://www.acrin.org/pdf_file2.html?file=protocol_docs/A6654partial_summary.pdf. Accessed October 15, 2007.

[47] Cagnon CH, Cody DD, McNitt-Gray MF, et al. Description and implementation of a quality control program in an imaging-based clinical trial. Acad Radiol 2006;13:1431–41.

[48] NLST: National Lung Screening Trial. Available at: http://www.cancer.gov/nlst/what-is-nlst. Accessed October 25, 2007.

[49] American College of Radiology Imaging Network: Protocol 6654. Contemporary screening for the detection of lung cancer. Available at: http://www.acrin.org/pdf_file2.html?file=protocol_docs/A6654partial_summary.pdf. Accessed October 15, 2007.

[50] Kaneko M, Eguchi K, Ohmatsu H, et al. Peripheral lung cancer: screening and detection with low dose spiral CT versus radiography. Radiology 1996;210: 798–802.

[51] Fontana RS, Sanderson DR, Taylor WF, et al. Lung cancer screening: the Mayo Program. J Occup Med 1986;28:746–50.

[52] Bota S, Auliac JB, Paris C, et al. Follow-up of bronchial precancerous lesions and carcinoma-in-situ using fluorescence endoscopy. Am J Respir Crit Care Med 2001;164:1688–93.

[53] Breuer RH, Pasic A, Emit EF, et al. The natural course of preneoplastic lesions in bronchial epithelium. Clin Cancer Res 2005;11:537–43.

[54] Morandi L, Asioli S, Cavassa A, et al. Genetic relationships among atypical adenomatous hyperplasia, bronchioloalveolar carcinoma and adenocarcinoma of the lung. Lung cancer 2007;56:35–42.

[55] Kitamura H, Kameda Y, Ito T, et al. Atypical adenomatous hyperplasia of the lung: implications for the pathogenesis of peripheral lung adenocarcinoma. Am J Clin Pathol 1999;111:610–22.

[56] Yokose T, Ito Y, Ochiai A. High prevalence of atypical adenomatous hyperplasia of the lung in autopsy specimens from elderly patients with malignant neoplasms. Lung Cancer 2000;29:125–30.

[57] Sekido Y, Fong KM, Minna JD. Molecular genetics of lung cancer. Annu Rev Med 2003;54:73–87.

[58] Greenberg AK, Lee MS. Biomarkers for lung cancer: clinical uses. Curr Opin Pulm Med 2007;13:249–55.

[59] Kennedy TC, Hirsch FR. Using molecular markers in sputum for the early detection of lung cancer: a review. Lung Cancer 2004;45:S21–7.

[60] Aviel-Ronen S, Blackhall F, Shepherd F, et al. K-*ras* mutations in nonsmall cell lung carcinoma: a review. Clin Lung Cancer 2006;30:211–4.

[61] Belinsky SA, Liechty KC, Gentry FD, et al. Promoter hypermethylation of multiple genes in sputum precedes lung cancer incidence in a high-risk cohort. Cancer Res 2006;66:3338–44.

[62] Russo AL, Thiagalingam A, Pan H, et al. Differential DNA hypermethylation of critical genes mediates the stage-specific tobacco smoke-induced neoplastic progression of lung cancer. Clin Cancer Res 2005;11(7):2466–70.

[63] Bremnes RM, Sirera R, Camps C. Circulating tumor-derived DNA and RNA markers in blood: a tool for early detection, diagnostics, and follow-up? Lung Cancer 2006;49:1–12.

[64] Bharti A, Ma PC, Salgia R. Biomarker discovery in lung cancer: promises and challenges of clinical proteomics. Mass Spectrom Rev 2007;26:451–66.

[65] Lee CI, Forman HP. CT screening for lung cancer: implications on social responsibility. AJR Am J Roentgenol 2007;188:297–8.

ELSEVIER
SAUNDERS

Clin Chest Med 29 (2008) 15–38

CLINICS
IN CHEST
MEDICINE

Imaging Evaluation of the Solitary Pulmonary Nodule

Jeffrey S. Klein, MD[a,b,*], Samuel Braff, MD[a,b]

[a]University of Vermont College of Medicine, Burlington, VT 05401, USA
[b]Fletcher Allen Health Care, 111 Colchester Avenue, Patrick 105, Burlington, VT 05401, USA

The evaluation and management of the solitary pulmonary nodule (SPN) is an increasingly common problem for pulmonologists, radiologists, and thoracic surgeons. The primary goal of the physician evaluating patients who have SPNs is to distinguish benign from potentially malignant lesions, a task that requires the incorporation of environmental and patient related factors and the results of imaging tests used to evaluate SPNs. Whereas before the advent of multi-detector row CT (MDCT) technology these lesions were most commonly encountered as incidental findings on chest radiography, now the widespread use of MDCT for the evaluation of lung and cardiovascular disease, with its inherent rapid scan acquisition and thin-section technique, has resulted in a significant increase in the detection of SPNs. A recent study using annual low-dose CT for lung cancer screening in 1520 high risk patients has shown that 74% of these patients have one or more nodules detected after five annual examinations [1]. The proper evaluation of these lesions requires careful consideration of a variety of patient-related imaging and logistical and socioeconomic factors. The purpose of this article is to review the current radiologic approach to the solitary pulmonary nodule with a focus on the use of thin-section CT and PET imaging for analysis.

Definition

A solitary pulmonary nodule is described as a well-circumscribed round or oval lung opacity less than 3 cm in diameter, which is completely surrounding by parenchyma and unassociated with lymph node enlargement, atelectasis, or pneumonia (Box 1) [2]. Opacities larger than 3 cm in diameter are termed pulmonary masses and are distinguished from SPNs, because they have a considerably higher likelihood of malignancy.

In the evaluation of focal opacities as seen on CT, it is important to distinguish those opacities that reflect SPNs (ie, have a relatively spherical shape) versus densities that are actually flat or pancake-like and are relatively two-dimensional in nature. Whereas this distinction usually is apparent for lesions that are oriented craniocaudally within the lungs, flat lesions that lie primarily in the axial plane can appear round on axial CT images, and coronal and sagittal reconstructions can help demonstrate their flat nature. The three-dimensional ratio is a measure of the spherical nature of focal opacities seen on CT, and it refers to the ratio of greatest in-plane (axial) diameter divided by the maximum craniocaudal dimension. Lesions with a relatively high three-dimensional ratio are typically benign, and they likely reflect benign plaque-like areas of fibrosis or intrapulmonary lymph nodes (Fig. 1). In one study of screening-detected SPNs, a measured three-dimensional ratio of greater than 1.78:1 showed 100% specificity for benign SPNs [3]. For this reason, it is useful to assess the three-dimensional nature of solitary pulmonary opacities to determine if one is dealing with a true solitary pulmonary nodule before embarking on a workup of these lesions.

Solitary pulmonary nodule mimics

Whereas the CT detection and characterization of a solitary pulmonary nodule is relatively

* Corresponding author. Fletcher Allen Health Care, 111 Colchester Avenue, Patrick 105, Burlington, VT 05401.
    E-mail address: jeffrey.klein@uvm.edu (J.S. Klein).

0272-5231/08/$ - see front matter © 2008 Elsevier Inc. All rights reserved.
doi:10.1016/j.ccm.2007.11.007

chestmed.theclinics.com

Box 1. Differential diagnosis of a solitary pulmonary nodule

Infectious
Granuloma (TB, fungus, sarcoidosis)
Organizing pneumonia
Lung abscess (or septic embolus)
Round pneumonia
Fungal infection (aspergillus)

Neoplastic
Benign-hamartoma
Malignant-carcinoma, metastasis,
  carcinoid tumor

Vascular
Arteriovenous malformation
Pulmonary infarct
Hematoma
Pulmonary artery aneurysm

Lymphatic
Intrapulmonary lymph node
Lymphoma

Congenital
Bronchogenic cyst

Inflammatory
Rheumatoid nodule
Wegener's granulomatosis

Airway
Mucoid impaction (bronchiectasis)

Miscellaneous
Rounded atelectasis
Amyloidosis

physical examination of the patient (usually following the chest radiograph) will reveal the surface lesion responsible for the "nodule" seen on chest film. One of the most troublesome skin "lesions" to distinguish from a true pulmonary nodule is the nipple shadow. This usually is identified by performing chest films with nipple markers. Occasionally, chest fluoroscopy or CT will be necessary for confident localization of a nodular opacity seen on conventional radiographs.

Clinical assessment

As with any test or series of diagnostic tests, the prevalence of the disease being evaluated (in this case lung cancer) in the population being studied and the presence of specific individual risk factors for malignancy will impact the overall accuracy of a particular test. Therefore it is important to incorporate a "pre-test" clinical probability for lung cancer and malignancy when interpreting diagnostic studies on patients with SPNs.

The most common recognized risk factor for lung cancer is current or recent cigarette smoking, with the risk proportional to the number of pack-years of smoking. Lung cancer incidence increases directly with advancing age, with cancer being very uncommon in patients less than 35 years old. Although approximately 85% of all cases of lung cancer in North America and Europe can be attributed to cigarette smoking, there are a number of additional risk factors that have been identified, most of which are environmental or occupational in nature. The most well recognized occupational exposure associated with lung cancer is asbestos, which produces a seven- to ten-fold increase in the risk of lung cancer and has a synergistic effect with cigarette smoke on lung cancer development. Other established exposures associated with an increased risk include silica, radiation (ie, Radon, x-rays, and gamma rays), air pollution, arsenic, cadmium, and chromium. Intrinsic risk factors for the development of lung cancer include the presence of chronic obstructive pulmonary disease and interstitial fibrosis. A genetic susceptibility to lung cancer has been postulated based on the observation that there is a higher risk of lung cancer among first degree relatives of lung cancer patients when smoking is accounted for. A history of previous malignancy, particularly lung cancer or head and neck cancer, also is associated with increased risk.

straightforward and will be discussed in detail in a subsequent section, a focal opacity on chest radiography may or may not represent an intrapulmonary lesion. Intrapulmonary lesions are discrete opacities that are completely circumscribed by aerated lung on frontal and lateral radiographs. A pleural or mediastinal lesion may be outlined by lung along that portion of the lesion that projects into the lung. However, the base of the lesion, which forms obtuse angles with the lung, is not outlined by lung where it arises from the pleura or mediastinum. Skin, chest wall, and pleural lesions including pleural plaques (Fig. 2), bone islands, and healing rib fractures also can mimic intrapulmonary nodules. Some skin lesions are circumscribed by air, but a careful

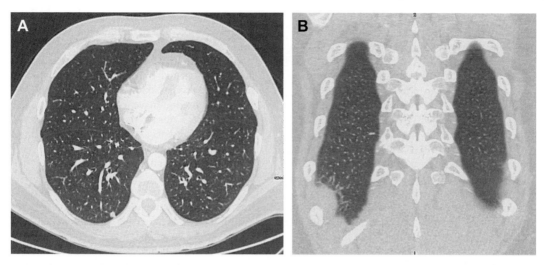

Fig. 1. Use of three-dimensional analysis for evaluation of nodular opacity. (*A*) Axial thin section CT scan at lung windows shows a nodular opacity in the right lower lobe. (*B*) Coronal reformation from CT at lung windows shows a plate-like density corresponding to the "nodule" as seen on the axial scan. The three-dimensional ratio for this opacity was 5:1, indicative of a benign lesion. The opacity has remained stable for more than 2 years.

Recently, investigators have created prediction models using known clinical risk factors to develop a pretest probability of lung cancer in patients who have solitary pulmonary nodules greater than 7 mm in diameter [4]. Gould and colleagues [4] identified four independent predictors of malignancy using multivariate logistic regression analysis in 375 patients, and they found that current or former smokers, increasing age, increasing nodule diameter, and decreasing interval since smoking cessation were all associated with increased risk of lung cancer. These authors suggested that use of their or similar clinical prediction models, when used in combination with the results of FDG-PET scanning, could help determine the post-test probability of malignancy and help guide appropriate clinical decision making. It is likely that many radiologists and

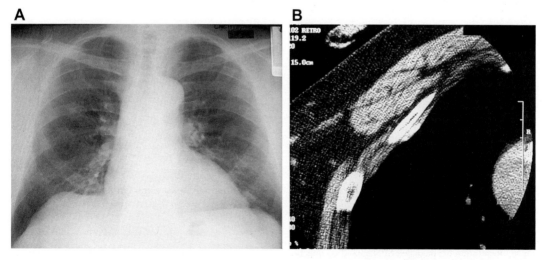

Fig. 2. Pleural plaque producing a "nodule" on chest radiography. (*A*) Frontal chest radiograph shows a nodular density projecting over the right upper lobe. (*B*) Coned down view of axial CT scan displayed at mediastinal windows obtained at the level of the density shows a partly calcified pleural plaque, which accounts for the "nodule."

pulmonologists use a subjective version of one of the validated clinical prediction models to help determine the proper role of imaging studies and biopsy in patients who have SPNs.

An important point to consider in the evaluation of patients who have SPNs, particularly lesions that have an ill-defined margin, is that with the increasing use of MDCT in the evaluation of chest disease, an increasing number of patients who have SPNs will have areas of resolving or organizing pneumonia that are indistinguishable radiologically from lung cancer (Fig. 3). For this reason, it is prudent for all patients who have a newly-detected SPN to obtain a thorough history and physical examination. If such an evaluation determines that a recent infection is considered likely as the possible cause of an SPN, a trial of broad-spectrum antibiotics and repeat CT examination in a short time interval (ie, 6–8 weeks) can be instituted, which will allow time for the majority of nongranulomatous infectious or inflammatory SPNs to resolve, thereby obviating the need for further diagnostic evaluation.

CT characterization of solitary pulmonary nodules

In patients found to have an SPN, CT remains the primary method for radiologic evaluation of such lesions. The use of chest CT for the evaluation of an SPN allows one to determine if the patient has one or multiple lung nodules, with the diagnostic evaluation of multiple nodules differing considerably from that for an SPN. In this regard, the use of multi-detector CT, in particular the use of thin-section and thin-slab maximum intensity projection reconstructions, provides a sensitive method of nodule detection. Additionally, thin-section MDCT forms the basis for the use of computer-aided detection and characterization of lung nodules.

With current multi-detector CT scanners that use 16–64 detector channels, thin-section (ie, 0.6–2.0 mm thick) analysis of SPN features readily are evaluated from retrospective reconstructions of the CT dataset through the nodule. These scans ideally should be reconstructed through the nodule with a targeted field-of-view to maximize the resolution of the scan. This is important not only for the analysis of thin-section CT features used to determine the likelihood of malignancy, but also it is particularly important, because this initial study serves as a high quality baseline examination that will be used to assess interval changes in size, shape, and density on follow-up thin-section CT studies.

The goal of assessing for various radiographic and thin-section characteristics of a solitary pulmonary nodule is to determine whether or not the lesion can be classified as benign. Those SPNs that do not meet specific benign criteria are considered indeterminate and almost always will require further evaluation.

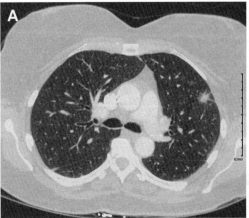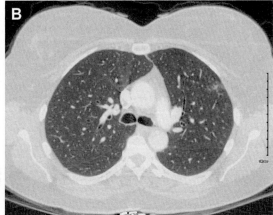

Fig. 3. Resolution of spiculated SPN caused by infection. (*A*) Axial CT scan at level of tracheal carina in a 52-year-old smoker who has fever, cough, and hemoptysis shows a spiculated nodule in the left upper lobe. (*B*) Repeat axial CT 5 weeks later shows marked decrease in the size of the nodule. The patient had been treated in the interval with broad spectrum antibiotics for a presumed infection.

Specific thin-section CT features of solitary pulmonary nodules

Size

It is clear that increasing diameter of a lung nodule is associated with a concomitant increasing risk for lung cancer: lesions greater than 3 cm in diameter have a greater then 90% likelihood of malignancy [5]. Conversely, small lesion size alone is not a reliable predictor of benignity, particularly if the lesion is detected initially by CT (Fig. 4). As a result of selection bias in many published studies, the reported prevalence of lung cancer in SPNs less than 10 mm varies widely. For example, in the 5-year Mayo Clinic CT screening study of 1520 subjects, during which 92% of nodules detected were less than 8 mm in diameter, only 4% of all nodules detected were found to be malignant [1]. In particular, less than 1% of nodules less than 4 mm in diameter detected in the same Mayo Clinic study were malignant. This has led to the recommendation that nodules <4 mm in diameter in low-risk patients require no further follow-up, and that high risk patients who have lesions less than 4 mm in diameter be followed by thin-section CT in 12 months to assess for growth. Alternatively, studies in which SPNs are diagnosed by thoracoscopic surgery tend to show a much higher incidence of cancer; one study of CT detected SPNs ≤ 1 cm, showing malignancy in 58% of resected lesions [6].

Shape and margins

The shape and marginal characteristics of an SPN can provide important clues to the nature of the lesion. In general, smooth round nodules are benign (Fig. 5), whereas lesions with spiculated margins (corona radiata) are much more likely to be malignant (Fig. 6). A lobulated margin can indicate either benign or malignant etiology, and is most often seen in hamartomas, peripheral carcinoid tumors, and adenocarcinomas. Although a smooth margin typically indicates benignancy, solitary hematogenous metastases (as seen in lung, colorectal, renal cell, or breast cancer) will be smoothly marginated (Fig. 7), as will peripheral carcinoid tumors. Similarly, while an irregular or spiculated margin in an SPN is highly suspicious for malignancy, irregular margins can be seen in benign nodules, particularly in patients who have focal areas of organizing or resolving pneumonia, and therefore is not specific for malignancy (see Fig. 3). For these reasons, a smooth or irregular margin to an SPN is not specific for benign or malignant etiology respectively, and additional characterization is required. Satellite lesions surrounding a larger central nodule usually indicates a granulomatous process, most often tuberculosis or histoplasmosis (Fig. 8). A pleural tail, seen as a linear opacity extending from a lung nodule toward the pleural surface, can be seen in either benign or malignant SPNs, but when associated with malignancy is seen most often in pulmonary adenocarcinoma. The recognition of feeding and draining pulmonary vessels extending from the hilum toward the medial aspect of a round or lobulated nodule allows a confident diagnosis of a pulmonary arteriovenous

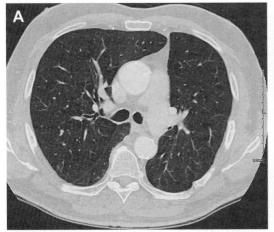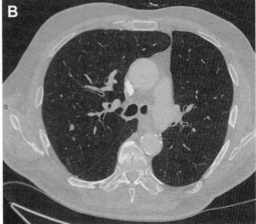

Fig. 4. Small adenocarcinoma detected on screening CT. (*A*) Initial axial thin section CT at the level of the right upper lobe bronchus shows a 4 mm nodule in the right upper lobe. (*B*) Repeat CT scan 3 months later at the same level shows slight enlargement of the nodule. Biopsy revealed adenocarcinoma.

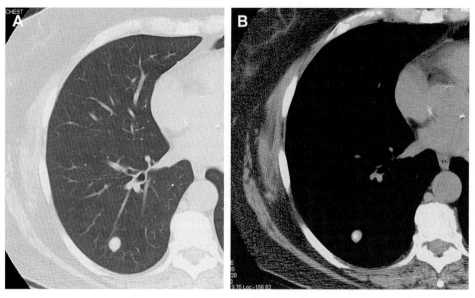

Fig. 5. Smoothly marginated granuloma presenting as an SPN. (*A*) Coned down axial thin-section CT shows a right lower lobe nodule with smooth margins. (*B*) Same image at mediastinal windows shows central calcification indicative of a granuloma.

malformation, which is most often associated with hereditary hemorrhagic telangiectasia but can occur as an isolated finding (Fig. 9). A bundle of curvilinear bronchi and vessels extending into the hilar aspect of a peripheral nodule or mass that lies adjacent to pleural thickening has been

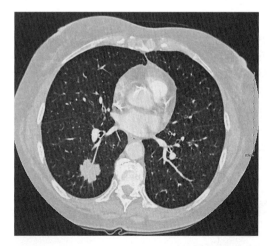

Fig. 6. Spiculated SPN from adenocarcinoma. Axial CT at lung windows in a 67-year-old woman who has biopsy-proven adenocarcinoma shows a lobulated and spiculated nodule in the superior segment of the right lower lobe.

termed the "comet tail sign" and is characteristic of rounded atelectasis. A tubular or branching opacity should suggest a dilated pulmonary artery or vein or mucus within an ectatic bronchus (ie, a mucocele), because tumors rarely grow longitudinally within a central airway. A lesion that shows only concave interface with the surrounding lung is described as polygonal in shape, and is highly specific for benignancy [3].

Internal density

Calcification

The presence of calcification in a specific pattern within an SPN is indicative of a benign lesion. These patterns include central (Fig. 10), laminated (see Fig. 8), diffuse, or popcorn calcification, and when seen within a smooth or lobulated nodule, reflect a granuloma (or in the case of popcorn calcification, a pulmonary hamartoma) (Fig. 11) [7]. However, the presence of eccentric or amorphous calcification can represent a calcified granuloma engulfed by a malignancy or dystrophic malignant calcification respectively and should not be taken as evidence of benignancy (Fig. 12). Rarely, lung metastases in patients who have osteogenic sarcoma or chondrosarcoma can show calcification of the bone- or cartilage-containing portions of the

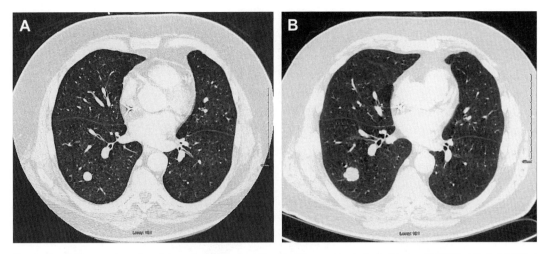

Fig. 7. Smoothly marginated nodule caused by metastatic primitive neuroectodermal tumor (PNET). (*A*) Axial CT at lung windows shows a smoothly-marginated right lower lobe nodule. (*B*) Repeat CT scan 6 weeks later shows interval enlargement of the nodule which now has a lobulated margin. Transthoracic needle biopsy confirmed a solitary metastasis from the patient's PNET, which was treated with CT-guided radiofrequency ablation.

nodules respectively. While the presence and pattern of calcification can sometimes be determined on conventional radiography, approximately 1/3 of noncalcified SPNs will have calcification on CT. For this reason, definitive identification of calcium usually requires review of thin-section CT scans using 1–2 mm collimation (Fig. 13).

In lesions where calcification is not visible on thin-section CT scans, CT densitometry can be performed to detect the presence of microscopic calcification within the nodule. Most thoracic radiologists no longer use a reference CT phantom for this purpose and calculate the average attenuation value through the central portion of the nodule. A value of 200 Hounsfield units (HU) or greater within a smoothly-marginated nodule is reliable evidence of microscopic calcification and therefore benignity.

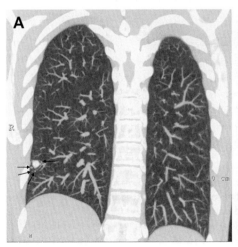
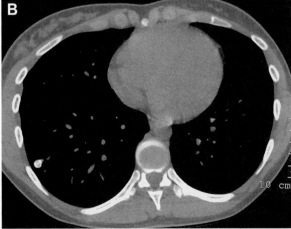

Fig. 8. Satellite nodules caused by prior granulomatous infection from histoplasmosis. (*A*) Coronal maximum intensity projection image displayed at lung windows from a MDCT scan shows a smooth right lower lobe nodule with surrounding smaller "satellite" nodules. (*B*) Axial thin-section CT scan at mediastinal windows through the central nodule which shows laminated calcification indicative of prior histoplasmosis.

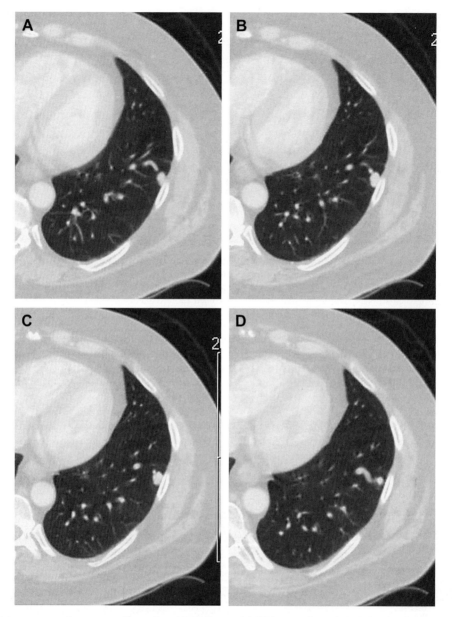

Fig. 9. Pulmonary arteriovenous malformation. (*A–D*) Sequential CT images through the left lower lung from superior to inferior displayed at lung windows show an artery branch feeding a pleural-based nodule with a draining vein seen inferiorly characteristic of a pulmonary arteriovenous malformation.

Fat

The detection of fat within an SPN with smooth or lobulated margins is diagnostic of a pulmonary hamartoma. Approximately 60% of hamartomas have fat, with a minority also showing coarse calcification (Fig. 14) [8]. Rarely, metastatases from renal cell carcinoma or liposarcoma will show fat attenuation, but for practical purposes, the confident identification of fat on thin-section CT analysis of an SPN is diagnostic of a hamartoma and does not warrant further evaluation. This is particularly important since FDG-PET activity has been described in pulmonary hamartomas, and a positive PET scan in such a setting might prompt unnecessary biopsy or resection.

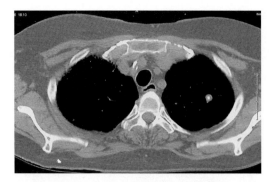

Fig. 10. Central calcification in a granuloma. Thin section axial CT at bone windows shows a left upper lobe nodule with central calcification representing a granuloma.

Cavitation

Cavitation may occur in necrotic malignant SPNs but does not allow distinction of benign lesions as inflammatory lesions, such as abscesses, infectious granulomatous lesions, and Wegener's granulomatosis and pulmonary infarcts can cavitate. Cavitation within a malignant SPN is most typical of a squamous cell carcinoma. However, the thickness of the cavity wall is helpful in distinguishing benign from malignant lesions. Cavities with a maximum wall thickness of less than 5 mm most often are benign, wheras the vast majority of those with a wall thickness of greater than 15 mm are malignant (Fig. 15) [9,10].

Nevertheless, cavity wall thickness is not a reliable distinguishing feature of an SPN, and additional evaluation of cavitary SPNs usually will be necessary.

Air bronchograms, air bronchiolograms, or "bubbly" lucencies

The presence of air bronchograms or cystic or "bubbly" lucencies within an SPN is highly suggestive of pulmonary carcinoma (Fig. 16) [11], although lymphoma and occasional benign lesions, such as organizing pneumonia and mass-like sarcoidosis, can have air bronchograms. Bubbly lucencies are common in adenocarcinomas with bronchioloalveolar cell features, and on histopathologic examination of resected lesions, have been shown to reflect distended distal air spaces surrounded by areas of fibrosis that are induced by the tumor [12].

Mixed solid/ground glass lesions

The widespread use of MDCT with thin-section reconstructions for the evaluation of chest disease, particularly as a screening modality for lung cancer in current or recent former smokers, has led to a significant increase in the detection of so-called subsolid SPNs, in which the nodule has a component of ground-glass attenuation. While subsolid lesions are detected with increasing frequency on MDCT, it is important to remember that the majority of malignant SPNs are

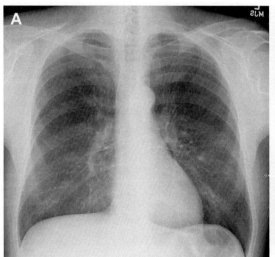

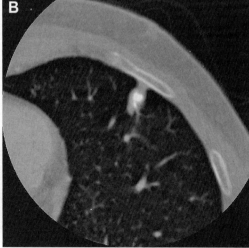

Fig. 11. Pulmonary hamartoma with "popcorn" calcification. (*A*) Frontal chest radiograph shows a dense nodule in the left mid lung. (*B*) Coned down axial CT scan through the lingular nodule shows characteristic popcorn calcification indicative of a hamartoma.

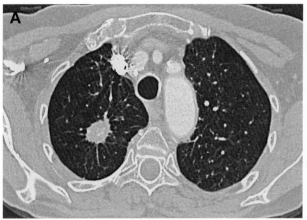
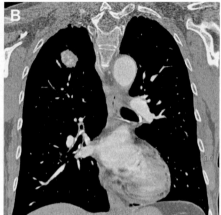

Fig. 12. Dystrophic calcification in lung cancer. (*A*) Axial CT scan through the upper lobes at lung windows shows a spiculated right upper lobe nodule. (*B*) Coronal CT reformation through the nodule shows multiple foci of calcification. Surgical resection revealed an adenocarcinoma.

completely solid in nature, whereas the majority of solid SPNs are benign and represent granulomas.

Subsolid nodules either can be mixed ground glass and solid (also termed part-solid) or pure ground glass (also termed nonsolid) in attenuation. The identification of subsolid SPNs has particular clinical import, because CT screening studies have shown that 34%–43% of subsolid nodules are malignant, with the majority of these lesions reflecting pure bronchioloalveolar cell carcinoma or adenocarcinoma with a bronchioloalveolar cell component of tumor growth (see Fig. 16) [13,14]. Pure ground-glass attenuation or nonsolid SPNs reflect one of three conditions: focal interstitial fibrosis, atypical adenomatous hyperplasia (which is typically seen in older patients and in patients who have lung cancer) or adenocarcinoma (most often bronchioloalveolar cell carcinoma [BAC]) [15]. The radiologic distinction amongst these entities is difficult. In general, pure ground-glass nodules less than 1 cm in diameter

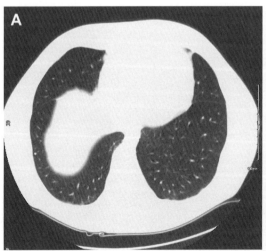
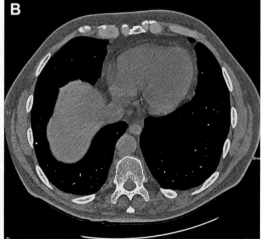

Fig. 13. 3 mm versus 1 mm CT scans for the detection of calcification. (*A*) CT scan at lung windows reconstructed at 3 mm collimation shows a small right lower lobe nodule. No definitive calcification could be seen on the mediastinal windows (not shown). (*B*) 1 mm reconstruction through the nodule shows dense calcification allowing definitive detection of calcification in a granuloma.

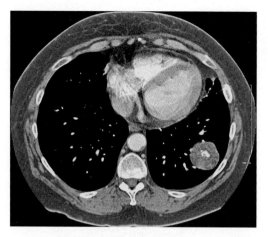

Fig. 14. Pulmonary hamartoma with fat and calcification. Axial CT scan through the lower lobes at mediastinal windows shows a left lower lobe nodule with multiple foci of fat and in addition popcorn-like calcification centrally, findings diagnostic of a hamartoma.

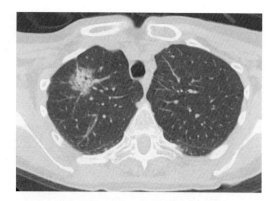

Fig. 16. Mixed solid/ground glass attenuation nodule caused by adenocarcinoma. Thin-section axial CT scan through the upper lobes at lung windows shows a nodule with peripheral ground glass attenuation and more central solid components. Note the presence of air bronchiolograms and small cystic lucencies within the lesion. Surgical resection confirmed an adenocarcinoma with bronchioloalveolar cell features.

either can be benign or malignant, whereas a significant percentage of solitary persistent ground-glass nodules greater than 1 cm in size are BACs [16] In addition to size, another useful distinguishing feature in pure ground-glass nodules is the identification of a round shape on axial thin-section scans, which, in one study, was seen in 65% of malignant screening-detected SPNs less than 2 cm in diameter as compared with 17% of benign SPNs [17]. The rate of malignancy within mixed-attenuation or part-solid SPNs is

particularly high, with 63% of such lesions in one CT screening study seen to reflect adenocarcinoma [13].

The imaging evaluation of nonsolid nodules poses particular challenges, because advanced imaging modalities, such as contrast CT nodule densitometry and FDG-PET scanning, are inaccurate, and invasive diagnostic techniques including CT-guided needle biopsy and video-assisted thoracoscopic diagnosis are difficult to perform for these lesions. Most patients who have small (<1 cm) pure ground-glass attenuation nodules will require thin-section CT follow-up. The identification of an increase in size, change in internal attenuation (ie, the development of solid foci within a ground-glass lesion), or change in marginal characteristics (ie, development of spiculation or adjacent architectural distortion) that could indicate the presence of malignancy should prompt biopsy for definitive diagnosis (Fig. 17) [16]. Given that subsolid lesions are often PET negative as a result of intrinsic low metabolic activity, subsolid lesions that exceed 10 mm in diameter are best biopsied or resected, particularly in high-risk patients.

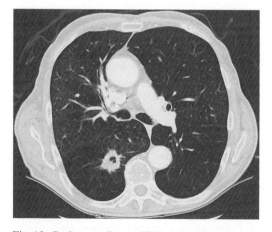

Fig. 15. Cavitary malignant SPN. Axial CT scan at the level of the right upper lobe bronchus at lung windows shows a spiculated superior segment right lower lobe nodule with cavitation and a thick posterolateral wall exceeding 15 mm. Biopsy revealed squamous cell carcinoma.

Growth

The assessment of the growth of an SPN is a useful feature that can help distinguish benign from malignant SPNs. Traditionally, the absence of growth of an SPN over a minimum 2 year

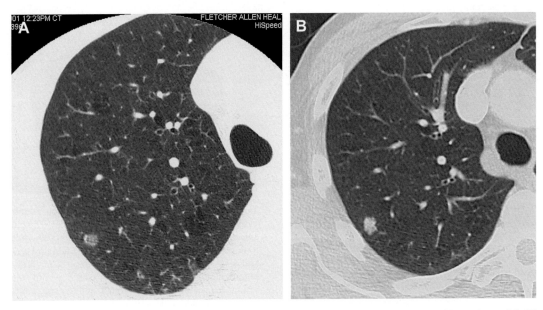

Fig. 17. Evolution of pure ground glass nodule reflecting adenocarcinoma. (*A*) Coned down thin-section axial CT through the right upper lobe shows a pure ground-glass attenuation nodule. (*B*) Repeat scan 3 years later shows the nodule is predominantly solid with irregular margins, but its size has not changed significantly. Transthoracic biopsy and subsequent surgical resection revealed an adenocarcinoma.

period as determined from a review of prior chest radiographic or CT studies is accepted as a reliable indicator of benignity, and these patients do not typically require further evaluation or follow-up. Those patients who lack prior radiographic examinations for comparison or in whom prior studies show no evidence of a nodule or an apparent enlargement in the SPN should proceed to further investigation with thin-section CT.

For solid nodules less than 1 cm in diameter, the accuracy of FDG-PET and image-guided transthoracic needle biopsy is limited somewhat, and most patients, unless at particularly high risk for lung cancer, will undergo follow-up thin-section CT to assess for nodule growth (Fig. 18). Some radiologists will calculate nodule volume doubling times (VDTs) in an attempt to distinguish benign from malignant SPNs, because most malignant SPNs have VDTs of between 30–450 days [18]. Doubling time (T_d) is calculated with the following equation:

$$T_d = T_i \times \log 2/3 \times \log(D_i/D_o),$$

where T_i is interval time, D_i is initial diameter, and D_o is final diameter. Nodule diameter represents the average of two orthogonal measurements through the center of the nodule [19]. A diameter increase of 26% in an SPN reflects a doubling or 100% increase in nodule volume. Recent studies that provide estimates of the volume doubling time of malignant SPNs detected at screening CT show a long mean VDT exceeding 450 days and as long as 928 days in screening-detected cancers [14,20]. These studies show significant positive correlations between VDT and tumor histology (ie, predominance of bronchioloalveolar cell features), the presence of ground-glass attenuation on thin-section CT, and female gender. Given the prolonged calculated doubling times of some slow-growing adenocarcinomas, most radiologists who detect any growth in the size of an SPN will recommend a more definitive diagnostic procedure, usually biopsy or surgical resection (see Fig. 18), so as not to miss these lesions, although the almost uniformly favorable prognosis for slow-growing adenocarcinomas with a predominant or uniform ground-glass attenuation component has raised the possibility of overdiagnosis of these probably nonfatal lung cancers.

There currently is significant investigation into the optimal method of determining growth, and therefore VDT, of an SPN on CT. The ability of a radiologist to accurately measure the diameter of an SPN and then discern an increase in volume is limited, because changes of less than 2 mm in

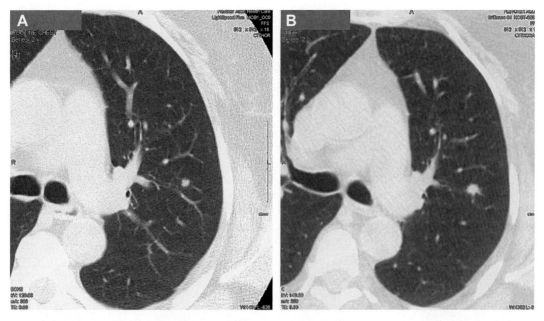

Fig. 18. Growth of small nodule on followup CT. (*A*) Initial thin-section axial CT coned to the left lung shows a small left upper lobe nodule measuring approximately 4 mm in diameter. (*B*) Repeat scan 6 months later shows interval growth of the lesion . The patient opted for surgical resection, and an invasive adenocarcinoma was found at surgery.

diameter are not measured reliably [21,22]. This is a particular problem for nodules 5–8 mm in diameter, because a doubling of volume would correspond to only a 1–2 mm increase in diameter for nodules in this size range. The widespread availability of MDCT, with its inherent volumetric capabilities, has spurred interest in its use for determining lung nodule volumes, and it has provided VDTs for small nodules using computer-aided segmentation and analysis of MDCT datasets through small SPNs obtained a short time apart, typically 90–180 days (Fig. 19). An early article describing the use of a software program that segments SPNs from a helical CT dataset found accurate measurement of synthetic lung nodule volume to within ±3%, which, when applied to a small series of patients, provided accurate discrimination of all malignant nodules (calculated doubling time less than 177 days) from benign lesions (calculated doubling time more than 396 days) [23]. A subsequent study similarly found that a software-calculated doubling time of more than 500 days for 63 solid nodules had a 98% negative predictive value for the diagnosis of malignancy [24]. Despite these encouraging preliminary results, the use of volumetric software in practice has remained limited. Recognized limitations of the technique include

interobserver variability in volume measurements of nodules. Additionally, measured nodule volumes may vary because of differences in CT slice thickness, nodule morphology, nodule attenuation (ie, the difficulty in accurately measuring the volume of part-solid or ground-glass attenuation nodules), nodule location within the chest, and the patient's lung volume during CT acquisition [25,26]. In addition, there are several disparate software programs requiring varying degrees of user manipulation, few of which have been integrated seamlessly into the picture archiving and communication system environment to allow easy access during routine study interpretation. Finally, there are no published outcome studies that validate the use of these software programs. Nevertheless, it is very likely that within the near future, computer-aided analysis of nodule volume will become an important part of the evaluation of small SPNs by helping to sensitively detect growth of small SPNs, and thereby help distinguish benign from malignant SPNs. The technique should prove useful particularly for irregularly-shaped small lesions and lesions that grow in the cephalocaudal plane, which are difficult to assess on axial images alone given differences in scan planes and patient positioning between baseline and followup CT studies.

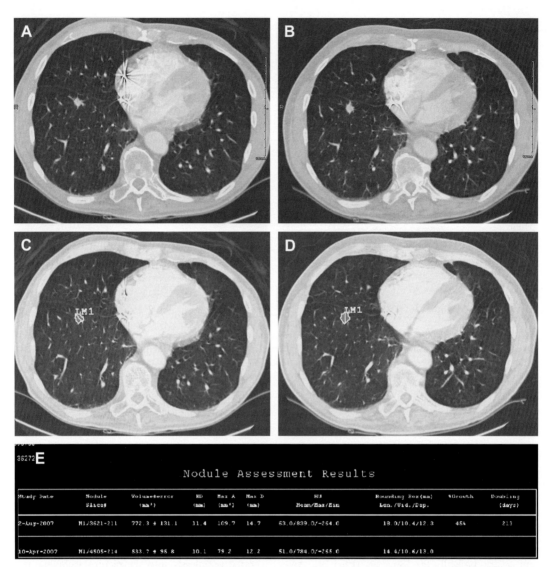

Fig. 19. Computer aided volumetric analysis of nodule growth on CT. (*A*) Initial thin-section axial CT through the lower lungs shows an irregular right lower lobe nodule. (*B*) A repeat axial scan 3.5 months later at the same level shows no apparent change in the appearance of the nodule. (*C, D*) Image of segmentation (removal) of nodule from surrounding lung for volume measurement shows the computer-generated demarcation of the nodules at baseline (*C*) and at 3.5 months (*D*). (*E*) Computer readout of the measurement of nodule volume at baseline and follow-up shows a change in nodule volume from 554 mm^3 to 772 mm^3, with a calculated doubling time of 213 days, which is in the range of a malignant lesion. Surgical resection revealed a non-small cell carcinoma.

Regarding the use of thin-section CT followup to assess for growth of SPNs, it is important to recognize that not all malignant SPNs will grow on follow-up examinations, and as many as 5%–10% of small malignant SPNs will become smaller between short interval scans (Fig. 20) [14,27]. It is important to continue to follow indeterminate lesions for at least 2 years so as not to mischaracterize a malignant SPN as benign based upon a single follow-up short-term CT examination.

Contrast enhancement

Dynamic contrast-enhanced CT and dynamic contrast-enhanced MRI have been used to characterize SPNs based on the observation that

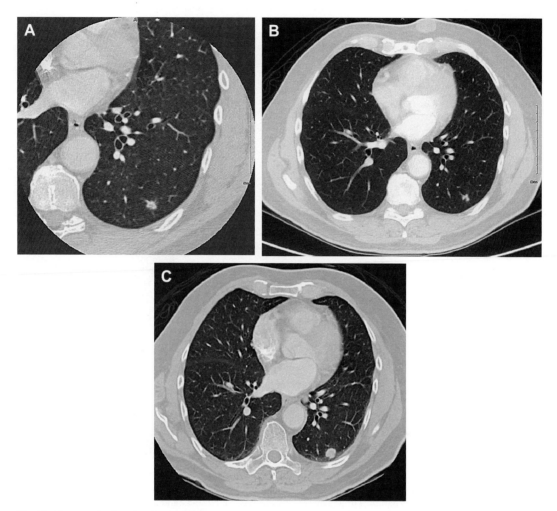

Fig. 20. Decrease in size of malignant SPN on short term follow-up CT. (*A*) Coned down axial CT scan through the left lower lobe shows an irregular nodule. (*B*) Repeat CT scan 4 months later shows a slight decrease in the size of the nodule, which still has an irregular margin. (*C*) Repeat CT scan 6 months after (*B*) shows a increase in size of the nodule, which has a lobulated margin. Transthoracic biopsy showed an adenocarcinoma.

malignant tumors are relatively hypervascular as compared with benign lesions [28,29]. Studies have shown a direct correlation between the presence of increased microvessel density as determined by the measurement of vascular endothelial growth factor within resected malignant SPNs and an increase in attenuation value of SPNs on contrast-enhanced CT studies.

Thin-section CT nodule enhancement following intravenous contrast administration now easily is accomplished with the use of power injectors and the rapid scan acquisition times of MDCT. The most common employed protocol involves overlapping 2–3 mm scans through a solid SPN

that measures 6–30 mm in diameter before and after intravenous contrast injection. The postcontrast scans are obtained at 1, 2, 3, and 4 minutes after contrast injection and are compared with the baseline unenhanced scans. An enhancement value is determined by calculating the mean attenuation value through the center of the nodule at peak contrast enhancement and subtracting the baseline attenuation value. A prospective multicenter study has shown that an enhancement value of 15 HU or less is virtually diagnostic of a benign lesion (ie, the test has a high sensitivity and high negative predictive value for malignancy) (Fig. 21) [30]. Whereas lack of significant

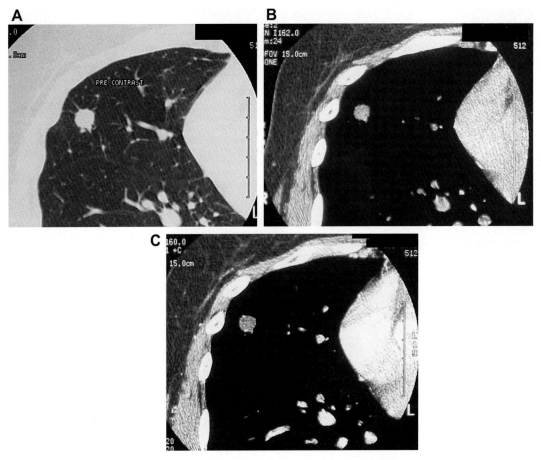

Fig. 21. Negative contrast CT enhancement of a benign nodule. (*A*) Axial CT through the middle lobe shows an irregular nodule. (*B, C*) Scans at mediastinal windows before (*B*) and (*C*) 1 minute after intravenous contrast injection shows
no visible change in nodule attenuation. The enhancement value was 2 HU Transthoracic biopsy showed a granuloma.

enhancement on the contrast CT nodule study has
a high sensitivity for malignant SPNs, its specificity for malignancy is only 50%–60%, because
active granulomas also can show enhancement
at CT. More recent studies using this technique
have measured not only the increase in attenuation of SPNs (ie, wash-in) but also the washout
or decrease in attenuation over the 15 minutes
following contrast injection, in an attempt to
improve on the relatively low specificity of the
technique. These studies have shown that, when
combined with the identification of contrast CT
wash-in, the presence of contrast washout of between 5–31 HU within an SPN was associated
with a relatively high specificity (90%) and overall
accuracy (92%) for malignant nodules [31]. Similar findings have been shown for dynamic MR of
solid pulmonary nodules [32].

Because of the rapid image acquisition with
MDCT, CT nodule enhancement can be performed following routine scanning of the chest
without need for additional contrast administration and little additional time and radiation.
However, the technique requires meticulous attention to detail and may be less accurate in larger
SPNs (ie, those larger than 2.5 cm), because these
lesions are more often necrotic and may produce
false negative studies. The technique may prove to
be most useful for evaluation of probably benign
SPNs when FDG-PET is unavailable or transthoracic needle biopsy cannot be performed. An
additional group in which contrast-CT nodule
densitometry may be preferable to FDG-PET is
patients who have a suspected peripheral carcinoid tumor (Fig. 22). In such patients, an abnormal contrast CT nodule enhancement study

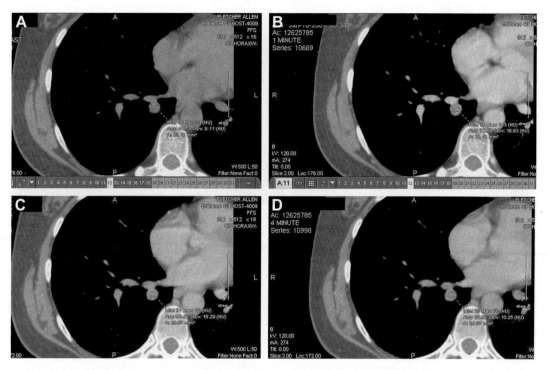

Fig. 22. True positive contrast CT nodule densitometry. Scans obtained through a right lower lobe nodule precontrast (*A*) and at 1 (*B*), 3 (*C*), and 4 (*D*) minutes after contrast injection show a significant increase in attenuation, with an enhancement value of 54 HU (69-15). Biopsy revealed a carcinoid tumor.

should prompt biopsy, because FDG-PET can be false negative in approximately 25% of these lesions.

Nuclear medicine imaging

Positron emission tomography

There is a large experience describing the use of PET and PET-CT using the radiopharmaceutical fluoro-2-deoxy-D-glucose (FDG) in the evaluation of focal lung lesions including SPNs. FDG uptake in focal lesions is measured semiquantitatively by calculating a standardized uptake ratio. In current practice, FDG-PET has a sensitivity of 97% and a specificity of 78% in the characterization of malignant SPNs greater than 10 mm in diameter (Fig. 23) [33]. The low false negative rate of PET makes this a useful adjunct to thin-section CT in excluding malignancy and allows clinical follow-up of probably benign lesions.

While PET has a high negative predictive value for characterizing SPNs as benign, there are two malignant lesions that can present as SPNs and produce a false negative PET study. The most common of these is well-differentiated adenocarcinoma of the lung, particularly those with a bronchioloalveolar cell component (Fig. 24). The relatively low metabolic activity of these lesions leads to false negative PET results in a significant percentage of cases, so if a lesion as seen on thin-section CT has a density and morphology that makes it concerning for an adenocarcinoma (such as mixed solid ground-glass attenuation, irregular or lobulated margins, or cystic lucencies), particularly in a high risk patient, PET may not prove particularly useful for accurate characterization. In a recent retrospective review of the results of FDG-PET in 22 non-small cell lung cancers detected in a lung cancer CT screening trial of high risk patients, 7 of 22 (32%) lesions were PET negative, with 6 of the 7 reflecting pure bronchioloalveolar cell carcinoma or true adenocarcinoma [34]. The peripheral carcinoid tumor, is encountered less, has low metabolic activity, and gives false negative results on PET scans in approximately 25% of cases (Fig. 25) [35]. These lesions can be difficult to distinguish radiologically from benign SPNs, although they often have a lobulated margin, are related to an airway

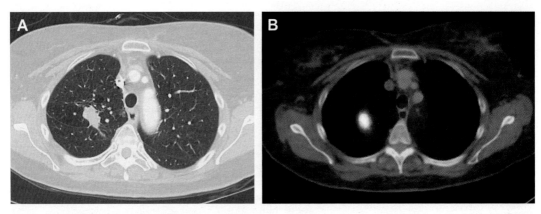

Fig. 23. PET positive non-small cell carcinoma. (*A*) Axial CT scan at lung windows through the lower trachea shows an irregular right upper lobe nodule. (*B*) Fused image from PET-CT shows marked increase in metabolic activity in the nodule. CT-guided biopsy revealed non-small cell carcinoma.

on thin-section analysis, and occasionally can be seen associated with peripheral parenchymal lucency or air trapping on expiratory scans caused by obstruction of the airway from the endobronchial component of the tumor. An additional clue to the diagnosis is the identification of dense enhancement on contrast CT because of the hypervascularity of the lesion (see Fig. 22).

False positive PET studies are more common than false negative studies and account for the lower specificity than sensitivity of PET. Common causes of false positive PET include granulomas with active inflammation (Fig. 26), focal areas of

organizing or resolving pneumonia, and occasionally hamartomas. In these cases, needle biopsy or resection often will be necessary for definitive diagnosis.

Although FDG-PET has become an important part of the noninvasive diagnostic armamentarium in the evaluation of the SPN, it is important that, as with any diagnostic test, it is employed thoughtfully in the evaluation of each patient. Because of its low sensitivity for lesions less than 1 cm in diameter, the use of PET in this setting is limited, but if positive, it would almost certainly prompt biopsy or resection. PET appears to be

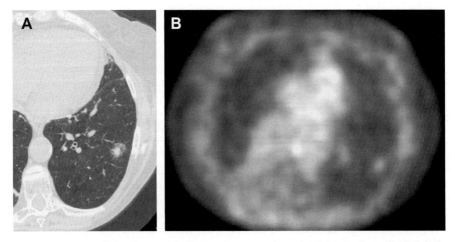

Fig. 24. PET negative adenocarcinoma of lung. (*A*) Axial CT through the left lower lobe in a 76-year-old former smoker demonstrates a 16 mm in diameter mixed solid/ground-glass attenuation nodule. (*B*) Axial image from PET scan at the level of the nodule shows no increase in metabolic activity within the nodule. Trnasthoracic needle biopsy showed adenocarcinoma.

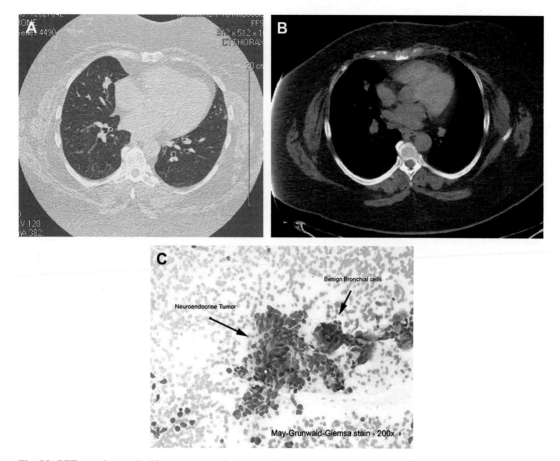

Fig. 25. PET negative carcinoid tumor presenting as an SPN. (*A*) Thin-section axial CT scan at lung windows shows an irregular middle lobe nodule. (*B*) Fused image from PET-CT shows no discernable metabolic activity in the nodule. (*C*) Photomicrograph of cytologic specimen obtained from CT-guided aspiration biopsy shows CT-guided biopsy revealed a cluster of neoplastic spindle-shpaed cells that stained positive for synaptophysin, indicative of a neuroendocrine tumor (May-Grunwald-Giemsa stain, 100x). Subsequent middle lobectomy confirmed the diagnosis of a pulmonary carcinoid tumor.

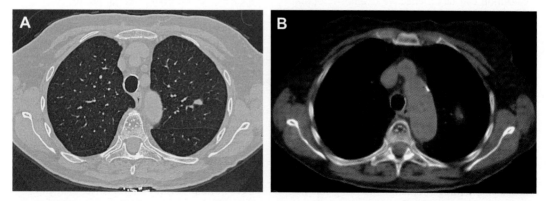

Fig. 26. False positive PET in patient with tuberculosis. (*A*) Thin-section axial CT scan through the upper lobes at lung windows shows a left upper lobe nodule with irregular margins. (*B*) Fused image from PET-CT shows increased metabolic activity within the nodule. Surgical resection revealed a granuloma with cultures positive for Mycobacterium tuberculosis.

most useful when its result is expected to change the management of the patient. In a patient who has a very low (<5%) likelihood of malignancy based upon an assessment of the clinical findings and imaging features of the lesion, the results of a PET study would be unlikely to change the post-test likelihood of malignancy significantly to alter the diagnostic approach to the patient. Similarly, the patient who has a high likelihood of lung cancer invariably will proceed to tissue sampling or resection of the lesion in question, and the false negative rate of PET in this setting would be unacceptably high to change management. Patients who have a low to intermediate likelihood of malignancy (range of 5%–80%), and whose lesions are greater than 1 cm would benefit most from PET imaging, because the result of the PET will usually guide further management [36].

Tissue sampling techniques

Despite the use of CT and FDG-PET imaging in the evaluation of SPNs, a minority of SPNs will require tissue diagnosis as the concern for malignancy based on clinical and imaging characterization remains unacceptably high. Biopsy of SPNs can be performed in several ways, including image-guided transthoracic needle biopsy (TNB), bronchoscopic biopsy with or without elecrtromagnetic navigation systems, video-assisted thoracoscopic surgery (VATS), or open thoracotomy. Patients who have small SPNs (less than 5–6 mm in diameter) that are situated within the peripheral lung that require biopsy for definitive diagnosis, VATS resection with preoperative needle and wire localization can be an effective diagnostic option (Fig. 27). For patients in whom the likelihood of malignancy is very high and are good surgical candidates, VATS or open resection of potentially malignant SPNs are appropriate and cost-effective approaches to definitive diagnosis and in the case of thoracotomy curative resection.

Transthoracic needle biopsy

TNB using image guidance with CT has great diagnostic use for the definitive characterization of SPNs that, after evaluation of clinical risk factors and imaging findings, remain concerning for malignancy, and for patients who have suspected opportunistic infection where a specific organism must be identified to guide appropriate antimicrobial therapy. The majority of these procedures are

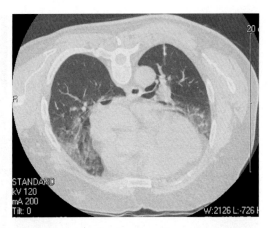

Fig. 27. Wire localization for video-assisted thoracoscopic (VATS) resection of a small peripheral nodule. Prone CT scan at lung windows shows a guidewire percutaneously placed through a 3 mm left lower lobe subpleural nodule in a patient who has a history of renal cell carcinoma. Histopathologic examination of the resected nodule revealed a granuloma.

performed on an outpatient basis using CT or CT-fluoroscopic guidance. Patients who have peripheral lesions well seen on orthogonal radiographic projections can be biopsied using fluoroscopic guidance, whereas those with pleural-based lesions that can be seen sonographically can be biopsied under ultrasound. The primary contraindications to TNB include an uncooperative patient, irreversible bleeding diathesis, severe bullous emphysema, and prior pneumonectomy.

Transthoracic needle biopsy for the diagnosis of SPNs can be performed using a variety of biopsy needles that generally fall into one of two types: aspiration needles that typically range from 20–22-gauge diameter, and core biopsy needles, most of which range from 18–20 gauge diameter (the majority of which are used with an automated cutting technique to provide histologic samples). Lung cancer and epithelial malignancies in general can be diagnosed reliably by microscopic examination of cytologic specimens, and core needle biopsy typically is not necessary for diagnosis of these lesions. The use of core needle biopsies for diagnosis of SPNs usually is not necessary and is reserved for potentially benign lesions, such as granulomas and hamartomas and particularly larger nodules greater than 2 cm in diameter.

Sensitivity rates of TNB for the diagnosis of malignant SPNs greater than 5 mm in diameter are generally above 90% (Fig. 28) [37], although the yield for specific benign lesions is considerably

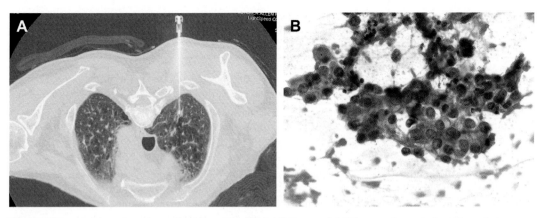

Fig. 28. CT-guided transthoracic needle biopsy of an SPN. (*A*) Prone axial CT scan at lung windows through the upper lobes shows a biopsy needle with its tip in an 8 mm right upper lobe nodule. (*B*) Photomicrograph of the aspirated specimen shows a cluster of large neoplastic cells with a high nuclear-to-cytoplasmic ratio indicative of non-small cell carcinoma (Papanicolaou's stain, 250x).

lower, approximately 60%–70%. While highly accurate in the diagnosis of malignancy, TNB has lower sensitivity and specificity for benign lung lesions, in part because of the nonspecific pathologic appearance of many common benign lesions, such as resolving pneumonia and granulomas. This issue has great significance, because the needle biopsy diagnosis of benign lesions in operable patients can have the greatest impact on management of solitary pulmonary nodules; thoracoscopic or open biopsy can be obviated when a specific benign diagnosis (defined as the detection on TNB of a specific entity that allows confident withholding of further diagnostic procedures [eg, a hamartoma]) is made (Fig. 29) [38]. It is important to keep benign lesions in mind when performing biopsies for suspected malignancy, and clearly, plans should be made in advance for aspirated material to be stained and cultured for microorganisms for patients who are at higher risk for opportunistic infections, (Fig. 30). In all patients, finding inflammatory changes on real-time interpretation of aspirated specimens will lead to aspiration of further material for stains and cultures. The use of core biopsy specimens in patients who have potentially benign lesions is of great use in providing material for specific benign histologic diagnoses, and they

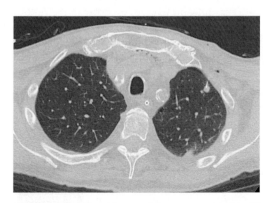

Fig. 29. CT-guided biopsy of hamartoma. Axial CT scan during transthoracic needle biopsy of a solitary left upper lobe nodule in a patient recently status-post laryngectomy for laryngeal cancer shows the biopsy needle within the nodule. Cytopathologic examination of the aspirated material revealed a hamartoma.

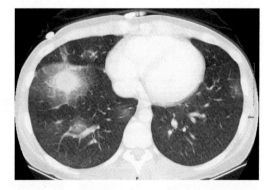

Fig. 30. Transthoracic needle biopsy of invasive aspergillosis complicating Hodgkin's disease. Axial CT scan through the lower lobes in a 32 year-old woman status post bone marrow transplantation for recurrent Hodgkin's disease shows a large nodule with a surrounding halo of ground-glass opacity. CT-guided biopsy revealed aspergillosis.

Table 1
Recommended follow-up of small (≤8 mm) incidental SPNs detected at CT

Nodule size	Low risk patient	High risk patient
≤4 mm	No follow-up needed	CT at 12 mos
>4–6 mm	CT at 12 mos	CT at 6–12, 18–24 mos
>6–8 mm	CT at 6–12, 18–24 mos	CT at 3–6, 9–12, and 24 mos

All recommendations assume no identifiable change on the initial follow-up scans.
Data from MacMahon H, Austin JHM, Gamsu G, et al. Guidelines for management of small pulmonary nodules detected on CT scans: a statement from the Fleischner Society. Radiology 2005;237:395–400.

can be particularly useful if on-site cytopathology is unavailable at the time of biopsy [39].

The main complications of TNB are pneumothorax (occurring in 20% of patients) and bleeding, which is self-limited almost invariably. Most large series of TNB of lung lesions report a chest tube insertion rate of approximately 3%–5% [40].

Fleischner society statement: management of small nodules detected at CT

In an attempt to help guide radiologists and clinicians in the proper evaluation of small, incidentally CT-detected lung nodules, the Fleischner Society recently published an evidence-based recommendation for the follow-up and management of these lesions [41]. These recommendations are summarized in Table 1, and apply to persons aged 35 years or older. Because PET, contrast-CT nodule enhancement, and biopsy are relatively accurate for the evaluation of nodules measuring more than 8 mm in diameter, the recommendations focus on SPNs measuring 8 mm in diameter or less. In general, the size of the nodule and the risk factors for malignancy guide the length and frequency of low-dose, limited CT follow-up. Beacause of the less than 1% likelihood of lung cancer in nodules measuring less than 4 mm in diameter

in low risk individuals, no follow-up of SPNs is recommended for these patients. All other patients who have indeterminate nodules 5–8 mm in diameter should be followed for 24 months. Those who have nodules 7–8 mm in diameter and who are at high risk for malignancy, including smoking history or history of malignancy with a propensity to metastasize to the lung, should undergo follow-up CT 3–6 months from initial detection with further follow-up if no change is detected between 9–12 months and then finally at 24 months. It is likely that as we learn more from the evaluation of SPNs in lung cancer screening studies and as technological advances in MDCT and computer aided diagnosis evolve, these recommendations will change.

Diagnostic algorithm for solitary pulmonary nodules

Based on the available evidence to date, a practical diagnostic algorithm for the evaluation and management of lung nodules is proposed (Fig. 31). It should be noted that local practice patterns, different levels of expertise in the various diagnostic modalities, and medicolegal considerations and individual patient-related comorbidities preclude specific recommendations for each

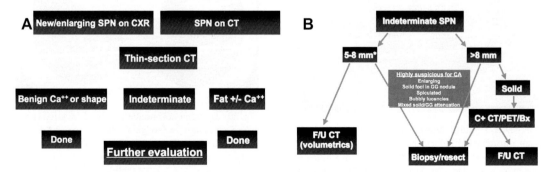

Fig. 31. (*A*, *B*) Algorithm for evaluation of an SPN. C+ CT, contrast nodule enhancement study; GG, ground glass; PET, positron emission tomography.

patient and may dictate disparate approaches for similar clinicoradiologic situations. Nevertheless, the illustrated algorithm reflects the approach to the SPN at the authors' institution and can be applied practically to the majority of patients who have SPNs.

References

[1] Swensen SJ, Jett JR, Hartman TE, et al. CT screening for lung cancer: five-year prospective experience. Radiology 2005;235:259–65.

[2] Austin JH, Muller NL, Friedman PJ, et al. Glossary of terms for CT of the lungs: recommendations of the Nomenclature Committee of the FLeischner Society. Radiology 1996;200:327–31.

[3] Takashima S, Sone S, Li F, et al. Small solitary pulmonary nodules (< or = 1 cm) detected at population-based CT screening for lung cancer: reliable high-resolution CT features of benign lesions. AJR Am J Roentgenol 2003;180:955–64.

[4] Gould MK, Ananth L, Barnett PG. A clinical model to estimate the pretest probability of lung cancer in patients with solitary pulmonary nodules. Chest 2007;131:383–8.

[5] Zerhouni EA, Stitik FP, Siegelman SS, et al. CT of the pulmonary nodule: a cooperative study. Radiology 1986;160:319–27.

[6] Munden RF, Pugatch RD, Liptay MJ, et al. Small pulmonary lesions detected at CT: clinical importance. Radiology 1997;202:105–10.

[7] Siegelman SS, Khouri NF, Leo FP, et al. Solitary pulmonary nodules: CT assessment. Radiology 1986;160:307–12.

[8] Siegelman SS, Khouri NF, Scott J, et al. Pulmonary hamartoma: CT findings. Radiology 1986;160:313–7.

[9] Woodring JH, Fried AM, Chuang VP. Solitary cavities of the lung wall: diagnostic implications of cavity wall thickness. AJR Am J Roentgenol 1980;135:1269–71.

[10] Woodring JH, Fried AM. Significance of wall thickness in solitary cavities of the lung: a follow-up study. AJR Am J Roentgenol 1983;140:473–4.

[11] Kui M, Templeton PA, White CS, et al. Evaluation of the air bronchogram sign on CT in solitary pulmonary lesions. J Comput Assist Tomogr 1996;20:983–6.

[12] Lee KS, Kim Y, Han J, et al. Bronchioloalveolar cell carcinoma: clinical, histopathologic, and radiologic findings. Radiographics 1997;17:1345–57.

[13] Henschke CI, Yankelevitz DF, Mirtcheva R, et al. CT screening for lung cancer: frequency and significance of part-solid and nonsolid nodules. AJR Am J Roentgenol 2002;178:1053–7.

[14] Lindell RM, Hartman TE, Swensen SJ, et al. Five-year lung cancer screening experience: CT appearance, growth rate, location, and histologic features of 61 lung cancers. Radiology 2007;242:555–62.

[15] Park CM, Goo JM, Lee HJ, et al. Nodular ground-glass opacity at thin-section CT: histologic correlation and evaluation of change at follow-up. Radiographics 2007;27:391–408.

[16] Ohtsuka T, Watanabe K, Kaji M, et al. A clinicopathological study of resected pulmonary nodules with focal pure ground-glass opacity. Eur J Cardiothorac Surg 2006;30:160–3.

[17] Li F, Sone S, Abe H, et al. Malignant versus benign nodules at CT screening for lung cancer: comparison of thin-section CT findings. Radiology 2004;233:793–8.

[18] Lillington GA, Caskey CI. Evaluation and management of solitary pulmonary nodules. Clin Chest Med 1983;14:111–9.

[19] Winer-Muram HT. The solitary pulmonary nodule. Radiology 2006;239:34–49.

[20] Hasegawa M, Sone S, Takashima S, et al. Growth rate of small lung cancers detected on mass CT screening. Br J Radiol 2000;73(876):1252–9.

[21] Jennings SG, Winer-Muram HT, Tarver RD, et al. Lung tumor growth: assessment with CT-comparison of diameter and corss-sectional area with volumetric measurements. Radiology 2004;231:866–71.

[22] Revel M-P, Bissery A, Bienvenu M, et al. Are two-dimensional measurements of small noncalcified pulmonary nodules reliable? Radiology 2004;231:453–8.

[23] Yankelevitz DF, Reeves AP, Kostis WJ, et al. Small pulmonary nodules: volumetrically determined growth rates based on CT evaluation. Radiology 2000;217:251–6.

[24] Revel M-P, Merlin A, Peyrard S, et al. Software volumetric evaluation of doubling times for differentiating benign versus malignant pulmonary nodules. AJR Am J Roentgenol 2006;187:135–42.

[25] Petrou M, Quint LE, Nan B, et al. Pulmonary nodule volumetric measurement variability as a function of CT slice thickness and nodule morphology. AJR Am J Roentgenol 2007;188:306–12.

[26] Petrovska I, Brown MS, Goldin JG, et al. The effect of lung volume on nodule size on CT. Acad Radiol 2007;14:476–85.

[27] Jennings SG, Winer-Muram HT, Tann M, et al. Distribution of stage I lung cancer growth rates determined with serial volumetric CT measurements. Radiology 2006;241:554–63.

[28] Swensen S, Brown LR, Colby TV, et al. Lung nodule enhancement on CT: prospective findings. Radiology 1996;201:447–55.

[29] Ohno Y, Hatabu H, Takenaka D, et al. Solitary pulmonary nodules: potential role of dynamic MR imaging in management-Initial experience. Radiology 2002;224:503–11.

[30] Swensen S, Viggiano RW, Midthun DE, et al. Lung nodule enhancement at CT: multicenter study. Radiology 2000;214:73–80.

[31] Jeong YJ, Lee KS, Jeong SY, et al. Solitary pulmonary nodule: characterization with combined wash-
in and washout features at dynamic multi-detector
row CT. Radiology 2005;237:675–83.

[32] Schaefer JF, Vollmar J, Schick F, et al. Solitary pulmonary nodules: dynamic contrast-enhanced MR
imaging-Perfusion differences in malignant and
benign lesions. Radiology 2004;232:544–53.

[33] Gould MK, Maclean CC, Kuschner WG, et al. Accuracy of positron emission tomography for diagnosis of pulmonary nodules and mass lesions. J Am
Med Assoc 2001;285:914–24.

[34] Lindell RM, Hartman TE, Swensen S, et al. Lung
cancer screening experience: a retrospective review
of PET in 22 non-small-cell lung carcinomas
detected on screening chest CT in a high risk population. AJR Am J Roentgenol 2005;185:126–31.

[35] Daniels CE, Lowe VJ, Aubry M-C, et al. The utility
of fluorodeoxyglucose positron emission tomography in the evaluation of carcinoid tumors presenting
as pulmonary nodules. Chest 2007;131:255–60.

[36] Detterbeck FC, Falen S, Rivera MP, et al. Seeking
a home for a PET, part 1. Defining the appropriate
place for positron emission tomography imaging in
the diagnosis of pulmonary nodules or masses. Chest
2004;125:2294–9.

[37] Stanley JH, Fish GD, Andriole JG, et al. Lung
lesions: cytologic diagnosis by fine-needle biopsy.
Radiology 1987;162:389–91.

[38] Fraser RS. Transthoracic needle aspiration. The benign diagnosis. Arch Pathol Lab Med 1991;115:
751–61.

[39] Salomon G, Stewart EA. Transthoracic needle biopsy with coaxially placed 20-gauge automated cutting needle: results in 122 patients. Radiology 1996;
198:715–72.

[40] Klein JS, Zarka MA. Transthoracic needle biopsy.
Radiol Clin North Am 2000;38:235–66.

[41] MacMahon H, Austin JHM, Gamsu G, et al. Guidelines for management of small pulmonary nodules
detected on CT scans: a statement from the Fleischner Society. Radiology 2005;237:395–400.

ELSEVIER SAUNDERS

Clin Chest Med 29 (2008) 39–57

CLINICS IN CHEST MEDICINE

CT, Positron Emission Tomography, and MRI in Staging Lung Cancer

Jeremy J. Erasmus, MBBCh*, Bradley S. Sabloff, MD

Division of Diagnostic Imaging, University of Texas, MD Anderson Cancer Center, 1515 Holcombe Boulevard, Unit 0371, Houston, TX 77030, USA

Lung cancer is a common malignancy and, although the number of new cases in men has decreased from a high of 102 per 100,000 in 1984 to 73.6 in 2004 and is approaching a plateau in women, with 50.2 per 100,000 new cases in 2004, it remains the leading cause of cancer-related deaths in both men and women in the United States [1]. The American Cancer Society estimates that 213,380 new cases of lung cancer will be diagnosed in the United States in the year 2007. In these patients, imaging has an important role in the detection, diagnosis, and staging of the disease as well as in assessing response to therapy and monitoring for tumor recurrence after treatment. This article reviews the staging of the two major histologic categories of lung cancer [2,3]—non–small-cell lung carcinoma (NSCLC) and small-cell lung carcinoma (SCLC)—and emphasizes the appropriate use of CT, MRI, and positron emission tomography (PET) imaging in patient management.

Non–small-cell lung cancer

Staging

The treatment and prognosis of patients with NSCLC depend on staging (ie, the determination of the anatomic extent of disease at initial presentation [4–7]). Uniform criteria for reporting the findings of clinical and or pathologic evaluation are important in the initial management of patients with NSCLC. In this regard, the sixth

edition of the Union Internationale Contre le Cancer and the American Joint Committee on Cancer (AJCC) is currently used to describe the extent of NSCLC in terms of the primary tumor (T status), lymph nodes (N status), and metastases (M status) (Table 1) [4]. Although this sixth edition has been used for the TNM staging system for lung cancer since 1997, a new staging project was initiated in 1999 by the International Association for the Study of Lung Cancer (IASLC). Recently, a proposal for the revision of the T, N, and M descriptors in the forthcoming seventh edition has been published by the IASLC's Lung Cancer Staging Project and are discussed below [5–7].

In terms of the T, N, and M descriptors, radiologic imaging is usually directed at detecting nonresectable disease (T4 or N3 or M1). The differentiation of T1-3 from T4 lung cancer and the detection of contralateral nodal (N3) and/or extrathoracic metastases (M1) are important as these typically preclude surgical resection or require additional chemotherapy or radiotherapy. However, there is currently little consensus on the imaging that should be performed for appropriate staging evaluation in patients presenting with NSCLC. Recently, the American Society of Clinical Oncology (ASCO) published evidence-based guidelines for the diagnostic evaluation of patients with NSCLC [8]. In the staging of locoregional disease, these guidelines recommend that a chest radiograph and contrast-enhanced chest CT that includes the liver and adrenals should be performed. In addition, the ASCO recommendations are that whole-body PET imaging with [18F]-fluoro-2-deoxy-D-glucose positron emission tomography (FDG-PET) should be performed when there is no evidence of distant metastatic

* Corresponding author.

E-mail address: jerasmus@di.mdacc.tmc.edu (J.J. Erasmus).

0272-5231/08/$ - see front matter © 2008 Elsevier Inc. All rights reserved.
doi:10.1016/j.ccm.2007.11.004

chestmed.theclinics.com

Table 1
International staging system for lung cancer TNM descriptors

Primary tumor (T)

TX—primary tumor cannot be assessed, or tumor proven by the presence of malignant cells in sputum or bronchial washings but not visualized by imaging or bronchoscopy

TO—no evidence of primary tumor

T is carcinoma in situ

T1 tumor ≤3 cm in greatest dimension, surrounded by lung or visceral pleura, without bronchoscopic evidence of invasion more proximal than the lobar bronchus[a] (ie, not in the main bronchus)

T2 tumor with any of the following features of size or extent:
- >3 cm in greatest dimension
- involves main bronchus, ≥2 cm distal to the carina
- invades the visceral pleura
- associated with atelectasis or obstructive pneumonitis that extends to the hilar region but does not involve the entire lung

T3 tumor of any size that directly invades any of the following: chest wall (including SSTs), diaphragm, mediastinal pleura, parietal pericardium; or tumor in the main bronchus <2 cm distal to the carina but without involvement of the carina; or associated atelectasis or obstructive pneumonitis of the entire lung

T4 tumor of any size that invades any of the following: mediastinum, heart, great vessels, trachea, esophagus, vertebral body, carina; or tumor with a malignant pleural or pericardial effusion[b], or with satellite tumor nodule(s) in the ipsilateral primary-tumor lobe(s) of the lung

Regional lymph nodes (N)

NX—regional lymph nodes cannot be assessed

N0—no regional lymph node metastasis

N1—metastasis to ipsilateral peribronchial and/or ipsilateral hilar lymph nodes, and intrapulmonary nodes involved by direct extension of the primary tumor

N2—metastasis to ipsilateral mediastinal and/or subcarinal lymph node(s)

N3—metastasis to contralateral mediastinal, contralateral hilar, ipsilateral or contralateral scalene, or supraclavicular lymph node(s)

Distant metastasis

MX—presence of distant metastasis cannot be assessed

M0—no distant metastasis

M1—distant metastasis present[c]

---

[a] The uncommon superficial tumor of any size with its invasive component limited to the bronchial wall, which may extend proximal to the main bronchus, is also classified T1.

[b] Most pleural effusions associated with lung cancer are due to tumor. However, there are a few patients in whom multiple cytopathologic examinations of pleural fluid show no tumor. In these cases, the fluid is nonbloody and is not an exudate. When these elements and clinical judgment dictate that the effusion is not related to the tumor, the effusion should be excluded as a staging element and the patient's disease should be staged T1, T2, or T3. Pericardial effusion is classified according to the same rules.

[c] Separate metastatic tumor nodule(s) in the ipsilateral nonprimary-tumor lobe(s) of the lung are also classified M1.

From Mountain CF. Revisions in the international system for staging lung cancer. Chest 1997;111:1710–7; with permission.

disease on CT [8]. This recommendation is based on the fact that FDG-PET imaging improves the detection of nodal and distant metastases and frequently alters patient management [9–14]. At present, FDG-PET is usually used together with CT because the relatively poor spatial resolution of FDG-PET limits its utility in the evaluation of the primary tumor (T descriptor) and in the determination of the precise anatomic location of regions of focal increased FDG-uptake (N and M descriptors). The introduction of integrated PET-CT scanners with coregistration of PET and CT images overcomes limitations inherent to both modalities when used separately. In fact, staging of NSCLC has been reported to be more accurate with integrated PET-CT than when using visual correlation of PET and CT performed separately [10,15].

Primary tumor (T status)

The T status defines the size, location, and extent of the primary tumor (see Table 1). The seventh edition of the TNM classification of lung cancer proposed by the IASLC Lung Cancer

Staging Project includes the following changes to the T descriptor that are based on differences in survival:

- To subclassify T1 as T1a (≤ 2 cm) or T1b ($>2-\leq 3$ cm)
- To subclassify T2 as T2a ($>3-\leq 5$ cm or T2 by other factor [see Table 1] and ≤ 5 cm) or T2b ($>5-\leq 7$ cm)
- To reclassify T2 tumors >7 cm as T3
- To reclassify T4 tumors with additional nodule(s) in the lung (primary lobe) as T3
- To reclassify M1 tumors with additional nodule(s) in the ipsilateral lung (different lobe) as T4
- To reclassify T4 pleural dissemination (malignant pleural effusions, pleural nodules) as M1 [5]

Because the extent of the primary tumor determines therapeutic management (surgical resection or palliative radiotherapy or chemotherapy), imaging is often performed to assess the degree of pleural, chest-wall, and mediastinal invasion. CT is useful in confirming gross chest-wall invasion, but is inaccurate in differentiating between anatomic contiguity and subtle invasion (Fig. 1). Findings suggestive of chest wall invasion include tumor-pleura contact extending over more than 3 cm, an obtuse angle at the tumor-pleura interface, and thickening of the pleura or increased attenuation of the extrapleural fat adjacent to the tumor [16]. Although MRI offers superior soft-tissue contrast resolution, the sensitivity (63%–90%) and specificity (84%–86%) in

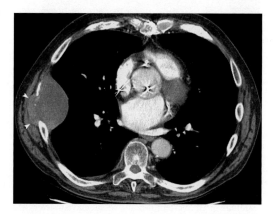

Fig. 1. A 78-year-old man with NSCLC and chest-wall invasion. Contrast-enhanced CT shows an 8 cm mass with tumor invasion into chest wall (*arrowheads*) and destruction of the adjacent rib. The T descriptor is T3 (tumor of any size that directly invades the chest wall).

identifying chest-wall invasion are similar to those of CT [17,18]. Imaging with CT or MRI is also useful in confirming gross invasion of the mediastinum, but these modalities, similar to chest-wall assessment, are inaccurate in determining subtle invasion (56%–89% and 50%–93%, respectively) (Fig. 2) [18–21]. CT and MRI findings that can be useful in suggesting subtle mediastinal invasion include tumor-mediastinal contact extending over more than 3 cm, obliteration of the fat plane between the mediastinum and tumor, and tumor contacting more than 90° of the aortic circumference [20,22,23].

Although MRI has limited accuracy in determining subtle invasion of the chest wall and mediastinum, it is particularly useful in the evaluation of cardiac invasion (see Fig. 2) and superior sulcus (Pancoast) tumors. Superior sulcus tumors (SSTs) are usually classified as T3 or higher because invasion of extrathoracic soft tissues is invariably present. MRI is usually used to evaluate this invasion and is particularly useful in the assessment of the degree of involvement of the brachial plexus, subclavian vessels, and vertebral bodies (Fig. 3) [18,24,25]. Although involvement of the brachial plexus or subclavian vessels is not defined by the standard AJCC staging system for lung cancer, limited involvement of the lower trunk or roots (C8, T1) of the brachial plexus is generally regarded as T3 disease, whereas more extensive invasion into the brachial plexus trunks or roots (C5–C7), subclavian vessels, vertebral bodies, spinal cord, trachea, or esophagus constitutes T4 disease. Nevertheless, it is important to be aware that a T4 classification for a superior sulcus lung carcinoma does not always imply nonresectability. In this regard, invasion of the subclavian vessels, which is often difficult to establish by imaging before surgery, is a relative contraindication to resection. Furthermore, tumors that invade less than 50% of a vertebral body may be resectable, but these tumors often require a combined thoracic and neurosurgical approach [26–28]. Lastly, invasion of the common carotid artery or vertebral artery represents another relative contraindication to surgery. These vessels will often have to be ligated to achieve complete resection of a locally invasive carcinoma. However, if there is significant atherosclerotic disease of the contralateral vessels, resection may not be feasible [29]. In such instances, CT or MRI may be the first examination to alert the surgeon to contralateral atherosclerosis. Importantly, absolute contraindications to surgery (invasion of the brachial plexus roots or trunks

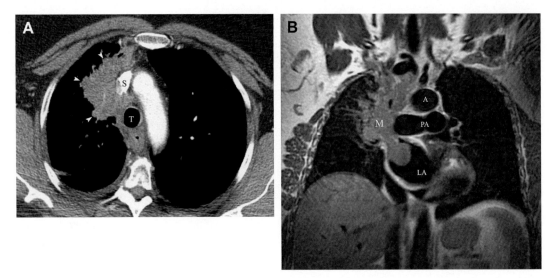

Fig. 2. A 64-year-old woman with NSCLC invading the left atrium. (*A*) Contrast-enhanced CT shows a poorly margin-ated right upper-lobe lung mass (*arrowheads*) that abuts and is inseparable from the adjacent mediastinum. Note oblit-eration of the fat plane between the mediastinum and tumor suspicious for mediastinal invasion and gross invasion of tumor into the mediastinum anterior to the trachea (*T*). Mediastinal invasion is classified as T4 and precludes resection. S, superior vena cava. (*B*) Double inversion recovery single breath-hold coronal MRI shows a right upper-lobe mass (*M*) that extends via the right superior pulmonary vein into the left atrium. A, aorta; LA, left atrium; PA, pulmonary artery.

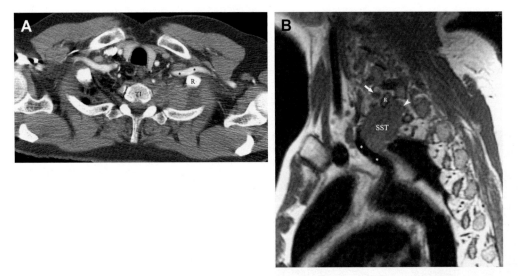

Fig. 3. A 68-year-old man with a superior sulcus NSCLC presenting with pain involving the medial aspect of the left arm and forearm and Horner's syndrome (ptosis, miosis, anhidrosis). Clinical presentation is indicative of involvement of the T1 nerve root and stellate ganglion (lower cervicothoracic sympathetic nerve plexus), respectively. (*A*) Axial CT image shows a soft-tissue mass in the left lung apex. There are no CT findings of rib, vertebral body, or subclavian artery (*) invasion. R, first rib; T1, first thoracic vertebral body. (*B*) Sagittal T1-weighted MR scan shows the left SST extending posteriorly into the T1/T2 neurovertebral foramen (*arrowhead*) and causing obliteration of the exiting T1 nerve root. The C8 nerve root is preserved (*arrow*). Limited involvement of the brachial plexus does not preclude surgical resection and patient underwent complete resection. (*Courtesy of* Clifton F. Mountain, MD, San Diego, CA; with permission. Copyright © 1996, Mountain and Dresler.)

above the level of T1 [26,29], invasion of greater than 50% of a vertebral body [27,29], and invasion of the esophagus or trachea) are often accurately assessed by MRI [25,29].

The International Staging System for Lung Cancer combines the T descriptors with the N and M descriptors into subsets or stages that have similar treatment options and prognosis (Table 2). However, it is important to realize that, although a T4 descriptor generally precludes resection, patients with cardiac, great-vessel, tracheal, and vertebral body invasion (all designated as T4 or nonresectable disease) can occasionally be completely resected (Fig. 4) [30,31]. Complete surgical resection has been reported to be possible in many of these patients (typically after induction therapy) who, on initial staging, would have been denied surgery. Besides an improvement in locoregional control, patients who could be completely resected also showed improvement in long-term survival rates that were unforeseen considering their initial clinical staging [30]. Additionally, primary tumors associated with satellite nodules in the same lobe are currently classified as T4 disease. However, because the survival of these patients is better than those with other T4 descriptors, the IASLC Lung Cancer Staging Project for the seventh edition of the TNM classification of lung cancer proposes to reclassify T4 tumors with additional nodule(s) in the same lobe as the primary tumor as T3 (Fig. 5) [5]. This T3 designation reflects the current clinical practice in which many patients with satellite

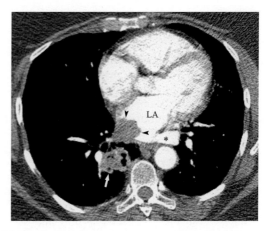

Fig. 4. A 76-year-old woman with NSCLC presenting with palpitations. Contrast-enhanced CT shows a cavitary mass (*arrow*) in the right lower lobe that extends into the left atrium (*arrowheads*). Clinical and pathologic staging was T4N0 and patient underwent surgical resection. Patient received adjuvant chemotherapy and remained disease-free for 10 months before developing a brain metastasis. LA, left atrium; *, left inferior pulmonary vein.

nodules in the same lobe undergo definitive resection if there are no other contraindications to surgery. Primary lung cancers associated with malignant pleural effusions or pleural metastases are also currently classified as T4. The diagnosis is important in patient management because the

Table 2
Stage grouping—TNM subsets

Stage	TNM Subset		
IA	T1	N0	M0
IB	T2	N0	M0
IIA	T1	N1	M0
IIB	T2	N1	M0
	T3	N0	M0
IIIA	T1–2	N2	M0
	T3	N1–2	M0
IIIB	T4	N0–2	M0
	T1–4	N3	M0
IV	any T any N M1		

From Mountain CF. Revisions in the international system for staging lung cancer. Chest 1997;111:1710–7; with permission.

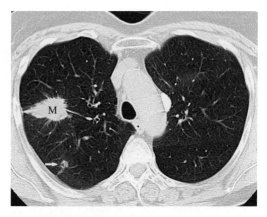

Fig. 5. A 63-year-old woman with NSCLC. Contrast-enhanced CT shows a spiculated mass (*M*) and a small satellite nodule in the right upper lobe (*arrow*). Although the classification is T4 (nonresectable), the IASLC Project has recently proposed a T3 (resectable) designation when the additional nodule(s) are in the same lobe as the primary tumor.

median overall survival is poor (8 months) [5,7]. In fact, the survival is similar to patients with disseminated extrathoracic metastases and, consequently, the IASLC Lung Cancer Staging Project proposal is to reclassify pleural dissemination (malignant pleural effusions, pleural nodules) as M1 disease [7]. It is important to be aware that pleural metastases are common at presentation and that the diagnosis of pleural metastases or malignant effusion can be difficult to confirm [4,32]. Pleural thickening and nodularity on CT scans suggest metastatic pleural disease, but these abnormalities may not be present in association with a malignant effusion (Fig. 6). Furthermore, cytologic evaluation is positive in only approximately 66% of patients with a malignant pleural effusion at presentation [32].

Regional lymph nodes (N status)

The presence and location of pleural metastases are of major importance in determining management and prognosis in patients with NSCLC [6,33]. To enable a consistent and standardized description of N status, nodal stations are defined by the American Thoracic Society in relation to anatomic structures or boundaries that can be identified before and during thoracotomy (Tables 3 and 4) [4,33]. The IASLC Lung Cancer Staging Project has proposed that the current N descriptors should be maintained as there were no significant survival differences in analysis by station [6]. However, it proposes that lymph node stations be grouped together in six zones within the current N1 and N2 patient subsets for further evaluation.

For N1 nodal status, zones were defined as peripheral (stations 12, 13, 14) or hilar (stations 10, 11). N2 nodes were classified as upper mediastinal (stations 1, 2, 3, 4), lower mediastinal (stations 8, 9), aortopulmonary (stations 5, 6), and subcarinal (station 7) [6]. This proposal is based on survival analysis by anatomic location (or zone) of involved nodes, the number of zones involved, and presence of skip metastases.

Lymph node size is the only imaging criterion used to diagnose nodal metastases, with nodes greater than 1 cm in short-axis diameter considered abnormal [34]. However, lymph node size is not a reliable parameter for the evaluation of nodal metastatic disease in patients with NSCLC [35–37]. Prenzel and colleagues [35] recently reported that in 2891 resected hilar and mediastinal nodes obtained from 256 patients with NSCLC, 77% of the 139 patients with no nodal metastases had at least one node greater than 1 cm in diameter. Furthermore, 12% of the 127 patients with nodal metastases had no nodes greater than 1 cm. In a meta-analysis of 20 studies (3438 patients) evaluating CT accuracy for staging the mediastinum, there was a pooled sensitivity of 57%, specificity of 82%, positive predictive value of 56%, and negative predictive value of 83% [38].

Because surgical resection and potential use of adjuvant therapy are dependent on the patient's N descriptor, attempts have been made to improve the accuracy of detection of nodal metastases. FDG-PET complements CT findings and provides information on locoregional nodal staging that impacts management (Fig. 7) [12,13,39,40]. In

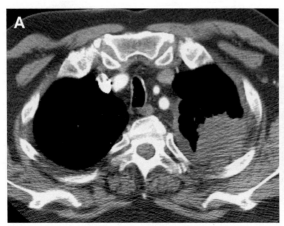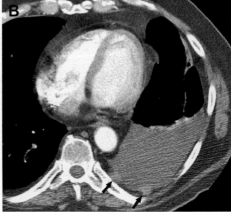

Fig. 6. (*A*) A 75-year-old man with primary NSCLC and a malignant pleural effusion at presentation manifesting as shortness of breath. (*B*) Contrast-enhanced CT shows a left upper-lobe lung mass, left pleural effusion, and nodular pleural lesions consistent with metastases (*arrows*).

Table 3
Regional lymph node stations for lung cancer staging

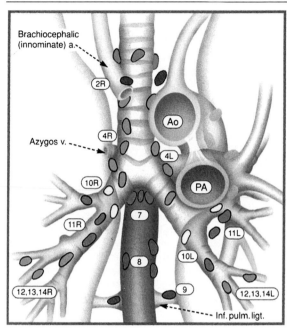

Superior Mediastinal Nodes

- **1** Highest Mediastinal
- **2** Upper Paratracheal
- **3** Pre-vascular and Retrotracheal
- **4** Lower Paratracheal
  (including Azygos Nodes)

N_2 = single digit, ipsilateral
N_3 = single digit, contralateral or supraclavicular

Aortic Nodes

- **5** Subaortic (A-P window)
- **6** Para-aortic (ascending
  aorta or phrenic)

Inferior Mediastinal Nodes

- **7** Subcarinal
- **8** Paraesophageal
  (below carina)
- **9** Pulmonary Ligament

N_1 Nodes

- **10** Hilar
- **11** Interlobar
- **12** Lobar
- **13** Segmental
- **14** Subsegmental

From Mountain CF, Dresler CM. Regional lymph node classification for lung cancer staging. Chest 1997;111:1718–23; with permission.

Table 4
Lymph node map definitions

Nodal station	Anatomic landmarks
N2 nodes—all N2 nodes lie within the mediastinal pleural envelope	
Highest mediastinal nodes	Nodes lying above a horizontal line at the upper rim of the brachiocephalic (left innominate) vein where it ascends to the left, crossing in front of the trachea at its midline
Upper paratracheal nodes	Nodes lying above a horizontal line drawn tangential to the upper margin of the aortic arch and below the inferior boundary of No. 1 nodes
Prevascular and retrotracheal nodes	Prevascular and retrotracheal nodes may be designated 3A and 3P; midline nodes are considered to be ipsilateral
Lower paratracheal nodes	The lower paratracheal nodes on the right lie to the right of the midline of the trachea between a horizontal line drawn tangential to the upper margin of the aortic arch and a line extending across the right main bronchus at the upper margin of the upper-lobe bronchus, and contained within the mediastinal pleural envelope; the lower paratracheal nodes on the left lie to the left of the midline of the trachea between a horizontal line drawn tangential to the upper margin of the aortic arch and a line extending across the left main bronchus at the level of the upper margin of the left upper-lobe bronchus, medial to the ligamentum arteriosum and contained within the mediastinal pleural envelope
Subaortic (aortopulmonary window)	Subaortic nodes are lateral to the ligamentum arteriosum or the aorta or left pulmonary artery and proximal to the first branch of the left pulmonary artery and lie within the mediastinal pleural envelope
Para-aortic nodes (ascending aorta or phrenic)	Nodes lying anterior and lateral to the ascending aorta and the aortic arch or the innominate artery, beneath a line tangential to the upper margin of the aortic arch
Subcarinal nodes	Nodes lying caudal to the carina of the trachea but not associated with the lower-lobe bronchi or arteries within the lung
Paraesophageal nodes (below carina)	Nodes lying adjacent to the wall of the esophagus and to the right or left of the midline, excluding subcarinal nodes
Pulmonary ligament nodes	Nodes lying within the pulmonary ligament, including those in the posterior wall and lower part of the inferior pulmonary vein
N1 nodes—all N1 nodes lie distal to the mediastinal pleural reflection and within the visceral pleura	
Hilar nodes	The proximal lobar nodes, distal to the mediastinal pleural reflection and the nodes adjacent to the bronchus intermedius on the right; radiographically, the hilar shadow may be created by enlargement of both hilar and interlobar nodes
Interlobar nodes	Nodes lying between the lobar bronchi
Lobar nodes	Nodes adjacent to the distal lobar bronchi
Segmental nodes	Nodes adjacent to the segmental bronchi
Subsegmental nodes	Nodes around the subsegmental bronchi

From Mountain CF, Dresler CM. Regional lymph node classification for lung cancer staging. Chest 1997;111:1718–23; with permission.

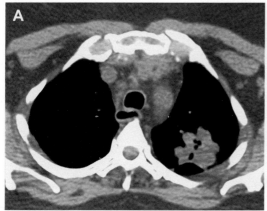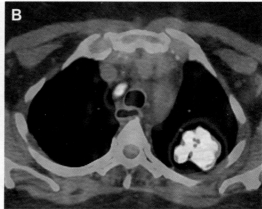

Fig. 7. A 73-year-old woman with a primary squamous cell carcinoma of the left upper lobe presenting with cough and hemoptysis. Axial CT (*A*) and integrated CT-PET (*B*) show increased uptake of FDG in the primary malignancy and in a right paratracheal node. Biopsy of nodes confirmed metastatic disease (N3) and patient was treated palliatively.

a recent meta-analysis (17 studies, 833 patients) comparing PET and CT in nodal staging in patients with NSCLC, the sensitivity and specificity of FDG-PET for detecting mediastinal lymph node metastases ranged from 66% to 100% (overall 83%) and 81% to 100% (overall 92%), respectively, compared with sensitivity and specificity of CT of 20% to 81% (overall 59%) and 44% to 100% (overall 78%), respectively [39]. In addition, significant improvements in the accuracy of overall tumor staging have been reported when using integrated CT-PET compared with CT and PET interpreted separately [15]. Because of the improvements of nodal staging when CT-PET is incorporated into the imaging algorithm of those patients with potentially resectable NSCLC, the performance of CT-PET should be considered in all patients without CT findings of distant metastasis regardless of the size of mediastinal nodes, to direct nodal sampling as well as to detect distant occult metastasis.

It is important to emphasize that in terms of invasive nodal staging, the role of FDG-PET should be considered an adjunct rather than an alternative [8,12]. In this regard, a meta-analysis evaluated the association between the size of mediastinal lymph nodes and the probability of malignancy [41]. The authors reported a 5% post-test probability for N2 disease in patients with a negative FDG-PET if the mediastinal nodes were 10 to 15 mm on CT and suggested that these patients should proceed directly to thoracotomy. In patients with a negative FDG-PET and lymph nodes larger than 16 mm on CT, the posttest

probability for N2 disease was 21%, suggesting that these patients should have mediastinoscopy before thoracotomy. Furthermore, although FDG-PET for nodal staging is cost effective and can reduce the likelihood that a patient with mediastinal nodal metastases (N3) that would preclude surgery will undergo attempted resection, the number of false-positive results due to infectious or inflammatory etiologies is too high to remove the need for invasive sampling [42,43]. Invasive sampling of FDG-avid nodes should be performed to confirm nodal metastatic disease in all patients where this will have an impact on management (Fig. 8).

Metastatic disease (M status)

Patients with NSCLC commonly have metastases to the lung, adrenals, liver, brain, bones, and extrathoracic lymph nodes at presentation [4,7]. The IASLC Lung Cancer Staging Project has proposed that the M1 descriptor should be subclassified into M1a (additional nodules in the contralateral lung) and M1b (distant metastases outside the lung and pleura) [7]. Additionally, on the basis of survival analysis, the current M descriptor should be modified to reclassify pleural metastases (malignant pleural effusions, pleural nodules) from T4 to M1a [7].

The role of imaging in detecting extrathoracic metastases is not clearly defined. However, because staging performed based on clinical findings and conventional radiologic imaging incorrectly stages some patients with NSCLC, whole-body FDG-PET is increasingly being used to improve

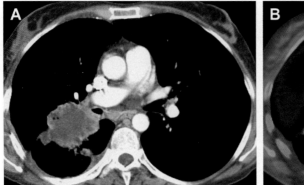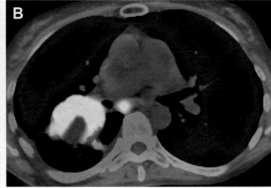

Fig. 8. A 42-year-old woman with a primary squamous cell carcinoma of the left upper lobe presenting with cough. Axial CT (*A*) and integrated CT-PET (*B*) show a large necrotic right lung mass with increased uptake of FDG. There is increased FDG uptake in a paraesophageal node that, by both PET and CT criteria, (short-axis diameter > than 1 cm) is suspicious for nodal metastatic disease. Bronchoscopy and endobronchial ultrasound-guided biopsy of mediastinal nodes were negative for malignancy.

the accuracy of staging (Fig. 9). FDG-PET has a higher sensitivity and specificity than CT in detecting metastases to the adrenals, bones, and extrathoracic lymph nodes (Fig. 10). In this regard, the American College of Surgeons Oncology Trial reports a sensitivity, specificity, positive predictive value, and negative predictive value of 83%, 90%, 36%, and 99%, respectively, for PET in identification of M1 disease [12]. Whole-body PET imaging stages intra- and extrathoracic disease in a single study and detects occult extrathoracic metastases in up to 24% of patients selected for curative resection [9,12,14,44]. The incidence of detection of occult metastases has been reported to increase as the staging T and N descriptors increase—from 7.5% in early-stage disease to 24% in advanced-stage disease [44]. In a recent randomized controlled trial of the role of PET in early-stage lung cancer (in which more than 90% of patients had T1-2N0 disease), Viney and colleagues [45] showed that distant metastases were rarely detected (less than 2.5%), although PET improved the accuracy of staging. However, Viney and colleagues have acknowledged that, subsequent to the study, patients with stage IIIA N2 disease at the participating hospitals now routinely receive neoadjuvant chemotherapy and, in this scenario, PET would have had an impact on the management in up to 20% of the patients. Two studies with a higher proportion of more advanced lung cancers considered resectable by standard clinical staging showed that PET imaging prevented nontherapeutic surgery in 1 in 5 patients [9,12]. It is

important to emphasize that although whole-body FDG-PET imaging improves the accuracy of staging, false-positive uptake of FDG can mimic distant metastases and, therefore, all focal lesions with increased FDG-uptake should be biopsied if they potentially would alter patient management [46].

Metastases to the adrenal glands are common and can occur as an isolated site of disease in up to 6% of patients [7]. CT and MRI can be useful in the evaluation of adrenal masses, and features favoring malignancy include size greater than 3 cm, poorly defined margins, irregularly enhancing rim, invasion of adjacent structures, and high signal intensity on T2-weighted MRI sequences [47]. A confident diagnosis of benignity can be made if an adrenal mass has an attenuation value less than 10 HU on a non–contrast-enhanced CT scan [47,48]. A meta-analysis of 10 studies to determine an optimal threshold for differentiating benign from malignant lesions yielded a sensitivity of 71% and a specificity of 98% for characterizing adrenal masses with a threshold of 10 HU [48]. Although the finding of low attenuation is useful to characterize an adenoma, up to 30% of adenomas do not contain sufficient lipid to demonstrate low attenuation at CT [49]. In these cases, MRI, the use of chemical shift analysis, and dynamic gadolinium enhancement can also be used to determine whether an adrenal mass is benign [50–52].

A decision analysis model to determine the most cost-effective way to evaluate an adrenal mass in patients with newly diagnosed NSCLC showed that unenhanced CT using a 10-HU

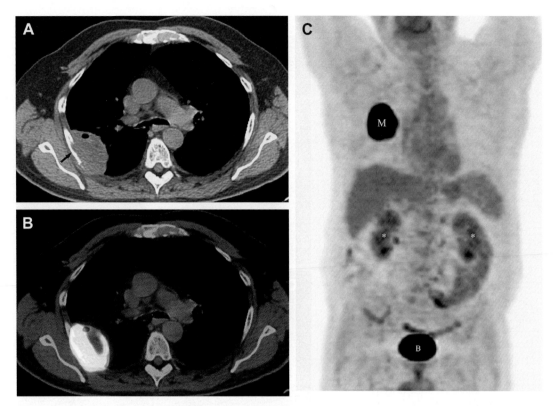

Fig. 9. A 64-year-old man with primary cell lung cancer presenting with chest pain. Axial CT (*A*) and integrated CT-PET (*B*) show a cavitary right lung mass with increased uptake of FDG. There is focal destruction of the adjacent rib (*arrow*). Locoregional chest-wall invasion is classified as T3. (*C*) Coronal whole-body PET scan shows increased FDG uptake within the primary malignancy (*M*). FDG uptake in the mediastinum is normal and there is no focal abnormal extrathoracic FDG uptake, findings indicative of the absence of nodal and distant metastases. Right upper-lobe and chest-wall resection with en bloc resection of the 4th, 5th, and 6th ribs was performed. B, accumulation of FDG in the bladder; *, renal excretion of FDG.

threshold followed by MRI, if needed, was the most cost-effective strategy [53]. However, FDG-PET was not included as a diagnostic option in this analysis. In fact, FDG-PET is useful in distinguishing benign from malignant adrenal masses detected on CT, and is particularly advocated when the adrenal mass is small. Two series have shown a sensitivity of 100% and specificities of 80% to 90% of PET in identifying adrenal metastases [54,55]. Consequently, if FDG uptake by an adrenal mass is normal in a patient with potentially resectable NSCLC, curative resection should be considered without further evaluation. Patients with NSCLC and an isolated adrenal mass with increased FDG uptake should have the adrenal lesion biopsied before being denied surgery.

Central nervous system (CNS) metastases are detected in up to 9% of patients as the sole site of metastatic disease at presentation (Fig. 11) [7].

Because these patients can be asymptomatic, it has been suggested that routine CT of the brain should be performed in the initial staging evaluation of all patients with NSCLC [56–60]. However, typically CNS metastases are usually associated with neurologic signs and symptoms, and consequently imaging for CNS metastases in asymptomatic patients with NSCLC is not considered cost effective and is not generally recommended [61,62]. This approach has been questioned as it is based on data that may be skewed by a high proportion of patients with early-stage disease who are at lower risk for brain metastases. In patients with resected lung cancer, there is a substantial incidence of early postoperative recurrence of tumor in the brain, particularly in patients with large-cell carcinomas and adenocarcinomas and stage of disease higher than T1N0, suggesting that undetected metastases were

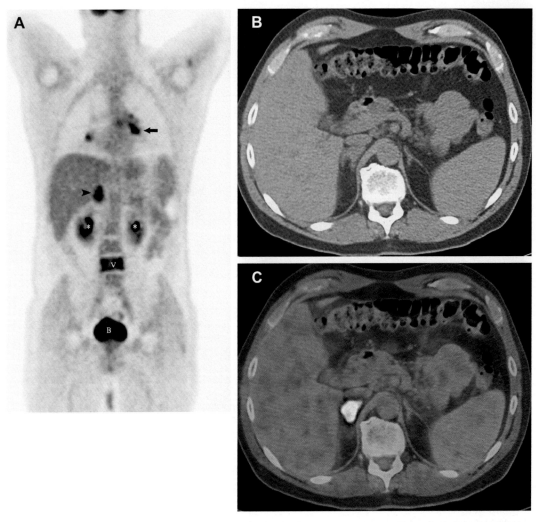

Fig. 10. A 52-year-old man who has NSCLC presenting with cough and hoarseness. (*A*) Coronal whole-body PET scan shows increased uptake of FDG within the primary malignancy (*arrow*). There is focal increased FDG uptake in mediastinal and contralateral hilar nodes and in the region of the right adrenal (*arrowhead*), left humerus, and in a lumbar vertebral body (*V*) suspicious for metastases. B, accumulation of FDG in the bladder; *, renal excretion of FDG. Axial CT (*B*) and integrated CT-PET (*C*) confirm an FDG-avid right adrenal mass. Biopsy revealed metastatic adenocarcinoma.

present at the time of surgical resection of the primary lung malignancy [63–65]. Additionally, Earnest and colleagues [66] have reported that occult brain metastases were identified in 6 of 27 (22%) patients with potentially resectable NSCLC (excluding early-stage lung caner) on contrast-enhanced MR images. These articles suggest that there may be a selective role for imaging in the detection of occult brain metastases. In particular, imaging of the brain may be indicated for the exclusion of brain metastases in patients

with clinically resectable, locally advanced NSCLC with nonsquamous histology. In fact, the 2003 ASCO recommendations are that asymptomatic patients with stage III disease being considered for aggressive local therapy (thoracic surgery or radiation) should have CT or MR imaging of the brain [8].

Patients with skeletal metastases are usually symptomatic or have laboratory abnormalities indicating bone metastases [60]. Because occult skeletal metastases are only occasionally detected

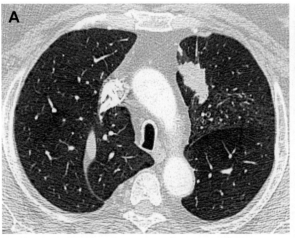
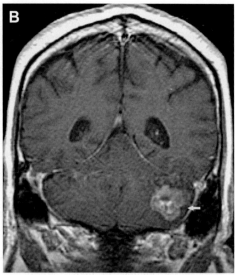

Fig. 11. A 64-year-old man with NSCLC presenting with an 8-month history of cough, dizziness, and ataxia. (*A*) Contrast-enhanced CT shows a 3.5-cm spiculated left upper-lobe mass. Linear and tubular opacity in the right lung is an azygos fissure containing the azygos vein. (*B*) Coronal contrast-enhanced cranial T1-weighted MRI scan shows an enhancing metastasis in the cerebellum (*arrow*).

in asymptomatic patients by radiologic imaging and technetium 99m-methylene diphosphonate (^{99m}Tc-MDP) bone scintigraphy, it is recommended that bone radiographs, MRI, and ^{99m}Tc-MDP bone scintigraphy be performed only to evaluate a history of focal bone pain or elevated alkaline phosphatase [60,62,67,68]. However, FDG-PET is a substitute for ^{99m}Tc-MDP bone scan imaging in the detection of skeletal metastases and may have utility in detecting occult osseous metastases. Compared with radionuclide ^{99m}Tc-MDP bone scans, FDG-PET has been reported to reduce the number of false-negative and -positive findings and to be more accurate in detecting skeletal metastases (accuracy of FDG-PET, 93.5%–96%; accuracy of ^{99m}Tc-MDP, 66%–72.5%) [69,70].

Limitations of the current TNM staging system

Clinical and surgical-pathologic staging is important in the management of patients with NSCLC. The TNM classification has undergone numerous revisions since its inception to improve the stratification of patients into groups with similar management and prognosis. The 1997 revisions have been criticized for inconsistencies in prognosis within the subsets of the different stages and for the imprecise definitions of T, N,

and M descriptors [71–73]. An attempt has been made to address some of these issues in the recently published proposal for the revision of the T, N, and M descriptors by the IASLC Lung Cancer Staging Project [5–7]. However, some of the concerns raised could not be evaluated because of the small number of patients, the inconsistent clinical and pathologic results, or the lack of validation.

In terms of T staging, a threshold of 3 cm diameter tumor has historically been arbitrarily selected to distinguish between T1 and T2 tumors. However, survival is significantly worse when the tumor is larger than 5 cm in diameter [5,71,74]. Consequently, the new staging system proposes to classify tumors larger than 5 cm in diameter as T2b, and to reclassify T2 tumors greater than 7 cm as T3 [5].

Naruke and colleagues [73], after a thorough single-institution staging analysis of the 1997 TNM staging classification, recommended that the broad categorization of T3 tumors should be redefined. This recommendation was based on the observation that tumors with limited parietal pleural invasion had a significantly better prognosis than those invading the chest wall, superior sulcus, diaphragm, and ribs. Consequently, it was suggested that the latter tumors should be reclassified as T4. Additionally, tumors in the aortic or supra-aortic region that invade the phrenic or vagus nerves may need to be staged as T4 because of their very poor prognosis [71]. However, these issues have not been resolved by the new IASLC Lung Cancer Staging Project proposals. Furthermore, it has also been suggested that the prognosis of patients with tracheal invasion and satellite nodes in the ipsilateral lobe warrant reclassification as T3 rather than T4 [72,73]. This suggestion has been partially addressed by the IASLC Lung Cancer Staging Project proposal to reclassify T4 tumors with additional nodule(s) in the same lobe as the primary tumor as T3 [5].

Controversy regarding N descriptors concerns the precise definition of what constitutes ipsilateral (potentially resectable) and contralateral (nonresectable) nodal metastases, the prognostic impact of the number of nodes, and/or nodal stations involved, as well as the arbitrary practice of using the midline as a reference point for anatomic description of nodal metastases rather than the normal lymphatic drainage of the lungs [71]. For instance, the presence of nodal metastases anywhere within the subcarinal space is designated N2 by some and N3 by others if the involved nodes involve the medial wall of the contralateral main bronchus. In terms of considering lymphatic drainage, Ginsberg suggests that because right-sided lung cancers drain to nodes as far as the left tracheal border in the superior mediastinum, this could be considered ipsilateral rather than contralateral disease [71]. In this regard, the left anterior border of the trachea rather than the midline is proposed as the dividing point between N2 and N3 nodal descriptors for right-sided lung tumors. Accordingly, N3 nodes from a right-sided lung cancer would include only those lymph nodes along the left tracheo-esophageal groove and along the lateral border of the left mainstem bronchus. By contrast, because left-sided lung tumors drain into the superior mediastinum only along the tracheo-esophageal groove, any nodal metastasis to the right of the left paratracheal border should be considered N3 disease.

Furthermore, the current TNM and the IASLC Lung Cancer Staging Project proposals do not specifically address the important differences in nodal disease in patients with SSTs compared with those with nonapical tumors. Specifically, the management of patients with SSTs and nodal metastases can differ significantly from those patients with nonapical lung cancers.

For example, mediastinal lymph node metastases (N2) are reported to occur in up to 20% of patients with SSTs [75] and, in contradistinction to nonapical tumors, represent absolute contraindications to surgery. Additionally, in contradistinction to nonapical tumors, ipsilateral supraclavicular (N3) nodal metastases from SSTs do not necessarily preclude long-term survival and can be successfully resected with the primary tumor [76,77].

Small-cell lung cancer

SCLC is generally staged according to the Veteran's Administration Lung Cancer Study Group recommendations as *limited disease* (LD) or *extensive disease* (ED) [78]. LD defines tumor confined to a hemithorax and the regional lymph nodes (Fig. 12). Unlike the TNM classification for NSCLC, metastases to the ipsilateral supraclavicular, contralateral supraclavicular, and mediastinal lymph nodes are considered LD. ED includes tumor with noncontiguous metastases to the contralateral lung and distant metastases (Fig. 13) [78,79]. Most patients with SCLC have ED at presentation [80]. Common sites of metastatic disease include the liver, bone, bone marrow, brain, and retroperitoneal lymph nodes [80]. Although there is no consensus regarding the imaging and invasive procedures that should

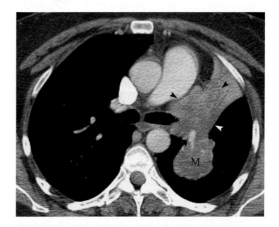

Fig. 12. A 49-year-old woman with LD small-cell lung cancer. Contrast-enhanced CT shows a left lower-lobe mass (*M*) and left hilar adenopathy (*arrowheads*). There is occlusion of the left upper-lobe bronchus and complete atelectasis of the left upper lobe. Clinical and pathologic staging was negative for distant metastases and patient received concurrent chemoradiation.

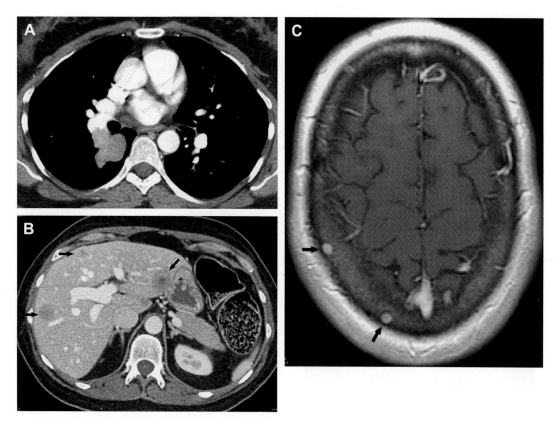

Fig. 13. A 36-year-old woman who has ED small-cell lung cancer presenting with hypokalemia and hypertension. (*A, B*) Contrast-enhanced CT shows a right lower-lobe mass contiguous with hilar adenopathy and multiple hepatic metastases (*arrows*). (*C*) Axial contrast-enhanced cranial T1-weighted MRI scan shows two, small enhancing metastases in the calvarium (*arrows*).

be performed in the staging evaluation of patients with SCLC, MRI has been advocated to assess the liver, adrenals, brain, and axial skeleton in a single study [80]. More recently, whole-body PET imaging has been reported to improve the accuracy of staging of patients with SCLC [81–84]. In this regard, Niho and colleagues [82] performed FDG-PET imaging in 63 patients diagnosed by conventional staging procedures as having limited-stage SCLC. Therapeutic management was changed in 5 patients (8%) owing to the detection of unsuspected distant metastases and change in stage from LD to ED (Fig. 14).

Evaluation of extrathoracic metastatic disease usually includes the following:

- *Bone marrow aspiration,* ^{99m}Tc-*MDP bone scintigraphy, and MRI.* Patients with bone (30%) and bone marrow (17%–34%) metastases are often asymptomatic, and blood alkaline phosphatase levels are frequently normal

[78,85–87]. Because isolated bone and bone marrow metastases are uncommon, however, routine bone marrow aspiration and radiologic imaging for occult metastases are usually performed only if there are other findings of ED.
- *Brain MRI.* CNS metastases are common (10%–27%) at presentation, and approximately 5% of patients are asymptomatic [78,85,88]. Because therapeutic CNS radiation and chemotherapy can decrease morbidity and improve prognosis, routine MRI of the brain is recommended in patients with SCLC [78,89,90].
- *CT or MRI of the abdomen.* Metastases to the liver (30%) and retroperitoneal nodes (11%) are common at presentation [78,85]. Because patients are often asymptomatic and liver function tests can be normal, staging evaluation routinely includes CT or MRI of the abdomen.

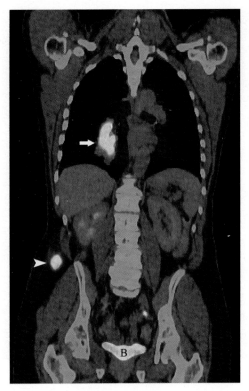

Fig. 14. A 58-year-old woman with ED small-cell lung cancer. Coronal integrated whole-body PET scan shows increased uptake of FDG within the primary malignancy (*arrow*). There is focal increased FDG uptake in a soft-tissue mass (*arrowhead*). Biopsy of the subcutaneous mass confirmed small-cell lung cancer and patient was treated with systemic chemotherapy. B, accumulation of FDG in the bladder; *, ureteric excretion of FDG.

Summary

TNM staging of lung cancer is important in determining therapeutic management and prognosis. CT, PET, and MR imaging are useful components of this evaluation. However, there is considerable variability in the imaging performed to evaluate for nodal and extrathoracic disease. Chest CT is almost universally used to stage patients with lung cancer and is typically performed to assess the primary tumor, direct mediastinoscopic nodal sampling, and detect intra- and extrathoracic metastases. MRI is particularly useful in the evaluation of SSTs. Otherwise, MRI is generally used as an adjunct to CT in evaluating patients whose CT findings are equivocal. PET complements conventional radiologic assessment of lung cancer and is routinely used to improve the detection of nodal and extrathoracic metastases.

References

[1] American Cancer Society on line. Available at: http//www.acs.org. August 2007.
[2] Travis WD, Brambilla E, Muller-Hermelink HK, et al. Pathology and genetics: tumours of the lung, pleura, thymus and heart. Lyon: IARC; 2004.
[3] Travis WD, Colby TV, Corrin B, et al. Histological typing of lung and pleural tumours. 3rd edition. Berlin, Germany: Springer-Verlag; 1999.
[4] Mountain CF. Revisions in the international system for staging lung cancer. Chest 1997;111:1710–7.
[5] Rami-Porta R, Ball D, Crowley J, et al. The IASLC Lung Cancer Staging Project: proposals for the revision of the T descriptors in the forthcoming (seventh) edition of the TNM classification for lung cancer. J Thorac Oncol 2007;2(7):593–602.
[6] Rusch VW, Crowley J, Giroux DJ, et al. The IASLC Lung Cancer Staging Project: proposals for the revision of the N descriptors in the forthcoming seventh edition of the TNM classification for lung cancer. J Thorac Oncol 2007;2(7):603–12.
[7] Postmus PE, Brambilla E, Chansky K, et al. The IASLC Lung Cancer Staging Project: proposals for revision of the M descriptors in the forthcoming (seventh) edition of the TNM classification of lung cancer. J Thorac Oncol 2007;2(8):686–93.
[8] Pfister DG, Johnson DH, Azzoli CG, et al. American Society of Clinical Oncology treatment of unresectable non-small-cell lung cancer guideline: update 2003. J Clin Oncol 2004;22(2):330–53.
[9] van Tinteren H, Hoekstra OS, Smit EF, et al. Effectiveness of positron emission tomography in the preoperative assessment of patients with suspected non-small-cell lung cancer: the PLUS multicentre randomised trial. Lancet 2002;359(9315):1388–93.
[10] Lardinois D, Weder W, Hany TF, et al. Staging of non-small-cell lung cancer with integrated positron-emission tomography and computed tomography. N Engl J Med 2003;348(25):2500–7.
[11] Verhagen AF, Bootsma GP, Tjan-Heijnen VC, et al. FDG-PET in staging lung cancer: how does it change the algorithm? Lung Cancer 2004;44(2):175–81.
[12] Reed CE, Harpole DH, Posther KE, et al. Results of the American college of surgeons oncology group Z0050 trial: the utility of positron emission tomography in staging potentially operable non-small cell lung cancer. J Thorac Cardiovasc Surg 2003;126(6):1943–51.
[13] Vansteenkiste JF, Stroobants SG, De Leyn PR, et al. Lymph node staging in non-small-cell lung cancer with FDG-PET scan: a prospective study on 690 lymph node stations from 68 patients. J Clin Oncol 1998;16:2142–9.
[14] Pieterman RM, van Putten JW, Meuzelaar JJ, et al. Preoperative staging of non-small-cell lung cancer with positron-emission tomography. N Engl J Med 2000;343(4):254–61.

[15] Antoch G, Stattaus J, Nemat AT, et al. Non-small cell lung cancer: dual-modality PET/CT in preoperative staging. Radiology 2003;229(2):526–33.

[16] Ratto GB, Piacenza G, Frola C, et al. Chest wall involvement by lung cancer: computed tomographic detection and results of operation. Ann Thorac Surg 1991;51:182–8.

[17] Padovani B, Mouroux J, Seksik L, et al. Chest wall invasion by bronchogenic carcinoma: evaluation with MR imaging. Radiology 1993;187(1):33–8.

[18] Webb WR, Gatsonis C, Zerhouni EA, et al. CT and MR imaging in staging non-small cell bronchogenic carcinoma: report of the Radiologic Diagnostic Oncology Group. Radiology 1991;178:705–13.

[19] Martini N, Heelan R, Westcott J, et al. Comparative merits of conventional, computed tomographic, and magnetic resonance imaging in assessing mediastinal involvement in surgically confirmed lung carcinoma. J Thorac Cardiovasc Surg 1985;90:639–48.

[20] McLoud TC. CT of bronchogenic carcinoma: indeterminate mediastinal invasion. Radiology 1989; 173:15–6.

[21] Musset D, Grenier P, Carette MF, et al. Primary lung cancer staging: prospective comparative study of MR imaging with CT. Radiology 1986;160: 607–11.

[22] Glazer HS, Kaiser LR, Anderson DJ, et al. Indeterminate mediastinal invasion in bronchogenic carcinoma: CT evaluation. Radiology 1989;173:37–42.

[23] Herman SJ, Winton TL, Weisbrod GL, et al. Mediastinal invasion by bronchogenic carcinoma: CT signs. Radiology 1994;190:841–6.

[24] Webb WR, Sostman HD. MR imaging of thoracic disease: clinical uses. Radiology 1992;182:621–30.

[25] Bruzzi J, Komaki R, Walsh G, et al. Comprehensive review of superior sulcus tumors. Part II: imaging: initial staging, assessment of resectability and therapeutic response. Radiographics 2007; in press.

[26] Bilsky MH, Vitaz TW, Boland PJ, et al. Surgical treatment of superior sulcus tumors with spinal and brachial plexus involvement. J Neurosurg 2002;97(3 Suppl):301–9.

[27] Gandhi S, Walsh GL, Komaki R, et al. A multidisciplinary surgical approach to superior sulcus tumors with vertebral invasion. Ann Thorac Surg 1999;68(5):1778–84 [discussion: 84–5].

[28] York JE, Walsh GL, Lang FF, et al. Combined chest wall resection with vertebrectomy and spinal reconstruction for the treatment of Pancoast tumors. J Neurosurg 1999;91(Suppl 1):74–80.

[29] Dartevelle P, Macchiarini P. Surgical management of superior sulcus tumors. Oncologist 1999;4(5):398–407.

[30] Galetta D, Cesario A, Margaritora S, et al. Enduring challenge in the treatment of nonsmall cell lung cancer with clinical stage IIIB: results of a trimodality approach. Ann Thorac Surg 2003;76(6):1802–8 [discussion: 8–9].

[31] Ichinose Y, Fukuyama Y, Asoh H, et al. Induction chemoradiotherapy and surgical resection for selected stage IIIB non-small-cell lung cancer. Ann Thorac Surg 2003;76(6):1810–4 [discussion: 5].

[32] Pretreatment evaluation of non-small-cell lung cancer. The American Thoracic Society and the European Respiratory Society. Am J Respir Crit Care Med 1997;156(1):320–32.

[33] Mountain CF, Dresler CM. Regional lymph node classification for lung cancer staging. Chest 1997; 111:1718–23.

[34] Glazer GM, Gross BH, Quint LE, et al. Normal mediastinal lymph nodes: number and size according to American Thoracic Society Mapping. Am J Roentgenol 1985;144:261–5.

[35] Prenzel KL, Monig SP, Sinning JM, et al. Lymph node size and metastatic infiltration in non-small cell lung cancer. Chest 2003;123(2):463–7.

[36] De Leyn P, Vansteenkiste J, Cuypers P, et al. Role of cervical mediastinoscopy in staging of non-small cell lung cancer without enlarged mediastinal lymph nodes on CT scan. Eur J Cardiothorac Surg 1997; 12(5):706–12.

[37] Choi YS, Shim YM, Kim J, et al. Mediastinoscopy in patients with clinical stage I non-small cell lung cancer. Ann Thorac Surg 2003;75(2):364–6.

[38] Toloza EM, Harpole L, Detterbeck F, et al. Invasive staging of non-small cell lung cancer: a review of the current evidence. Chest 2003;123(Suppl 1): 157S–66S.

[39] Birim O, Kappetein AP, Stijnen T, et al. Meta-analysis of positron emission tomographic and computed tomographic imaging in detecting mediastinal lymph node metastases in nonsmall cell lung cancer. Ann Thorac Surg 2005;79(1):375–82.

[40] Gould MK, Kuschner WG, Rydzak CE, et al. Test performance of positron emission tomography and computed tomography for mediastinal staging in patients with non-small-cell lung cancer: a meta-analysis. Ann Intern Med 2003;139(11):879–92.

[41] de Langen AJ, Raijmakers P, Riphagen I, et al. The size of mediastinal lymph nodes and its relation with metastatic involvement: a meta-analysis. Eur J Cardiothorac Surg 2006;29(1):26–9.

[42] Dietlein M, Weber K, Gandjour A, et al. Cost-effectiveness of FDG-PET for the management of potentially operable non-small cell lung cancer: priority for a PET-based strategy after nodal-negative CT results. Eur J Nucl Med 2000;27(11):1598–609.

[43] Scott WJ, Shepherd J, Gambhir SS. Cost-effectiveness of FDG-PET for staging non-small cell lung cancer: a decision analysis. Ann Thorac Surg 1998; 66:1876–85.

[44] MacManus MP, Hicks RJ, Matthews JP, et al. High rate of detection of unsuspected distant metastases by PET in apparent stage III non-small-cell lung cancer: implications for radical radiation therapy. Int J Radiat Oncol Biol Phys 2001;50(2):287–93.

[45] Viney RC, Boyer MJ, King MT, et al. Randomized controlled trial of the role of positron emission tomography in the management of stage I and II

non-small-cell lung cancer. J Clin Oncol 2004;22(12): 2357–62.

[46] Lardinois D, Weder W, Roudas M, et al. Etiology of solitary extrapulmonary positron emission tomography and computed tomography findings in patients with lung cancer. J Clin Oncol 2005;23(28):6846–53.

[47] Mayo-Smith WW, Boland GW, Noto RB, et al. State-of-the-art adrenal imaging. Radio Graphics 2001;21(4):995–1012.

[48] Boland GW, Lee MJ, Gazelle GS, et al. Characterization of adrenal masses using unenhanced CT: an analysis of the CT literature. Am J Roentgenol 1998;171:201–4.

[49] Pena CS, Boland GW, Hahn PF, et al. Characterization of indeterminate (lipid-poor) adrenal masses: use of washout characteristics at contrast-enhanced CT. Radiology 2000;217(3):798–802.

[50] Boland GW, Lee MJ. Magnetic resonance imaging of the adrenal gland. Crit Rev Diagn Imaging 1995;36:115–74.

[51] Outwater EK, Siegelman ES, Huang AB, et al. Adrenal masses: correlation between CT attenuation value and chemical shift ratio at MR imaging with in-phase and opposed-phase sequences. Radiology 1996;200(3):749–52.

[52] Schwartz LH, Ginsberg MS, Burt ME, et al. MRI as an alternative to CT-guided biopsy of adrenal masses in patients with lung cancer. Ann Thorac Surg 1998;65(1):193–7.

[53] Remer EM, Obuchowski N, Ellis JD, et al. Adrenal mass evaluation in patients with lung carcinoma: a cost-effectiveness analysis. Am J Roentgenol 2000;174(4):1033–9.

[54] Yun M, Kim W, Alnafisi N, et al. 18F-FDG PET in characterizing adrenal lesions detected on CT or MRI. J Nucl Med 2001;42(12):1795–9.

[55] Erasmus JJ, Patz EF, McAdams HP, et al. Evaluation of adrenal masses in patients with bronchogenic carcinoma by using 18F-fluorodeoxyglucose positron emission tomography. Am J Roentgenol 1997; 168:1357–60.

[56] Ferrigno D, Buccheri G. Cranial computed tomography as a part of the initial staging procedures for patients with non-small-cell lung cancer. Chest 1994;106:1025–9.

[57] Hooper RG, Tenholder MF, Underwood GH, et al. Computed tomographic scanning of the brain in initial staging of bronchogenic carcinoma. Chest 1984; 85:774–6.

[58] Mintz BJ, Tuhrim S, Alexander S, et al. Intracranial metastases in the initial staging of bronchogenic carcinoma. Chest 1984;86:850–3.

[59] Newman SJ, Hansen HH. Proceedings: frequency, diagnosis, and treatment of brain metastases in 247 consecutive patients with bronchogenic carcinoma. Cancer 1974;33(2):492–6.

[60] Salvatierra A, Baamonde C, Llamas JM, et al. Extrathoracic staging of bronchogenic carcinoma. Chest 1990;97:1052–8.

[61] Colice GL, Birkmeyer JD, Black WC, et al. Cost-effectiveness of head CT in patients with lung cancer without clinical evidence of metastases. Chest 1995; 108:1264–71.

[62] Silvestri GA, Littenberg B, Colice GL. The clinical evaluation for detecting metastatic lung cancer. A meta-analysis. Am J Respir Crit Care Med 1995; 152(1):225–30.

[63] Yokoi K, Kamiya N, Matsuguma H, et al. Detection of brain metastasis in potentially operable non-small cell lung cancer. A comparison of CT and MRI. Chest 1999;115:714–9.

[64] Figlin RA, Piantadosi S, Feld R. Intracranial recurrence of carcinoma after complete surgical resection of stage I, II, and III non-small-cell lung cancer. N Engl J Med 1988;318(20):1300–5.

[65] Robnett TJ, Machtay M, Stevenson JP, et al. Factors affecting the risk of brain metastases after definitive chemoradiation for locally advanced non-small-cell lung carcinoma. J Clin Oncol 2001; 19(5):1344–9.

[66] Earnest F IV, Ryu JH, Miller GM, et al. Suspected non-small cell lung cancer: incidence of occult brain and skeletal metastases and effectiveness of imaging for detection–pilot study. Radiology 1999;211(1): 137–45.

[67] Little AG, Stitik FP. Clinical staging of patients with non-small cell lung cancer. Chest 1990;97:1431–8.

[68] Michel F, Soler M, Imhof E, et al. Initial staging of non-small cell lung cancer: value of routine radioisotope bone scanning. Thorax 1991;46: 469–73.

[69] Bury T, Barreto A, Daenen F, et al. Fluorine-18 deoxyglucose positron emission tomography for the detection of bone metastases in patients with non-small cell lung cancer. Eur J Nucl Med 1998; 25(9):1244–7.

[70] Hsia TC, Shen YY, Yen RF, et al. Comparing whole body 18F-2-deoxyglucose positron emission tomography and technetium-99m methylene diophosphate bone scan to detect bone metastases in patients with non-small cell lung cancer. Neoplasma 2002;49(4): 267–71.

[71] Ginsberg RJ. Continuing controversies in staging NSCLC: an analysis of the revised 1997 staging system. Oncology (Huntingt) 1998;12(1 Suppl 2): 51–4.

[72] Kameyama K, Huang CL, Liu D, et al. Problems related to TNM staging: patients with stage III non-small cell lung cancer. J Thorac Cardiovasc Surg 2002;124(3):503–10.

[73] Naruke T, Goya T, Tsuchiya R, et al. Prognosis and survival in resected lung carcinoma based on the new international staging system. J Thorac Cardiovasc Surg 1988;96:440–7.

[74] Carbone E, Asamura H, Takei H, et al. T2 tumors larger than five centimeters in diameter can be upgraded to T3 in non-small cell lung cancer. J Thorac Cardiovasc Surg 2001;122(5):907–12.

[75] Vallieres E, Karmy-Jones R, Mulligan MS, et al. Pancoast tumors. Curr Probl Surg 2001;38(5):293–376.

[76] Ginsberg RJ, Martini N, Zaman M, et al. Influence of surgical resection and brachytherapy in the management of superior sulcus tumor. Ann Thorac Surg 1994;57(6):1440–5.

[77] Hilaris BS, Martini N, Wong GY, et al. Treatment of superior sulcus tumor (Pancoast tumor). Surg Clin North Am 1987;67(5):965–77.

[78] Darling GE. Staging of the patient with small cell lung cancer. Chest Surg Clin N Am 1997;7:81–94.

[79] Stitik FP. The new staging of lung cancer. Radiol Clin North Am 1994;32:635–47.

[80] Jelinek JS, Redmond J, Perry JJ, et al. Small cell lung cancer: staging with MR imaging. Radiology 1990;177:837–42.

[81] Kut V, Spies W, Spies S, et al. Staging and monitoring of small cell lung cancer using [18F]fluoro-2-deoxy-D-glucose-positron emission tomography (FDG-PET). Am J Clin Oncol 2007;30(1):45–50.

[82] Niho S, Fujii H, Murakami K, et al. Detection of unsuspected distant metastases and/or regional nodes by FDG-PET in LD-SCLC scan in apparent limited-disease small-cell lung cancer. Lung Cancer 2007;57(5):328–33.

[83] Brink I, Schumacher T, Mix M, et al. Impact of [18F]FDG-PET on the primary staging of small-cell lung cancer. Eur J Nucl Med Mol Imaging 2004;31(12):1614–20.

[84] Bradley JD, Dehdashti F, Mintun MA, et al. Positron emission tomography in limited-stage small-cell lung cancer: a prospective study. J Clin Oncol 2004;22(16):3248–54.

[85] Abrams J, Doyle LA, Aisner J. Staging prognostic factors, and special considerations in small cell lung cancer. Semin Oncol 1988;15:261–77.

[86] Stahel RA, Mabry M, Skarin AT, et al. Detection of bone marrow metastasis in small-cell lung cancer by monoclonal antibody. J Clin Oncol 1985;3(4):455–61.

[87] Stahel RA, Ginsberg R, Havemann K, et al. Staging and prognostic factors in small cell lung cancer: a consensus report. Lung Cancer 1989;5:119–26.

[88] Bunn PA Jr, Rosen ST. Central nervous system manifestations of small cell lung cancer. In: Aisner J, editor. Contemporary issues in clinical oncology: lung cancer. New York: Churchill Livingstone; 1985. p. 287–305.

[89] Elias AD. Small cell lung cancer. State-of-the-art therapy in 1996. Chest 1997;112:251S–8S.

[90] van de Pol M, van Oosterhout AGM, Wilmink JT, et al. MRI in detection of brain metastases at initial staging of small-cell lung cancer. Neuroradiology 1996;38:207–10.

ELSEVIER
SAUNDERS

Clin Chest Med 29 (2008) 59–76

CLINICS
IN CHEST
MEDICINE

ICU Imaging

Joshua R. Hill, MD[a],*, Peder E. Horner, MD[b],
Steven L. Primack, MD[a,c]

[a]Department of Radiology, Oregon Health and Science University, 3181 SW Sam Jackson Park Road, L340,
Portland, OR 97239, USA
[b]Vascular and Interventional Radiology, Dotter Interventional Institute, Oregon Health and Science University,
3181 SW Sam Jackson Park Road, L340, Portland, OR 97239, USA
[c]Division of Pulmonary Medicine, Oregon Health and Science University, 3181 SW Sam Jackson Park Road,
L340, Portland, OR 97239, USA

The chest radiograph is a crucial tool in the care of the critically ill. It serves to diagnose and to monitor a variety of cardiopulmonary disorders. In addition, it is used to evaluate a broad range of monitoring and support equipment, ensure proper positioning, and survey for complications. Daily rounds and prompt communication between the radiologist and the intensivist can help improve diagnostic accuracy and manage potential complications.

Indications for portable chest radiography

Indications for portable chest radiography include cardiopulmonary symptoms following cardiac or thoracic surgery, trauma, patients who have monitoring and life-support devices, and critically ill patients, according to the American College of Radiology (ACR) practice guidelines (revised 2006)[1]. There are no absolute guidelines dictating the frequency of chest radiography for ICU patients. Several studies assessing the benefit of daily chest radiography in the ICU have been performed, with varied findings [2–5]. The ACR recommends daily chest radiography for patients who have acute cardiopulmonary problems [6]. Chest radiographs should also be obtained immediately after the placement of endotracheal tubes, nasogastric tubes, vascular catheters, and chest tubes [6]. Follow-up is warranted when tube or catheter position is suspected to have changed or when otherwise clinically indicated.

Technical factors

Inherent challenges exist in ICU chest radiography, all of which limit diagnostic accuracy. Many patients are debilitated and not readily able to cooperate with the examination, precluding optimal upright (posteroanterior) positioning. Radiographs are usually obtained in a semiupright or supine anteroposterior (AP) position. A lateral radiograph is often impractical. External monitoring devices, overlying tubes, and electrocardiographic leads can obscure underlying disease, mimic radiographic pathology, and create ambiguity as to the positioning of other support equipment.

Role of CT

CT is another valuable imaging modality in assessing the ICU patient. CT is superior to chest radiography in the detection and characterization of pulmonary, pleural, and mediastinal abnormalities [7]. CT more accurately depicts the pattern and distribution of pulmonary parenchymal abnormalities. Contrast-enhanced CT is useful particularly in assessing pleural fluid collections and potentially for guiding interventional procedures. Pulmonary CT angiography is the primary method of evaluating for pulmonary embolus in the ICU patient.

* Corresponding author.
E-mail address: hilljo@ohsu.edu (J.R. Hill).

CT imaging of the ICU patient is not without its logistical limitations. Safe transport of the critically ill, along with support devices, is often difficult. In addition, renal failure may preclude the administration of intravenous contrast, diminishing diagnostic capabilities.

Monitoring and support devices

Evaluation of support equipment and monitoring devices is of utmost importance in the imaging of patients in the ICU. Early recognition of malpositioning reduces the likelihood of potentially serious complications. Radiologists often review the position of all support equipment in their initial appraisal of the radiograph. For this reason, and to underline its importance, the evaluation of monitoring and support devices is discussed first.

Endotracheal and tracheostomy tubes

Endotracheal tubes are seen in patients requiring short-term respiratory support with mechanical ventilation. With the patient's head in a neutral position, the endotracheal tube tip should be located 4 to 6 cm above the carina. Neck flexion results in caudal movement of the tube, up to 2 cm. Neck extension can cause 2 cm superior migration.

A malpositioned endotracheal tube is not an uncommon finding. Intubation of the main bronchi can occur when endotracheal tube position is too low, resulting in subsegmental atelectasis, segmental collapse, or complete collapse of the contralateral lung. The ipsilateral lung may be overventilated, increasing the risk of pneumothorax. Main bronchus intubation is most frequently right-sided, owing to a more direct angle of the trachea and right main bronchus (Fig. 1). When the endotracheal tube is too high, there may be inadvertent extubation or damage to the larynx. Esophageal intubation is a severe complication compromising ventilation and introducing excessive amounts of air into the gastrointestinal tract but is typically clinically apparent. Aspiration occurs in up to 8% of intubations [8].

The endotracheal balloon should not be inflated beyond the normal diameter of the trachea. Overinflation to 1.5 times the normal tracheal diameter frequently causes tracheal damage [9]. Tracheal rupture can occur acutely. Tracheal stenosis is a potential chronic complication (Fig. 2).

Tracheostomy tubes are placed when long-term intubation is necessary. The tracheostomy tube tip should be approximately at the T3 level. Position is maintained with neck flexion and extension. Tracheostomy tube diameter should be approximately two thirds that of the trachea's, and the cuff should not distend the tracheal wall. Mediastinal air can be seen after uncomplicated tube placement.

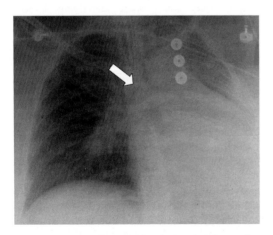

Fig. 1. Right main bronchus intubation. AP chest radiograph demonstrating endotracheal tube tip in the proximal right main bronchus (*arrow*) with resultant left upper and lower lobe atelectasis and mild leftward shift of the mediastinum.

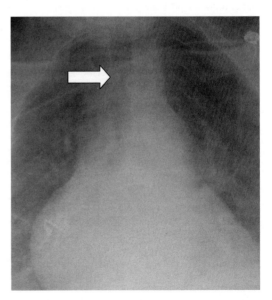

Fig. 2. Tracheal stenosis. Magnified AP view of the trachea of a 42-year-old man who had a history of prolonged intubation showing focal tracheal stenosis (*arrow*).

Enteric tubes

Oroenteric and nasoenteric tubes are used for feeding, medication administration, and suction. For feeding, ideal tip position is in the gastric antrum or the duodenum to reduce aspiration risk. When the enteric tube is used exclusively for suction or medication administration, placement within the stomach is adequate. Sideports, when present, should extend beyond the gastroesophageal junction to decrease aspiration risk.

Radiography is important in detecting aberrant tube location and in preventing potentially lethal complications. Tubes can coil within the pharynx or esophagus, creating a high risk of aspiration if nutrition is administered. Pharyngeal and esophageal perforations are rare complications. Occasionally, enteric tubes terminate in the trachea or bronchi, and ectopic feeding can result in direct bronchopulmonary injury and pneumonia. Pneumothorax, pulmonary laceration, and pulmonary contusion may be seen if the lung parenchyma is punctured. If an enteric tube has been placed in the airway and extends to the lung periphery or into the pleural space, then it is essential to obtain a follow-up radiograph because pneumothorax may only be apparent post removal (Fig. 3).

Venous catheters

Venous catheters are common in the ICU. Medications and intravenous fluids can be administered, blood withdrawn, and central venous pressure measurements obtained. Catheters may be inserted peripherally in upper-extremity veins (peripherally inserted central catheter [PICC]) or more proximally within the subclavian or internal jugular veins, depending on their intended use. The femoral vein is less commonly accessed. Tunneled catheters are often used for renal dialysis, and ports are placed in the chest wall in patients requiring repeated doses of intravenous pharmacotherapy for extended periods.

The venous catheter tip should be located within the superior vena cava (SVC), beyond venous valves, to reduce the risk of thrombosis. Positioning of the catheter tip in the lower SVC likely results in further reduction of thrombosis around the catheter tip [10]. When catheter position is too caudal, it may enter the right atrium, increasing the risk of dysrhythmia and, rarely, cardiac perforation. Thus, catheters should ideally terminate within the lower SVC or at the cavoatrial junction.

Aberrant positioning of venous catheters is quite common. Usually, the aberrantly located catheter is intravenous or within the right atrium. Peripherally inserted catheters can coil in the veins of the upper extremity, course cephalad within the internal jugular vein (Fig. 4), or traverse midline by way of the contralateral brachiocephalic vein. Catheter location within a persistent left-sided SVC, an anomalous vein occurring in 0.3% of the population [11], is occasionally seen (Fig. 5). When a catheter is located in a left-sided SVC, it may mimic an intra-arterial location on an AP chest radiograph. The catheter may also terminate

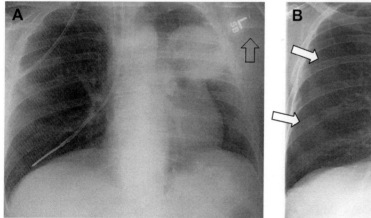
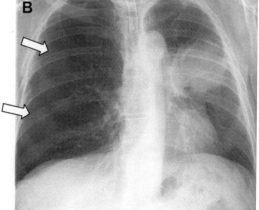

Fig. 3. Right lower lobe feeding tube placement. (*A*) AP chest radiograph of a 75-year-old man demonstrates aberrant enteric tube terminating in the right lower lobe. (*B*) Follow-up AP chest radiograph after enteric tube removal shows a visceral pleural line (*arrows*) indicative of right-sided pneumothorax. The left upper lobe mass proved to be poorly differentiated large cell carcinoma.

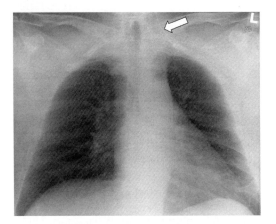

Fig. 4. Aberrant PICC. AP chest radiograph demonstrates aberrantly placed left PICC (*arrow*) coursing cephalad in the left internal jugular vein.

within smaller venous side branches, including the azygous vein.

Occasionally, arteries are inadvertently accessed, most often the subclavian artery or common carotid artery (Fig. 6). Arterial catheterization is usually clinically apparent with pulsatile flow of bright red oxygenated blood from the catheter. On the AP chest radiograph, subclavian artery placement should be suspected when the

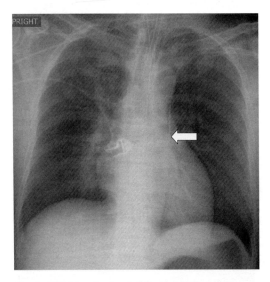

Fig. 5. PICC terminating in left-sided SVC. AP chest radiograph of a mechanically ventilated 53-year-old patient shows a left PICC coursing lateral to the descending aorta (*arrow*) within a persistent left-sided SVC. Right upper and lower lobe patchy consolidative opacities represent aspiration.

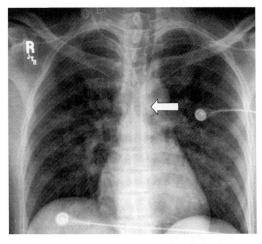

Fig. 6. Intra-arterial central venous catheter. AP chest radiograph demonstrates central venous catheter entering the right common carotid artery, traversing midline, and terminating at the aortic arch (*arrow*). The catheter deviates from the normal right paratracheal vertical course expected with right internal jugular venous catheter placement.

catheter travels above the clavicle. If uncertainty remains after radiographic analysis, the determination of wave form (arterial versus venous) can confirm location.

When the catheter tip is directed at and abuts the venous wall, the catheter should be repositioned or withdrawn to reduce the risk of vessel perforation. Vascular perforation causes hematoma in the surrounding soft tissues. Fluid and medications can accumulate in adjacent soft tissues or pleural space if extravascular catheter position (Fig. 7) is unnoticed. The chest radiograph should also be used to evaluate for hemothorax and pneumothorax following line placement. Pneumothorax occurs uncommonly with PICC placement and is most frequently seen when the subclavian vein is accessed.

Pulmonary artery catheters

Pulmonary artery catheters, or Swan-Ganz catheters, are used to measure pulmonary artery pressure, pulmonary capillary wedge pressure, and cardiac output. The catheter tip should be within the right main pulmonary artery, left main pulmonary artery, or the proximal interlobar pulmonary artery. When the catheter extends beyond the pulmonary hilum on the chest radiograph, the catheter should be retracted [12]. The pulmonary arteries narrow as they extend from

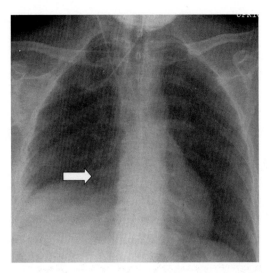

Fig. 7. Extravascular catheter placement. AP chest radiograph of a 55-year-old man shows extravascular catheter location after attempted placement of a right internal jugular central venous catheter. The tip (*arrow*) proved to be in the right pleural space.

the hila, and distal catheter location increases the risk of arterial occlusion and rupture. When measuring pulmonary wedge pressures, the balloon should be inflated for only a short period of time to prevent pulmonary infarction; on the chest radiograph it should be deflated. Pulmonary artery occlusion and subsequent pulmonary infarct can also be secondary to pericatheter thrombus.

Pulmonary hemorrhage (Fig. 8) and pseudoaneurysm are complications of pulmonary artery rupture. Intracardiac or intravascular knots may form (Fig. 9), limiting catheter motility and complicating its removal. In addition, pulmonary artery catheters are subject to the same complications as central venous catheters, including dysrhythmia, cardiac perforation, pneumothorax, and hemothorax.

Intra-aortic balloon pump

The intra-aortic balloon pump (IABP) is a 26 to 28 cm–long balloon device [10] that inflates during systole to assist coronary perfusion, and deflates during diastole to decrease cardiac afterload. It is radiolucent, except for its radio-opaque tip that assists in radiographic localization. The IABP tip should be within the proximal descending thoracic aorta just distal to the origins of the major branch arteries of the aortic arch (Fig. 10). Cerebral or left upper-extremity ischemia may result when the catheter is located too proximally. Too distal a location risks occlusion of the abdominal aortic branch arteries and renal and mesenteric ischemia. Aortic rupture, limb ischemia, and balloon rupture with air embolization are other rare potential complications.

Chest tubes

Chest tube malposition occurs in approximately 10% of placements [6]. Chest tube sideholes—radiographically evident as interruptions

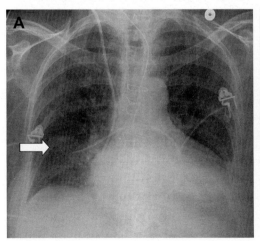
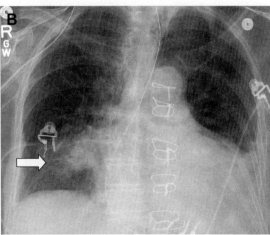

Fig. 8. Pulmonary hemorrhage, pulmonary artery catheter. (*A*) AP chest radiograph of a 90-year-old woman shows right lower lobe pulmonary hemorrhage (*arrow*) adjacent to pulmonary artery catheter tip. The pulmonary artery catheter is malpositioned distal to the interlobar pulmonary artery. (*B*) Follow-up radiograph after catheter removal shows increased conspicuity of the pulmonary hemorrhage (*arrow*).

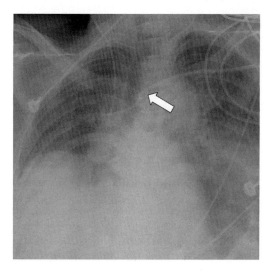

Fig. 9. Pulmonary artery catheter knot. AP chest radiograph demonstrates pulmonary artery catheter with knot (*arrow*) in the left brachiocephalic vein.

of the tube's radio-opaque line—should be located within the pleural space. Improper chest tube location may manifest as a poorly functioning or nonfunctioning tube. When a chest tube is inserted into the pulmonary parenchyma (Fig. 11), pulmonary contusion may be seen, manifested as a new opacity adjacent to the chest tube. Abnormal location in the pulmonary fissures may or may not affect tube function. Viscous debris

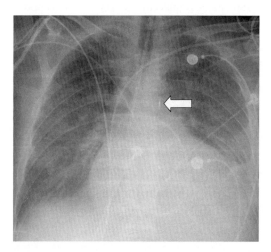

Fig. 10. Normal IABP. AP chest radiograph in a 57-year-old man shows normal location of an IABP with radio-opaque tip (*arrow*) in the proximal thoracic aorta, just distal to the origin of the left subclavian artery. The pulmonary artery catheter is appropriately positioned. Hydrostatic pulmonary edema is present.

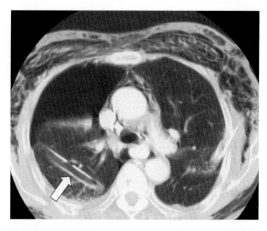

Fig. 11. Chest tube in right lung. Axial CT image of the mid chest demonstrates right-sided chest tube (*arrow*) aberrantly located within the right lung with persistent pneumothorax. Extensive chest wall emphysema and pneumomediastinum are also present.

within the chest tube is easily identified on chest CT but may be occult on conventional radiography. An inappropriately positioned chest tube can injure mediastinal and upper abdominal organs, major blood vessels, and the diaphragm.

Pneumothorax, pneumomediastinum, and pleural fluid

Pleural space abnormalities include pnuemothorax and pleural fluid and are extremely common in the ICU setting. Pneumomediastinum is less commonly encountered but important to recognize because it may be indicative of underlying tracheobronchial injury or alveolar rupture in a mechanically ventilated patient.

Pneumothorax

Underlying pulmonary disease, trauma, and iatrogenesis may result in pneumothorax (Fig. 12). The classic sign of a thin radiodense curvilinear pleural line, bordered by lung on one side and pleural air on the other, is often absent in the supine ICU patient. Detection can require a high degree of suspicion. In the ventilated patient, a small pneumothorax can rapidly progress to tension, and recognition is critical.

In the supine patient, pleural air initially accumulates in the anteromedial recess, the least-dependent location in the hemithorax [13]. Abnormal lucency at the lung base or projecting over the upper abdomen is suggestive of pneumothorax.

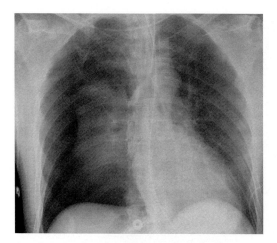

Fig. 12. Pneumothorax. AP chest radiograph showing large right pneumothorax with retraction of the radio-opaque, collapsed right lung toward the right hilum.

A lucent deep sulcus may be visualized in the medial or lateral hemithorax (Fig. 13). In addition, the mediastinum may be unusually well outlined [13]. The lateral decubitus position is the most sensitive for detecting pleural air but is often impractical. When pneumothorax is suspected, an upright radiograph should be obtained for confirmation.

Tension pneumothorax occurs when intrathoracic pressure is greater than atmospheric

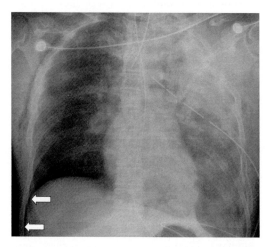

Fig. 13. Pneumothorax, "deep sulcus sign." AP chest radiograph in a supine trauma patient demonstrating lucent deep lateral costophrenic sulcus (arrows) and lucency of the right hemithoracic base, characteristic of pneumothorax. Left pulmonary contusion, subcutaneous emphysema, multiple displaced rib fractures, and left basilar pneumothorax are also seen.

pressure. Radiographically, tension pneumothorax is most reliably diagnosed by inversion or flattening of the hemidiaphragm. Mediastinal shift may also be seen but is less reliable and frequently less pronounced in patients who have acute respiratory distress syndrome (ARDS), because of reduced lung compliance.

Because skin folds can mimic pneumothoraces, important distinguishing features should be recognized. A skin fold is seen as a soft tissue–air interface, with radio-opacity on one side and normal lung on the other. In pneumothorax, a pleural line is often bordered by air on both sides: normal lung and pleural air (Fig. 14). The diagnosis may be more complex when the lung is abnormally opaque, creating the illusion of a soft tissue–air interface. If pulmonary vessels extend peripheral to the interface, then the opacity is a skin fold. If no pulmonary vessels are seen peripherally, then a pneumothorax is present.

Pneumomediastinum

Pneumomediastinum is extraluminal air within the mediastinum. It can be seen in tracheobronchial injury, tracheostomy tube placement, mechanically ventilated patients, asthmatics, and esophageal rupture (although this is a rare cause). Most commonly, pneumomediastinum occurs by way of the Macklin effect. The Macklin effect describes the process by which air from ruptured alveoli dissects along the bronchovascular interstitium to the mediastinum [14]. Pulmonary interstitial emphysema in the mechanically ventilated patient is a sign of alveolar rupture. Air may dissect cephalad to the subcutaneous tissues of the neck (Fig. 15), and caudad to the retroperitoneum.

The Mach band effect can mimic pneumomediastinum on the chest radiograph [15]. The Mach band effect is a perceptual error, creating the appearance of abnormal lucency adjacent to a radiodense convexity such as the heart. When paracardiac lucency is seen in the absence of an adjacent pleural line, the Mach band effect should be suspected.

Pleural fluid

Pleural fluid is common in ICU patients and is most frequently transudative. The supine radiograph is relatively insensitive in the detection of pleural fluid and often underestimates the amount of pleural fluid. On the upright lateral radiograph, blunting of the costophrenic angle usually occurs when 200 mL of fluid are present but may be

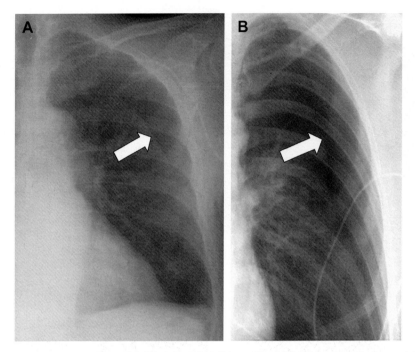

Fig. 14. Skin fold versus pneumothorax. (*A*) AP view of the left lateral hemithorax shows a soft tissue–air interface (*arrow*) representing a skin fold, mimicking a pleural line. Note the presence of pulmonary vessels peripheral to the skin fold. (*B*) AP view of the left lateral hemithorax of a different patient demonstrates a visceral pleural line (*arrow*) consistent with pneumothorax. Note the absence of pulmonary vessels peripheral to the pleural line.

absent with as much as 500 mL [16]. Layering pleural fluid is more difficult to detect on the supine radiograph. The costophrenic angle is often not blunted, and the supine radiograph may only demonstrate hazy "veil-like" opacification due to layering pleural fluid (Fig. 16). The apex is the most dependent location in the supine patient, and pleural effusion may manifest as an apical cap [16].

Consolidation, atelectasis, and pleural fluid cause opacities on the chest radiograph and frequently coexist, particularly at the thoracic base. CT is useful in differentiating pleural fluid from pulmonary parenchymal disease (Fig. 17). CT also better characterizes loculated pleural fluid collections. Empyema is suggested when pleural fluid is bordered by enhancing, thick pleura. Hemothorax is suggested by relatively high attenuation pleural fluid [17], commonly 35 to 70 Hounsfield units [18].

Pulmonary parenchymal abnormalities

Atelectasis, aspiration, pneumonia, hydrostatic pulmonary edema, and noncardiogenic pulmonary

edema present as opacities on chest radiography and CT. Although it is often difficult and sometimes impossible to distinguish between these entities, certain radiographic features can aid in their diagnoses.

Atelectasis

Atelectasis, a decrease in lung volume, is the most common cause of pulmonary opacities in the ICU population. It is frequently found after general anesthesia and thoracic or upper abdominal surgery, occurring in up to 64% of patients in one surgical investigation [19]. The most common location is the left lower lobe (66%), followed by the right lower lobe (22%), and right upper lobe (11%) [20]. Atelectasis is usually subsegmental and can mimic pneumonia, particularly when signs of volume loss such as crowding of air bronchograms, fissural deviation, mediastinal shift, and diaphragmatic elevation are absent. Flat, platelike opacities are characteristic of discoid atelectasis (Fig. 18). Complete lung collapse, lobar collapse (Fig. 19), or segmental collapse can also be seen. Atelectasis is categorized (according to mechanism) as obstructive, compressive,

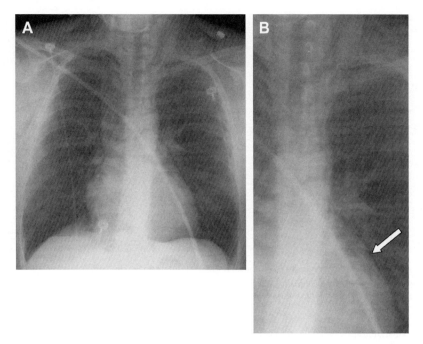

Fig. 15. Pneumomediastinum. (*A*) AP chest radiograph of an asthmatic 16-year-old patient who presented with spontaneous pneumomediastinum. Lucencies are seen in the mediastinum, the supraclavicular soft tissues, and the soft tissues at the base of the neck. (*B*) Magnified view of the mediastinum of the same patient demonstrates mediastinal air outlined by parietal pleura (*arrow*).

cicatricial, or adhesive. Adhesive atelectasis, common in premature neonates secondary to insufficient production of surfactant, is not discussed further.

Obstructive atelectasis is the most common type of atelectasis. Impaired mucociliary function, increased secretions, and altered consciousness are predisposing factors. When only the distal, small

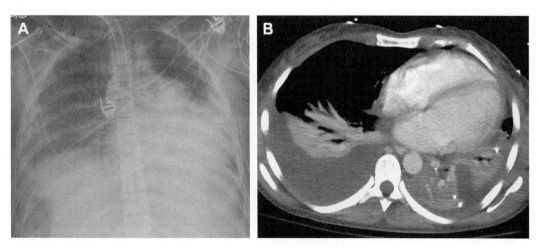

Fig. 16. Layering pleural fluid. (*A*) Supine AP chest radiograph of a 30-year-old woman demonstrates bibasilar atelectasis and "veil-like" opacity of the right lower hemithorax suggestive of layering pleural fluid. (*B*) Axial CT image through the lower chest in the same patient confirms layering right pleural effusion. There is a smaller left effusion, and both lower lobes show compressive atelectasis.

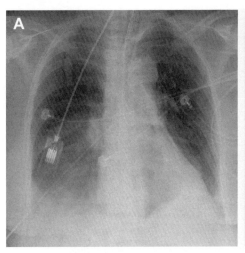
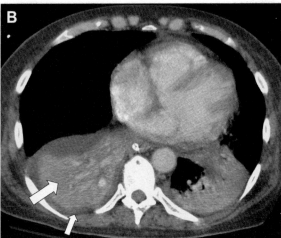

Fig. 17. Pleural effusion versus atelectasis. (*A*) Supine AP chest radiograph shows hazy, "veil-like" opacity of the right lower hemithorax. (*B*) Axial CT image through the lower chest in the same patient demonstrates only a small right pleural effusion (*small arrow*) but significant right lower lobe atelectasis (*large arrow*). There is also left lower lobe atelectasis.

airways are obstructed, crowded air bronchograms are seen. Air bronchograms are absent when the obstruction is more proximal, in larger airways. Mucous plugging is a common cause of acute segmental, lobar, and complete lung collapse (Fig. 20). The absence of air bronchograms in patients who have acute lobar collapse favors mucoid impaction as the etiology and predicts a higher rate of therapeutic success with bronchoscopy (79%–89% in favorable patients) [21].

Compressive atelectasis is volume loss secondary to mass effect exerted on the lung. In the ICU population, pleural fluid is usually the cause. Other potential causes are thoracic tumor,

pulmonary abscess, and severe cardiomegaly. Cicatricial atelectasis is volume loss secondary to pulmonary fibrosis and can be seen in patients who have underlying pulmonary disease or as a complication of ARDS.

On CT, atelectasis can often be identified by signs of volume loss. On contrast-enhanced CT, atelectasis results in relatively high attenuation of the lung parenchyma, a useful feature distinguishing it from relatively lower attenuating consolidative processes such as pneumonia.

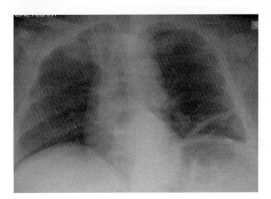

Fig. 18. Discoid atelectasis. AP chest radiograph of a 54-year-old man demonstrates low lung volumes and linear left basilar opacity characteristic of discoid atelectasis.

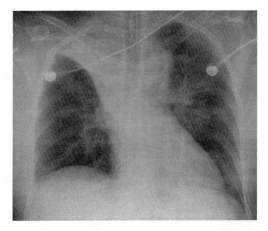

Fig. 19. Right upper lobe collapse. AP chest radiograph of a 72-year-old man demonstrates right upper lobe collapse with cephalad deviation of the minor fissure. Subsequent therapeutic bronchoscopy found viscous secretions within the right upper lobe bronchi.

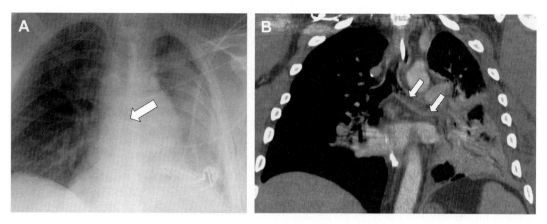

Fig. 20. Atelectasis, mucous plug. (*A*) AP chest radiograph demonstrates abrupt truncation of the left main bronchus (*arrow*) and significant left lung atelectasis suggestive of a mucous plug. (*B*) Coronal CT image through the chest in the same patient confirms presence of a mucous plug in the left main bronchus (*arrows*) with postobstructive atelectasis.

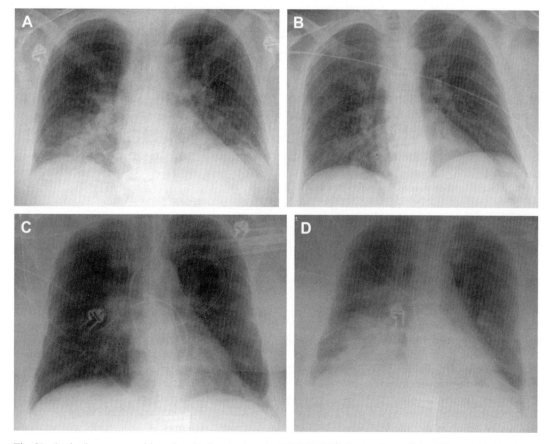

Fig. 21. Aspiration pneumonitis and aspiration pneumonia. (*A*) Initial AP chest radiograph in a 38-year-old man shows bilateral perihilar and lower lung nodular and consolidative opacities; (*B*) follow-up radiograph 1 week later shows marked improvement, consistent with resolving aspiration pneumonitis. (*C*) AP radiograph in a different patient demonstrates right greater than left perihilar and lower lung nodular and ill-defined consolidative opacities; (*D*) AP radiograph obtained 1 week later shows progression to dense right lower lobe consolidation, consistent with aspiration pneumonia.

Aspiration

Intubation, diminished cough reflex, sedation, and enteric tube feeds increase aspiration risk. Aspiration can occur in mechanically ventilated patients despite adequate inflation of the endotracheal tube cuff. Clinically, aspiration events may go unnoticed or may be severe, causing respiratory distress. Aspiration can result in airway obstruction, chemical pneumonitis, or infectious pneumonia, depending on the volume and type of aspirate. Small amounts of aspirated saliva may result in no radiographic abnormality, whereas aspiration of large amounts of food substance increases the likelihood of aspiration pneumonia.

Patchy, ill-defined ground-glass, consolidative, and nodular opacities are the most frequently encountered radiographic manifestations of aspiration. Opacities typically appear rapidly and are most commonly located in the dependent regions of the lungs: the posterior segment of the upper lobes and the superior and posterior basal segments of the lower lobes [22]. Opacities may increase in conspicuity over the first 1 to 2 days in aspiration pneumonitis but should resolve relatively rapidly thereafter. When opacities persist or increase over several days, aspiration pneumonia is likely present (Fig. 21).

Patchy, dependent ground-glass and consolidative opacities are also seen on CT. "Tree-in-bud" opacities [23] result from inflammation of the distal airways. Although tree-in-bud opacities are nonspecific, when present in a dependent distribution, they are highly suggestive of aspiration (Fig. 22).

Pneumonia

Pneumonia is another cause of pulmonary opacities in ICU patients. Aspiration and mechanical ventilation [24] are two important risk factors for pneumonia in the ICU population. Ventilator-associated pneumonia occurs in 9% to 24% of patients ventilated for more than 48 hours [25]. Most pneumonias are caused by mixed anaerobic or, more frequently in the ventilated patient, aerobic gram-negative bacteria such as *Pseudomonas aeruginosa* [26].

Pneumonia may present as a focal consolidation on the chest radiograph; however, it is often multifocal (Fig. 23). Pneumonia can be difficult to differentiate from other causes of pulmonary opacities such as atelectasis, aspiration, and pulmonary edema. Typically, pneumonia changes more slowly than these other entities. In addition,

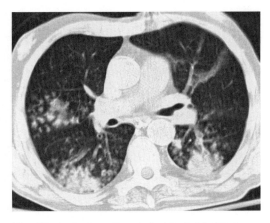

Fig. 22. Aspiration, "tree-in-bud." Axial CT image through the chest in a 59-year-old man shows tree-in-bud and consolidative opacities in the posterior segment of the right upper lobe and superior segments of both lower lobes, consistent with aspiration.

air bronchograms may be seen and can be differentiated from those seen in atelectasis by noting the absence of volume loss and crowding of bronchi.

When ARDS is present, the diagnostic accuracy of CT and chest radiography is diminished [27,28]. The presence of underlying consolidation in ARDS limits the ability to exclude the presence of pneumonia. The incidence of pneumonia in patients who have diffuse lung injury at autopsy has been reported to be 58% [29].

Noncardiogenic pulmonary edema

Pulmonary edema can be classified as hydrostatic pulmonary edema or noncardiogenic pulmonary edema, also referred to as increased permeability edema. These entities can be difficult to distinguish radiographically and may coexist, further complicating their diagnoses.

Noncardiogenic pulmonary edema is caused by primary pulmonary pathology such as pneumonia, aspiration, and pulmonary contusion [30]. Extrathoracic causes of increased permeability include drug toxicity, systemic inflammatory response syndrome, sepsis, shock, and extrathoracic trauma. Neurogenic, postpneumonectomy, and re-expansion pulmonary edema demonstrate radiographic features of hydrostasis and capillary leak [31]. Diffuse alveolar damage (DAD) results from injury to the alveolar capillaries and epithelium. The degree of DAD varies from severe (in cases of ARDS) to relatively nonexistent (as in many cases of heroin-induced pulmonary edema)

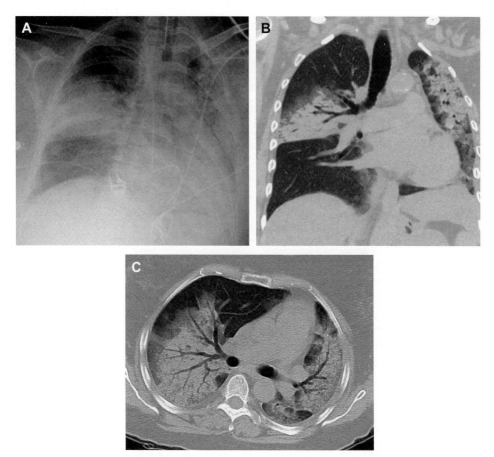

Fig. 23. Multifocal pneumonia. AP chest radiograph (*A*), coronal CT image through the chest (*B*), and axial CT image through the chest (*C*) show bilateral, multifocal consolidative opacities with air bronchograms, consistent with pneumonia. Note the absence of airway crowding that is seen in atelectasis.

[31]. When DAD is absent or minimal, radiographic abnormalities are likely to be relatively transient.

Respiratory symptoms may precede radiographic abnormalities in noncardiogenic pulmonary edema, and the initial radiograph is often normal. Within the first 24 hours, patchy, bilateral ground-glass and consolidative opacities typically appear. These opacities coalesce, forming diffuse pulmonary opacification (Fig. 24) that lasts for days to months depending on etiology, degree of DAD, complications such as aspiration and pneumonia, and treatment. Radiographic features typically associated with hydrostatic pulmonary edema, including septal lines, pleural fluid, and widening of the vascular pedicle, may also be seen with noncardiogenic pulmonary edema. Aberle and colleagues [32] found that a patchy, peripheral distribution is much more commonly

seen in noncardiogenic (50%) than in cardiogenic (13%) pulmonary edema and is the best discriminating radiographic feature. Radiographic change is typically slow, and monitoring of ARDS requires the comparison of multiple chest radiographs.

ARDS is a clinical syndrome characterized by hypoxemia resistant to oxygen therapy, the absence of clinically apparent left atrial hypertension, and bilateral pulmonary opacification on the chest radiograph [33]. It was originally described by Ashbaugh and colleagues [34] in 1967 and was previously known as "adult" respiratory distress syndrome. Acute lung injury (ALI) is on the same clinical spectrum as ARDS, and represents a syndrome of respiratory distress due to underlying pulmonary edema and inflammation [35]. The incidence of ARDS/ALI has not been well defined. A recent study conducted in the United

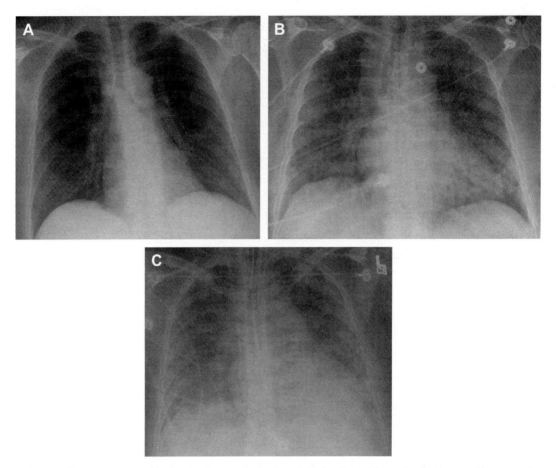

Fig. 24. Progression of noncardiogenic pulmonary edema. (*A*) Initial AP chest radiograph of a 53-year-old woman who had urosepsis is normal. (*B, C*) Follow-up radiographs over the next 2 days demonstrate progressive diffuse bilateral ground-glass and consolidative opacities, consistent with noncardiogenic pulmonary edema. Note the diminishing lung volumes, a feature frequently seen in ARDS.

States by Rubenfeld and colleagues [36] determined the age-adjusted incidence of ALI to be 86.2 per 100,000 person-years, with an in-hospital mortality rate of 38.5%.

Pulmonary opacities on CT are often more heterogeneous than on the chest radiograph. Goodman and colleagues [37] found that asymmetric ground-glass and consolidative opacities predominate when ARDS is secondary to pulmonary disease. When ARDS is due to extrapulmonary causes, a relatively symmetric ground-glass distribution predominates (Fig. 25). CT patterns in ARDS may be described as typical or atypical. In a typical pattern, dense consolidation involves the posterior lungs in a dependent distribution (Fig. 26). Ground-glass opacities are seen in a nondependent distribution. In the atypical pattern, dense consolidation is seen in nondependent

locations. The atypical distribution of consolidation is more likely to be found when ARDS is incited by pulmonary disease [38]. Air bronchograms are frequently seen in both forms. "Crazy-paving," a nonspecific CT appearance of interlobular septal thickening in a background of ground-glass attenuation [39], may also be seen.

DAD can be categorized into exudative, proliferative, and fibrotic phases on pathologic findings, although varying degrees of these phases may be occurring at any one time. The early exudative phase cannot be reliably identified using CT [40]; however, in the proliferative and fibrotic phases, traction bronchiectasis and bronchiolectasis may be seen [40]. Ichikado and colleagues [41] found that the presence of extensive fibroproliferative change early in the clinical course of ARDS is predictive of poor prognosis.

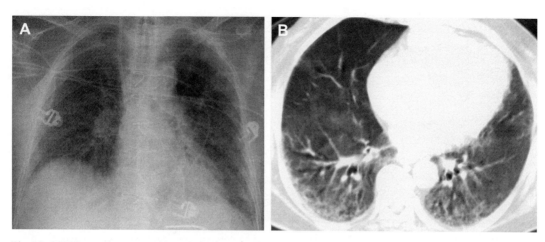

Fig. 25. ARDS secondary to extrathoracic disease. (*A*) AP chest radiograph of an 81-year-old woman who had sepsis shows diffuse ground-glass opacities with relative sparing of the left upper lobe. In addition, lung volumes are low. (*B*) Axial CT image through the lower chest demonstrates symmetric ground-glass opacities. Dependent atelectasis is also present.

Survivors of ARDS often show marked improvement over the first 6 months, with normal spirometric findings, although diffusion capacity often remains low after 1 year [42]. Anterior reticular opacities are the most frequent finding on follow-up CT in survivors of ARDS [43].

Hydrostatic pulmonary edema

Hydrostatic pulmonary edema may be due to cardiac disease, renal failure, or overhydration. The radiographic findings may not be temporally synchronous with clinical disease. Characteristic radiographic findings of hydrostatic pulmonary edema include interlobular septal thickening, manifested as Kerley B lines (1- to 2-cm linear opacities projecting horizontally from the lung periphery), and Kerley A lines (2–6-cm linear opacities projecting horizontally from the mediastinum). Pleural fluid and a widened vascular pedicle are also characteristically seen. Pleural effusions may be bilateral or unilateral. When unilateral, right-sided pleural effusions are more common. Indistinctness of the pulmonary vessels is often subtle but useful in diagnosing pulmonary

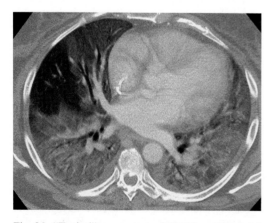

Fig. 26. "Typical" appearance of ARDS on CT. Axial CT image through the lower chest in a 48 year-old postoperative patient demonstrates the typical pattern of ARDS, manifested as dependent opacities with relative sparing of the nondependent regions. Small bilateral pleural effusions are also seen.

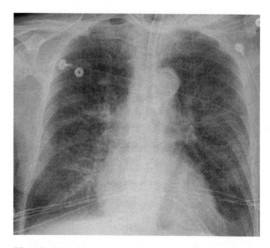

Fig. 27. Hydrostatic pulmonary edema. AP chest radiograph of an 87-year-old man shows airway thickening and pulmonary vascular indistinctness, consistent with hydrostatic pulmonary edema.

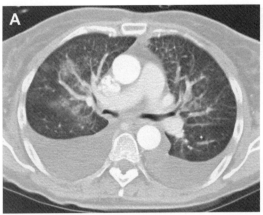
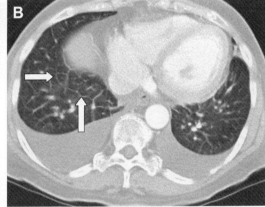

Fig. 28. Hydrostatic pulmonary edema, CT. (*A*, *B*) Axial CT images through the lower chest in a 59-year-old woman show findings characteristic of hydrostatic pulmonary edema including bilateral ground-glass opacities (predominantly in the perihilar regions), interlobular septal thickening (*arrows*), and bilateral pleural effusions.

edema (Fig. 27). Ground-glass opacities may be seen, and consolidative opacities are present in more advanced cases. Distribution is gravity dependent, and abnormalities are most notable at the lung bases; however, this gradient may be absent in the supine ICU patient. Radiographic changes typically occur much more rapidly than those of noncardiogenic pulmonary edema.

Cardiomegaly, with other findings of hydrostatic pulmonary edema, is suggestive of cardiogenic edema. Renal failure may present with similar findings in addition to characteristic perihilar opacities, sometimes referred to as "batwing edema." Aggressive hydration is often seen in settings of trauma and postoperative patients and may coincide with noncardiogenic pulmonary edema.

CT findings of hydrostatic pulmonary edema include smooth interlobular septal thickening, ground-glass and consolidative opacities, and pleural fluid (Fig. 28). When underlying pulmonary disease such as emphysema is present, hydrostatic pulmonary edema may have an atypical appearance and mimic other pathology such as aspiration pneumonitis or pneumonia. Mitral regurgitation can present as asymmetric opacification of the right upper lobe.

Summary

Chest radiography is a critical component in the evaluation of the ICU patient. Daily chest radiography is typically used in patients who have severe cardiopulmonary compromise and are mechanically ventilated. Atelectasis, aspiration, hydrostatic and noncardiogenic pulmonary edema, pneumonia, pneumothorax, and pleural fluid are frequently encountered abnormalities. Chest radiography is useful in diagnosing and evaluating the progression of these entities. Chest radiography is also paramount in ensuring the proper positioning of support and monitoring equipment and in evaluating potential complications. CT can be useful when clinical and radiologic presentations are discrepant, when the patient is not responding to therapy, and in further assessing pleural fluid collections.

Daily rounds involving critical care physicians and radiologists can assist in more accurate and expedient diagnoses.

References

[1] ACR practice guideline for the performance of pediatric and adult portable (mobile unit) chest radiography. In: Practice guidelines and technical standards. Reston (VA): American College of Radiology; 2006. p. 239–43.
[2] Hall JB, White SR, Karrison T. Efficacy of daily routine chest radiographs in intubated, mechanically ventilated patients. Crit Care Med 1990;19(5):689–93.
[3] Krivopal M, Shlobin OA, Schwartzstein RM. Utility of daily routine portable chest radiographs in mechanically ventilated patients in the medical ICU. Chest 2003;123(5):1607–14.
[4] Marik PE, Janower ML. The impact of routine chest radiography on ICU management decisions: an observational study. Am J Crit Care 1997;6(2): 95–8.

[5] Strain DS, Kinasewitz GT, Vereen LE, et al. Value of routine daily chest x-rays in the medical intensive care unit. Crit Care Med 1985;13(7):534–6.

[6] Aquino SL. Routine chest radiograph. ACR appropriateness criteria, 2006. American College of Radiology. Available at http://www.acr.org.

[7] Miller WT, Tino G, Friedburg JS. Thoracic CT in the intensive care unit: assessment of clinical usefulness. Radiology 1998;209:491–8.

[8] Wechsler RJ, Steiner RM, Kinori I. Monitoring the monitors: the radiology of thoracic catheters, wires, and tubes. Semin Roentgenol 1988;23:61–84.

[9] Khan F, Reddy NC. Enlarging intratracheal tube cuff diameter: a quantitative roentgenographic study of its value in the early prediction of serious tracheal damage. Ann Thorac Surg 1977;24(1): 49–53.

[10] Cadman A, Lawrance JAL, Fitzsimmons L, et al. To clot or not to clot? That is the question in central venous catheters. Clin Radiol 2004;59:349–55.

[11] Collins J, Stern EJ. Monitoring and support devices—"Tubes and Lines." In: Chest radiology: the essentials. Philadelphia: Lippincott Williams & Wilkins; 1999. p. 59–71.

[12] Kazerooni EA, Gross BH. Lines, tubes, and devices. In: Cardiopulmonary imaging. Philadephia: Lippincott Williams & Wilkins; 2004. p. 255–93.

[13] Tocino IM. Pneumothorax in the supine patient: radiographic anatomy. Radiographics 1985;5(4): 557–86.

[14] Wintermark M, Schnyder P. The Macklin effect. Chest 2001;120(2):543–6.

[15] Zylak CM, Standen JR, Barnes GR, et al. Pneumomediastinum revisited. Radiographics 2000;20: 1043–57.

[16] Müller N. Imaging of the pleura. Radiology 1993; 186:297–309.

[17] Kuhlman JE, Sinha NK. Complex disease of the pleural space: radiographic and CT evaluation. Radiographics 1997;17:63–79.

[18] Rivas LA, Fishman JE, Múnera F, et al. Multislice CT in thoracic trauma. Radiol Clin North Am 2003;41:599–616.

[19] Gale GD, Teasdale SJ, Sanders DE, et al. Pulmonary atelectasis and other respiratory complications after cardiopulmonary bypass and investigation of aetiological factors. Can Anaesth Soc J 1979;26(1): 15–21.

[20] Sheuland JE, Hireleman MR, Hoang KA, et al. Lobar collapse in the surgical intensive care unit. Br J Radiol 1983;56:531–4.

[21] Kreider ME, Lipson DA. Bronchoscopy for atelectasis in the ICU. A case report and review of the literature. Chest 2003;124(7):344–50.

[22] Franquet T, Giménez A, Rosón N, et al. Aspiration diseases: findings, pitfalls, and differential diagnosis. Radiographics 2000;20:673–85.

[23] Rossi SE, Franquet T, Volpacchio M, et al. Tree-in-bud pattern at thin-section CT of the lungs:

radiologic-pathologic overview. Radiographics 2005;25:789–801.

[24] Cunnion KM, Weber DJ, Broadhead WE, et al. Risk factors for nososcomial pneumonia: comparing adult critical-care populations. Am J Respir Crit Care Med 1996;153(1):158–62.

[25] Morehead RS, Pinto SJ. Ventilator-associated pneumonia. Arch Intern Med 2000;160:1926–36.

[26] Winer-Muram HT, Jennings SG, Wunderink RG, et al. Ventilator-associated *Pseudomonas aeruginosa* pneumonia: radiographic findings. Radiology 1995; 195:247–52.

[27] Winer-Muram HT, Rubin SA, Ellis JV, et al. Pneumonia and ARDS in patients receiving mechanical ventilation: diagnostic accuracy of chest radiography. Radiology 1993;188:479–85.

[28] Winer-Muram HT, Steiner RM, Gurney JW, et al. Ventilator-associated pneumonia in patients with adult respiratory distress syndrome: CT evaluation. Radiology 1998;208(1):193–9.

[29] Andrews CP, Coalson JJ, Smith JD, et al. Diagnosis of nosocomial bacterial pneumonia in acute, diffuse lung injury. Chest 1981;80(3):254–8.

[30] Miller PR, Croce MA, Bee TK, et al. ARDS after pulmonary contusion: accurate measurement of contusion volume identifies high-risk patients. J Trauma 2001;51(2):223–30.

[31] Gluecker T, Capasso P, Schnyder P, et al. Clinical and radiologic features of pulmonary edema. Radiographics 1999;19:1507–31.

[32] Aberle DR, Wiener-Kronish JP, Webb WR, et al. Hydrostatic versus increased permeability pulmonary edema: diagnosis based on radiographic criteria in critically ill patients. Radiology 1988;168: 73–9.

[33] Bernard GR, Artigas A, Brigham KL, et al. The American-European Consensus Conference on ARDS: definitions, mechanisms, relevant outcomes, and clinical trial coordination. Am J Respir Crit Care Med 1994;149:818–24.

[34] Ashbaugh DG, Bigelow DB, Petty TL, et al. Acute respiratory distress in adults. Lancet 1967;2: 319–23.

[35] Matthay MA, Zimmerman GA, Esmon C, et al. Future research directions in acute lung injury. Am J Respir Crit Care Med 2003;167:1027–35.

[36] Rubenfeld GD, Caldwell E, Peabody E, et al. Incidence and outcomes of acute lung injury. N Engl J Med 2005;353(16):1685–93.

[37] Goodman LR, Fumagalli R, Tagliabue P. Adult respiratory distress syndrome due to pulmonary and extrapulmonary causes: CT, clinical, and functional correlations. Radiology 1999;213:545–52.

[38] Desai SR, Suntharalingam G, Rubens MB, et al. Acute respiratory distress syndrome caused by pulmonary and extrapulmonary injury: a comparative CT study. Radiology 2001;218:689–93.

[39] Rossi SE, Erasmus JJ, Volpacchio M. "Crazy-paving" pattern at thin-section CT of the

lungs: radiologic-pathologic overview. Radio-graphics 2003;23:1508–19.

[40] Ichikado K, Suga M, Gushima Y, et al. Hyperoxia-induced diffuse alveolar damage in pigs: correlation between thin-section CT and histopathologic findings. Radiology 2000;216:531–8.

[41] Ichikado K, Suga M, Muranaka S, et al. Prediction of prognosis for acute respiratory distress syndrome

with thin-section CT: validation in 44 cases. Radiology 2006;238(1):321–9.

[42] Herridge MS, Cheung AM, Tansey CM, et al. One-year outcomes in survivors of the acute respiratory distress syndrome. N Engl J Med 2003;348(8):683–93.

[43] Desai SR, Wells AU, Rubens MB, et al. Acute respiratory distress syndrome: CT abnormalities at long-term follow-up. Radiology 1999;210:29–35.

ELSEVIER
SAUNDERS

Clin Chest Med 29 (2008) 77–105

CLINICS
IN CHEST
MEDICINE

Imaging Infection

Loren Ketai, MD[a],*, Kirk Jordan, MD[b], Edith M. Marom, MD[c]

[a]Department of Radiology, MSC10 5530, University of New Mexico Health Science Center,
Albuquerque, NM 87131–0001, USA
[b]Department of Radiology, University of Texas Southwestern Medical Center at Dallas,
5323 Harry Hines Boulevard, Dallas, TX 75390-8896, USA
[c]Department of Diagnostic Imaging, University of Texas, MD Andersen Cancer Center,
1515 Holcombe Boulevard, Houston, TX 77030, USA

The imaging of thoracic infection is usually split into separate discussions of immunocompetent patients, non-AIDS immunocompromised patients, and patients with AIDS. Although categorization is useful, it is also important to identify practical goals for thoracic imaging in each of these groups. In general terms, radiology is useful in detecting suspected pneumonias and identifying complications of pneumonia in all three groups [1,2]. In normal hosts, radiology is often called on to help differentiate infection from noninfectious intrathoracic disease, with variable success [3]. Only occasionally can imaging suggest specific pathogens. In patients with immunocompromise, whether caused by AIDS or other entities, radiologic findings can often be combined with clinical information (eg, the patient's CD4 counts or time elapsed since organ transplant) to focus on a specific organism or group of organisms. In some cases this can facilitate treatment decisions despite the absence of diagnostic cultures.

The first part of this article reviews the role of thoracic imaging in normal or minimally compromised hosts. Many of the observations regarding detection of infectious complications and differentiation of infection from noninfectious disease can also be generalized to immunocompromised hosts. The remaining two thirds of this article focus on immunocompromised hosts, particularly on combinations of imaging and clinical characteristics that may suggest bacterial, fungal, or viral pathogens.

* Corresponding author.
E-mail address: lketai@salud.unm.edu (L. Ketai).

Normal hosts

Detection of infection

Community-acquired pneumonia is usually readily diagnosed by chest radiographs. In a significant minority of such patients, however, the clinical diagnosis may be at odds with radiographic findings. Among 2000 patients hospitalized with a clinical diagnosis of pneumonia, subsequent review of chest radiographs failed to confirm radiographic findings of pneumonia in a third [4]. Most patients in which review of radiographs did not confirm pneumonia had other radiographic abnormalities, either congestive heart failure, atelectasis, or chronic obstructive lung disease. The latter has also been shown to confound the radiographic diagnosis of pneumonia in other series [5]. In populations without a high prevalence of confounding disease, interobserver agreement on presence or absence of pneumonia can be high, greater than 85%, but agreement on lobar pneumonia and bronchopneumonia patterns (see below) remains poor [6].

The accuracy of chest radiology for the detection of hospital-acquired pneumonia is less than that for community-acquired pneumonia, lower still in the subset of hospitalized patients receiving mechanical ventilation, and lowest in patients that have developed adult respiratory distress syndrome (ARDS). In the setting of ARDS, receiver operating curves have shown that chest radiographic findings are not useful in discriminating between patients with and without pneumonia [7]. Diagnostic accuracy remains elusive with the use of CT. CT imaging done early in the course of ARDS usually reveals ground glass opacities (GGO) and dependent consolidation, which is caused by a combination of true airspace filling and atelectasis of the diffusely edematous lung (Fig. 1) [8]. CT images of patients with ARDS that develop superimposed ventilator-acquired pneumonia are likely to show consolidation in the ventral, nondependent lung, a region that appears most normal on CT images of early ARDS [3]. These nosocomial pneumonias may contribute to the observed increase in nondependent consolidation as the duration of ARDS lengthens [9]. Unfortunately, development of nondependent consolidations is not sufficiently sensitive or specific to serve as an indication for antibiotic therapy.

Complications of pneumonia

After pneumonia is diagnosed, additional imaging is often performed if there is clinical or image-based suspicion of pleural disease, lung necrosis, or adenopathy. Both CT and ultrasound have advantages in evaluating suspected parapneumonic effusions. Ultrasound's principal advantages are its low cost, portability, and lack of ionizing radiation. Ultrasound images can also demonstrate septations within pleural fluid collections that are not visible on contrast-enhanced CT scanning [10]. These septations, however, are often fibrinous strands rather than dense adhesions between visceral and parietal pleura and are probably not a good predictor for the adequacy of catheter drainage. Potential pitfalls in ultrasound evaluation of pleural fluid include the

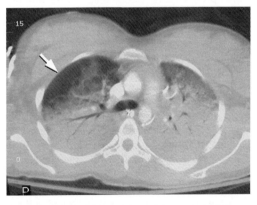

Fig. 1. CT section from patient with severe ARDS, uncomplicated by infection. Dorsal portions of the lung are densely consolidated. GGO and nearly normal-appearing parenchyma (*arrow*) are seen in ventral aspect of lung.

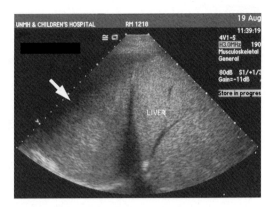

Fig. 2. Ultrasound of empyema shows markedly echogenic fluid (*arrow*) above the diaphragm adjacent to liver.

misclassification of diffusely echogenic fluid. Approximately 5% of parapneumonic effusions, usually empyema, may be sufficiently echogenic to be mistaken for solid tissue by inexperienced users (Fig. 2) [11]. In more experienced hands, Doppler demonstration of the lack of blood flow can differentiate loculated echogenic fluid from solid tissue.

CT scanning is superior to ultrasound in providing a "global" assessment of multiloculated pleural fluid including paramediastinal collections that do not have a good ultrasonographic window. Pleural enhancement is seen on contrast-enhanced CT in most uninfected parapneumonic effusions and in 85% to 100% of empyema [10,12]. Optimal detection of pleural enhancement requires a longer delay (60–90 seconds) after contrast administration than routinely performed (Fig. 3). Absence of parietal pleural enhancement in a properly performed CT argues strongly against the presence of an empyema. Thickening and increased attenuation of the extrapleural fat may be a more specific sign than pleural enhancement but only the presence of gas within previously uninstrumented pleural fluid is sufficiently specific to warrant proceeding directly to pleural drainage catheter without initially sampling the pleural fluid [13].

Lucencies within an area of lobar consolidation early in the course of pneumonia often represent underlying emphysema, whereas lucencies appearing later can indicate lung necrosis. Contrast-enhanced CT imaging in these patients may show geographic areas of nonenhancing lung parenchyma that are sufficiently hypodense that the margins between lung and adjacent pleural fluid are indistinct (Fig. 4). This finding presages

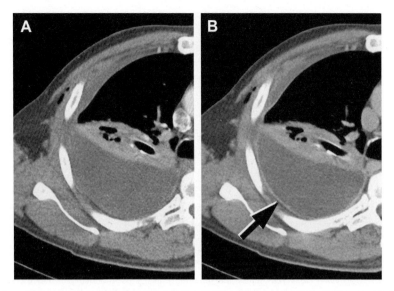

Fig. 3. CT sections from a patient with empyema. (*A*) Detail from CT image performed 25 seconds after intravenous contrast administration shows minimal pleural enhancement. (*B*) Image performed 90 seconds after contrast administered clearly shows pleural enhancement (*arrow*).

frank abscess formation and is a predictor of prolonged hospital stay [14]. In rare cases necrosis may extend into the pulmonary vasculature resulting in in situ thrombosis of a pulmonary artery or sufficient destruction of the arterial wall to form a pseudoaneurysm, both complications often requiring surgical resection (Fig. 5) [15].

Focal areas of necrosis most commonly result in lung abscesses; however, pneumatocele can occur when focal alveolar or bronchiolar necrosis

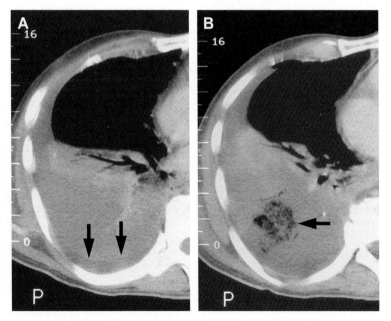

Fig. 4. CT sections from patient with necrotizing pneumonia. (*A*) Detail from CT with intravenous contrast shows that most of the right lower lobe is nonenhancing, with an attenuation barely greater than that of pleural fluid (*arrows*). (*B*) Detail from another level in the same patient shows air within an area of early necrosis (*arrow*).

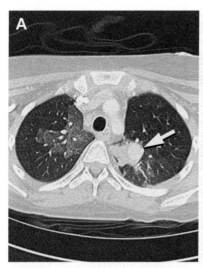
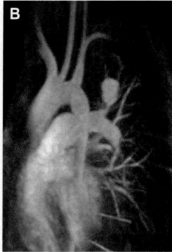

Fig. 5. Patient with *Staphylococcus aureus* sepsis and pulmonary artery pseudoaneurysm. (*A*) CT shows right-sided GGO and left apical consolidation with high-attenuation (*arrow*) center. (*B*) MRA of the thorax confirms presence of mycotic pseudoaneurysm arising from pulmonary artery.

allows air to dissect into the pulmonary parenchyma and create an air cyst. Because this cyst is formed by ball valve phenomena rather than excavation of necrotic tissue it can enlarge rapidly over several days and cause compression of adjacent structures [16]. Often thin-walled, pneumatocele may give rise to pneumothoraces [17]. Pneumatocele formation is more common in children than adults, and although classically associated with staphylococcal infections has been reported in pneumococcal and gram-negative pneumonia (Fig. 6).

In addition to pleural effusion and lung parenchymal necrosis, radiographs of patients with pneumonia occasionally reveal hilar or mediastinal adenopathy. Adenopathy that is apparent on chest radiograph suggests either an underlying disease, such as neoplasm or sarcoidosis, or a short list of infectious agents that include primary tuberculosis, endemic fungal infections, tularemia, and anthrax. The detection of enlarged lymph nodes on chest CT, however, is a nonspecific finding in the setting of pneumonia. Lymph nodes that exceed normal CT size criteria (1.5 cm short axis in the subcarinal area, 1 cm elsewhere) are found in about half of patients with either bacteremic pneumococcal pneumonia or an empyema [18]. Enlarged nodes with low-attenuation centers are much less common and in a non-immunocompromised patient suggest primary tuberculosis. Enlargement of lymph nodes in reactivation tuberculosis is rare [19].

Differentiation of pneumonia from noninfectious diseases

Among normal hosts with suspected pneumonia the radiologic pattern helps determine which noninfectious diseases might also be considered in a differential diagnosis (Table 1). A linear interstitial pattern is one of the most reliably recognized patterns, dominated by apparent Kerley's A and B lines, often accompanied by subpleural edema (thickening the fissures) and pleural effusions. The CT equivalent of this pattern is smooth thickening of the interlobular septa. These septa are 1 to 2 cm in length and represent the divisions

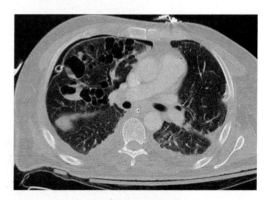

Fig. 6. CT of patient with *Staphylococcus aureus* pneumonia and pneumatoceles. CT section shows numerous thin-walled cysts and associated pneumothorax. Minimal consolidation is present.

Table 1
Radiologic patterns shared by infectious and noninfectious disease

CT Pattern	Infection	Noninfectious disease
Linear interstitial	Rare	CHF, drug reaction
Nodules		
Centrilobular	Common	HP, Respiratory bronchiolitis
Tree-in-bud	Common	Gastric aspiration
Random	Uncommon	Metastases
Lobular GGO or consolidation	Common	CHF, pulmonary hemorrhage, drug reaction
Consolidation		
Nonsegmental	Common	Atelectasis
Segmental	Common	Pulmonary infarction

Abbreviations: CHF, congestive heart failure; GGO, ground glass opacity; HP, hypersensitivity pneumonitis.

between secondary lobules, the smallest unit of lung surrounded by connective tissue (Fig. 7). Infectious agents, including viruses, rarely cause this pattern, with the notable exception of the North American hantaviruses and occasionally rickettsial diseases (Fig. 8) [20,21]. Although in most cases linear interstitial patterns are caused by hydrostatic edema, occasionally a drug reaction has a similar pattern.

Reticulonodular or nodular patterns are the most common "interstitial" appearance of pneumonia. In the setting of pneumonia this pattern is often the radiographic manifestation of bronchial wall thickening and bronchiolitis. Bronchiolitis results in small nodules that are individually too small to be seen on chest radiograph but become visible when multiple overlying nodules summate. On CT images the individual 1- to 3-mm nodules are readily seen. The nodules are caused by inflammation around the bronchioles, which are located in the center of the secondary lobule. Because bronchioles do not extend all the way to the pleura, the nodules that form around bronchioles (centrilobular nodules) characteristically spare the pleural surfaces (see Fig. 7).

If the bronchioles connecting centrilobular nodules are thickened or filled with secretions, they may become visible on CT. The resulting pattern of centrilobular nodules connected by branching structures is termed a "tree-in-bud" pattern. This subset of centrilobular nodules has strong association with infection or gastric aspiration (Fig. 9) [22]. The CT finding of simple centrilobular nodules (without features of tree-in-bud) is less specific. It may be caused by infection but also occurs commonly in other diseases caused by inhaled materials, most notably hypersensitivity pneumonitis.

CT is particularly useful in the evaluation of patients presenting with reticulonodular or

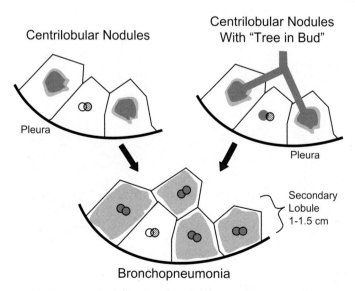

Fig. 7. Line drawing demonstrating disease patterns within secondary lobule. These include simple centrilobular nodules, centrilobular nodules as part of "tree-in-bud" pattern, and lobular opacities typical of progression to bronchopneumonia.

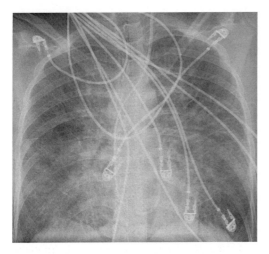

Fig. 8. Chest radiograph from patient with severe, early hantavirus pulmonary syndrome shows linear interstitial pattern. Numerous Kerley's A and B lines are present.

nodular opacities on chest radiograph. CT imaging can distinguish nodules with a simple centrilobular pattern from centrilobular nodules with a tree-in-bud pattern and, more important, can distinguish both types of centrilobular nodules from nodules with a random distribution. Randomly distributed nodules are often caused by blood-borne dissemination of disease. Unlike centrilobular nodules, random nodules can touch the pleural surfaces, including the fissures [23]. Miliary tuberculosis is the classic cause of randomly distributed micronodules. Disseminated fungal infections and metastatic neoplasms, such as renal cell, thyroid, and melanoma, may have the identical appearance (Fig. 10).

Rather than causing reticulonodular opacities, most pneumonias fill airspaces creating a bronchopneumonia or lobar pneumonia pattern. On chest radiographs bronchopneumonia appear as patchy opacities that may be accompanied by bronchial wall thickening. Because of the scattered distribution of inflammation, areas of consolidation are often not sufficiently confluent to create air bronchograms.

The CT appearance of bronchopneumonia may illustrate progression from an initial bronchiolitis, with infection spreading outward from the center of the secondary lobule. As entire lobules fill with inflammatory debris the opacities created conform to lobular architecture and are sharply marginated by interlobular lines (Fig. 11). Opacities that are sufficiently transparent to allow visualization of underlying vasculature are called "ground glass opacities," and those dense enough to obscure vessels are called "consolidation." In

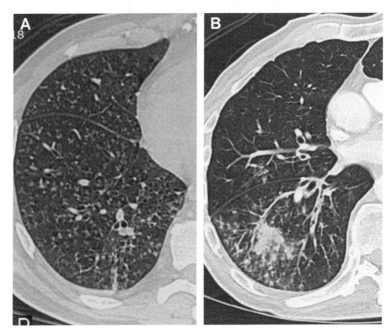

Fig. 9. CT of tree-in-bud pattern caused by two different etiologies. (A) Detail from CT of patient with diffuse tree-in-bud pattern caused with mycoplasma infection. (B) Detail from CT patient with acute aspiration shows tree-in-bud pattern in the dependent lung. Nodules in both Fig. 9A and B largely spare pleural surfaces.

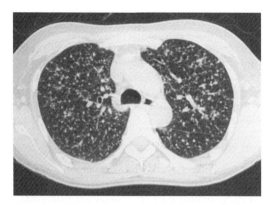

Fig. 10. CT from patient with miliary tuberculosis. Diffuse nodules are present, some of which abut the pleural surfaces, including the pleural fissures.

addition to bronchopneumonia, a lobular pattern of GGO or consolidation may be caused by drug toxicity, chronic infiltrative lung diseases, pulmonary hemorrhage, or pulmonary edema [24]. The presence of a tree-in bud configuration combined with lobular opacities on CT, however, favors pneumonia over these other diagnoses.

Lobar pneumonias characteristically begin in the lung periphery and then spread centrally. Consolidation is confluent rather than patchy and often sufficient to form air bronchograms. Although early in the course of infection consolidation may be confined to a single segment, over time it can spread through a lobe of the lung without regard for segmental boundaries (the

resulting opacities sometimes referred to as "nonsegmental"). Most of the organisms that cause lobar pneumonia, particularly pneumococcus, can also cause bronchopneumonia and examples of both patterns may be present in the same patient. Distinguishing bronchopneumonia from lobar pneumonia is not helpful in identifying a specific pathogen. Confluent consolidation, however, is associated with a different spectrum of noninfectious diseases than bronchopneumonia.

Lobar consolidation (with preserved lung volume) almost always represents pneumonia, but less extensive consolidation requires a broader differential diagnosis that includes pulmonary infarction and atelectasis. If atelectasis involves less than an entire lobe definitive signs of volume loss may not be evident on chest radiographs. CT often more clearly demonstrates displacement and crowding of fissures and bronchi. Contrast enhancement pattern may also help differentiate atelectasis from pneumonia. On contrast-enhanced CT the lung parenchyma in areas of passive atelectasis enhances markedly, often enough partially to obscure underlying vessels. Some pneumonias enhance to a similar degree, but a third or more of pneumonias and cases of obstructive atelectasis enhance less intensely, allowing clear delineation of pulmonary vasculature from surrounding lung parenchyma (Fig. 12) [25]. This relatively low attenuation of lung parenchyma likely represents retained fluid within alveoli. Its presence in conjunction with air-filled bronchi favors pneumonia. Relatively low-

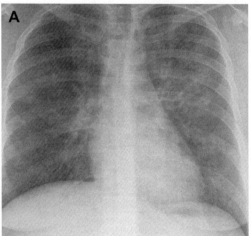
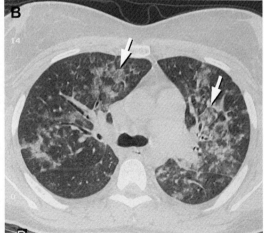

Fig. 11. Bronchopneumonia chest radiograph and CT. (*A*) Chest radiograph shows patchy bilateral opacities with few air bronchograms. (*B*) CT section shows lobular GGO (*arrows*) and scattered centrilobular nodules.

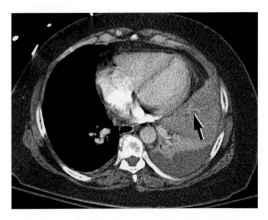

Fig. 12. CT scan of patient with atelectasis and pneumonia. Following intravenous contrast administration, an area of passive atelectasis in left lower lobe shows dense enhancement, obscuring pulmonary vessels. The lingula is lower in attenuation, however, and vessels are visible (*arrow*), with preservation of lingular volume, consistent with pneumonia or obstructive atelectasis.

attenuation lung in conjunction with fluid-filled bronchi suggests obstructive atelectasis.

Both pulmonary infarcts and early lobar pneumonia arise in the periphery of the lung and may appear similar on chest radiography. CT images of infarcts demonstrate a characteristic triangular opacity, with its broad base against the pleura and

its apex truncated and pointing centrally (Fig. 13). Central lucency within the opacity and absence of air bronchograms both strongly favor infarct over other causes of parenchymal lung disease [26]. Demonstration of opacities with this configuration on a noncontrast or thick-section contrasted CT may warrant further evaluation with a CT pulmonary angiogram.

Specific diagnosis: mycoplasma and mycobacterium

Mycoplasma is the most common cause of respiratory infection to present as a reticulonodular radiographic pattern, correlating with centrilobular nodules evident on CT imaging (see Fig. 9) [27]. Adults may be more likely to present with this bronchiolitis-bronchopneumonia pattern than children in whom segmental and lobar pneumonia may be more common, possibly because a more active immune response in adults limits the scope of infection [28].

Bacterial pathogens and *Chlamydia* can also cause centrilobular nodules, but do so less commonly than mycoplasma. Viral infections, such as influenza, metapneumovirus, and respiratory syncytial virus, can also cause bronchiolitis in adults but the infections are most often radiologically occult in normal hosts; imaging signs of bronchiolitis are much more common in immunocompromised patients. Viral bronchiolitis is very common in

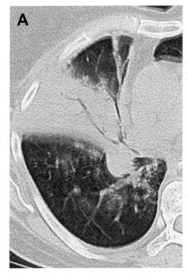 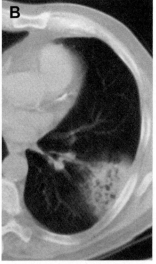

Fig. 13. Comparison of CT findings of lobar pneumonia and pulmonary infarction. (*A*) Detail of CT of patient with lobar pneumonia shows consolidation extending contiguously from pleura to the hilum. (*B*) Detail of CT pulmonary infarct shows opacity is truncated medially. Ill-defined low-attenuation is also seen developing with the center of the opacity but no air bronchograms are seen.

young children, but because of the smaller airway size radiologic findings are usually dominated by signs of air trapping rather than a reticulonodular or nodular interstitial pattern [29].

Upper lobe predominance of centrilobular nodules is a common early manifestation of reactivation tuberculosis, representing broncho-genic spread of disease [30]. These centrilobular nodules may be accompanied by macronodules (5–10 mm in diameter). Associated lobular con-solidation and small areas of cavitation may help distinguish tuberculosis from mycoplasma and most other causes of infectious bronchiolitis (Fig. 14). Increasing numbers of centrilobular nodules and cavities on CT imaging of tuberculo-sis also increase the likelihood that the infection is active and the likelihood that sputum smears are positive [19,31].

Centrilobular nodules are also associated with nontuberculous mycobacterial (NTMB) infec-tions. In normal hosts, NTMB infections can present as a classic form that mimics tuberculosis, as a bronchiectatic form, or as hypersensitivity pneumonitis [32]. All three forms of disease may have centrilobular nodules but the bronchiectatic form has the most distinctive radiologic pattern. This form of disease manifests as centrilobular nodules with or without tree-in-bud configuration accompanied by cylindric bronchiectasis [2]. Bronchiectasis characteristically occurs in the middle and lingular lobes, but positive cultures are most commonly obtained in patients with in-volvement of all lobes [33]. The bronchiectatic form of NTMB most commonly occurs in elderly women, who may be considered partially immu-nocompromised (see next section).

Non-AIDS immune compromised

Immune compromised patients may suffer from community-acquired pneumonia, which is undetectable by chest radiographs because of a combination of decreased immunologic host response and the limited sensitivity of the chest radiograph, reported to be normal in 10% of patients with early infections [34]. In addition, such patients may suffer from opportunistic infec-tions, some of which may show a characteristic radiographic pattern. Often, however, these char-acteristic patterns of disease are difficult to appre-ciate by chest radiography. Because early identification of opportunistic infections, such as fungal infections, results in increased survival [35], CT is now routinely used in assessment of im-munocompromised patients with a normal chest radiograph or when a nonspecific pattern of dis-ease is seen with chest radiography. Typical CT appearances of fungal pneumonia are now used to diagnose fungal pneumonia [36] because the likelihood of obtaining a positive culture in fungal

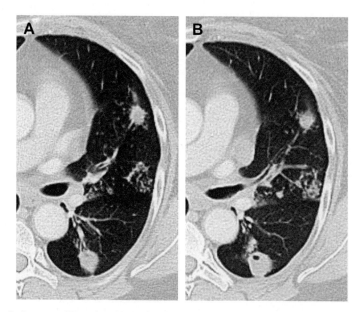

Fig. 14. (A, B) Details from two CT sections in patient with tuberculosis shows several macronodules, the most posterior with a developing cavity, and numerous centrilobular micronodules, the latter consistent with active disease.

pneumonia is unacceptably low, ranging from 30% to 54% [37,38]. CT patterns should be interpreted with caution, however, because they are not pathognomonic and any of the patterns encountered, whether nodules, masses, tree-in-bud opacities, or the halo sign, can be seen with bacterial, viral, or fungal infections [39]. Knowing the clinical history of the patient, specifically the type and level of immune suppression, is crucial in reaching the correct diagnosis.

For interpretive purposes, immune compromised patients can be divided into two major groups: severely immune compromised patients, such as bone marrow transplant recipients (BMT), solid organ recipients, or patients undergoing aggressive chemotherapy regimens, in which there is a high likelihood that imaging will discover fungal and viral pneumonias; and mild immunosuppression, which can be seen in the elderly, heavy smokers, or those with underlying lung disease, in which infection is usually limited to bacterial and mycobacterial pneumonias.

CT technique

Multidetector CT scans have replaced single detector ones and thin slices of the entire chest are performed within seconds. In many institutions, 2.5-mm slices are considered standard for imaging the chest. This has improved the quality of imaging and with such technique, high-resolution CT scan protocols are no longer needed for evaluation of pulmonary infections. High-resolution CT scans are now reserved for those patients in which prone imaging and expiratory imaging is needed, for example patients suspected of having air trapping (bronchiolitis obliterans, graft-versus-host disease) or early lung fibrosis. Despite the fact that low-dose CT can decrease the radiation 10-fold depending on technique, subtle parenchymal abnormalities are suboptimally visualized with low-dose technique, such as GGO, which in the immunocompromised patient may signify opportunistic infection. With current CT capabilities, evaluation of the severely immunocompromised patient for infection is performed with standard radiation dose. Using CT performed with a standard radiation, a slice thickness of 3 mm or less and a supine inspiratory acquisition should suffice.

Fungal infections

Invasive mold pulmonary infections are not encountered with mild immune suppression yet are responsible for more than 10% of pulmonary infections in BMT and in approximately 5% of pulmonary infections in solid organ transplant recipients [40,41]. When encountered in the BMT recipient they are more likely to be seen in the first month, before engraftment has occurred, and when profound prolonged neutropenia is present (Fig. 15). Even after engraftment, in the first 6 months patients who are treated with steroids for graft-versus-host disease continue to be vulnerable to mold infections. In solid organ recipients, particularly lung transplant recipients, fungal pneumonia is not common but usually seen within the first 2 months after transplantation when immune suppressive therapy is highest (Fig. 16) [42]. Mortality from fungal pneumonia is high and can approach 80% to 90% even with antifungal therapy [43].

The most common invasive mold is invasive aspergillosis. On CT it more commonly presents with findings related to its angioinvasiveness, although abnormalities related to airway spread are seen in up to 30%, where peribronchial consolidative nodules or masses can be seen and there is often overlap of findings [44]. More than 90% of patients with pulmonary invasive aspergillosis have either a nodule or mass on CT, which are usually multiple with no lobar predominance. The nodules are usually larger than 1 cm, can be round and solid or present as masslike consolidation, sometimes peripheral and wedge-like (Fig. 17). Other characteristic nodules have been described for aspergillus but can also be seen with other fungal infections. The halo sign, a solid nodule surrounded by peripheral GGO, is seen in more than half of the patients with invasive aspergillosis [45]. The central solid nodule is caused by consolidated, sometimes necrotic lung laden with fungi, whereas the surrounding GGO is caused by hemorrhage related to thrombosis from fungal angioinvasion (Fig. 18) [46]. The reversed halo sign is when GGO are surrounded by a rim of soft tissue and represent infarcted lung with hemorrhage greater at the periphery. The hypodense sign is a central region of lower attenuation surrounded by enhancing mass or consolidation (Fig. 19). With time, during the recovery phase of infection when neutropenia is resolving, necrosed material is digested, leaving cavitation (Fig. 20). When imaged early in the cavitary process the cavitation can be eccentric giving rise to the crescent sign. The halo sign and the reversed halo sign are early CT findings and can present at initial presentation even before specific

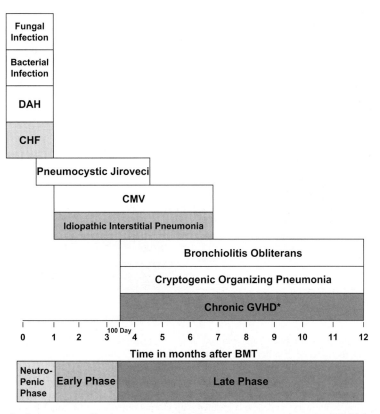

Fig. 15. Timeline of pulmonary complications occurring after bone marrow transplantation. BMT, bone marrow transplantation; CHF, congestive heart failure; CMV, cytomegalovirus; DAH, diffuse alveolar hemorrhage; GVHD, graftversus-host disease; *Vulnerability to fungal infections caused by treatment of GVHD. (*Data from* Boroja M, Barrie JR, Raymond GS. Radiographic findings in 20 patients with hantavirus pulmonary syndrome correlated with clinical outcome. AJR Am J Roentgenol 2002;178:159–63.)

respiratory symptoms predominate, may precede positive galactomannan results, and are important when seen in a severely immunocompromised patient because antifungal treatment is usually initiated and prognosis is improved [35,45]. The hypodense sign is a later sign seen 3 to 23 days (mean, 8 days) after initial CT findings of infections are documented and used for confirmation of fungal infection rather than initial diagnosis. Likewise, the crescent sign follows it, usually 2 to 3 weeks after initiation of treatment, associated with resolution of neutropenia and usually indicates a good prognosis [47]. Although the halo, hypodense, and crescent signs are suggestive of invasive aspergillosis, they can also be seen in other fungal infections or bacterial infections (eg, *Pseudomonas aeruginosa*). In addition, these signs should be interpreted as infectious only in the severely immune compromised patient because they can be mimicked by noninfectious

processes as hemorrhagic or cavitating metastases or cryptogenic organizing pneumonia. Pseudoaneurysm formation is a rare complication of invasive aspergillosis that necessitates resection to prevent fatal hemorrhage. If CT is performed with intravenous contrast careful investigation of the pulmonary arteries is necessary to discover these pseudoaneurysms because they change clinical management.

Fusarium infection is the second most common mold infection, after invasive aspergillosis, in severely immunocompromised patients [48], because of the increasing use of highly immunosuppressive chemotherapeutic regimens and the broad use of antifungal agents targeting aspergillus species. Distinguishing between fusariosis and aspergillosis is important because *Fusarium* species are more resistant to amphotericin B and some of the oral antifungals, but this cannot be done by radiology. Most patients with fusariosis

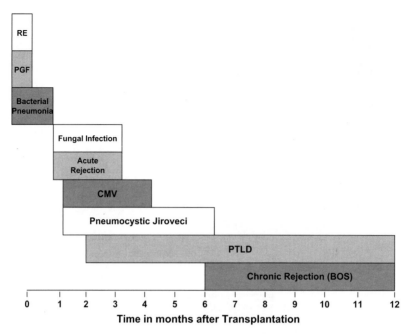

Fig. 16. Timeline of pulmonary complications occurring after lung transplantation. The timeline of the infectious complications is similar to the timeline of other solid organ transplantations. CMV, cytomegalovirus; PGF, primary graft failure; PTLD, post-transplant lymphoproliferative disease; RE, reperfusion edema. (*Data from* Desai SR, Wells AU, Suntharalingam G, et al. Acute respiratory distress syndrome caused by pulmonary and extrapulmonary injury: a comparative CT study. Radiology 2001;218:689–93; and Boroja M, Barrie JR, Raymond GS. Radiographic findings in 20 patients with hantavirus pulmonary syndrome correlated with clinical outcome. AJR Am J Roentgenol 2002;178:159–63.)

present with a pulmonary nodule or mass but this is often difficult to appreciate by chest radiography, and CT is helpful for early identification. These nodules or masses may coexist with consolidation or GGO but the halo sign or reversed halo sign have yet to be described with fusariosis.

The reported radiologic manifestations of mucormycosis (zygomycosis) are identical to those reported for aspergillosis and include consolidation, cavitation, the crescent sign, the halo sign, reversed halo sign (Fig. 21), solitary or multiple pulmonary nodules, bronchopleural fistula, and pulmonary artery pseudoaneurysm [49]. Chest wall invasion or direct extension through fissures is sometimes seen (Fig. 22). Antifungal agents with anti-*Aspergillus* activity, such as voriconazole, are sometimes used empirically to treat patients with suspected fungal infection. Voriconazole has no activity against mucormycosis, and this may account for the recently increased incidence of mucormycosis in heavily immunocompromised patients. Multiple nodules (≥10) and the presence of a pleural effusion when seen at the time of initial CT are more commonly associated with mucormycosis

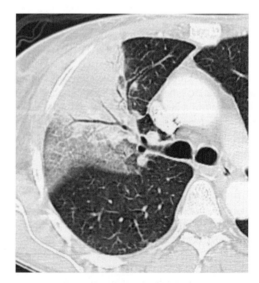

Fig. 17. Sixty-year-old woman with history of relapsed acute myelogenous leukemia after BMT, currently undergoing salvage chemotherapy. Contrast-enhanced chest CT shows a peripheral consolidative wedge-shaped mass with some adjacent GGO. Culture from the right upper lobe lesion grew *Aspergillus fumigatus*.

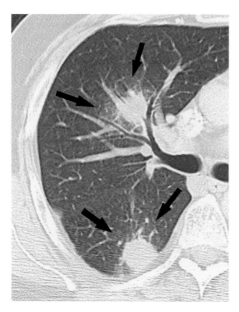

Fig. 18. Forty-one-year-old man following two cycles of chemotherapy for newly diagnosed acute myelogenous leukemia presents with neutropenic fever with no respiratory symptoms. Contrast-enhanced chest CT shows 2.5-cm solid pulmonary nodules surrounded by GGO: the halo sign. Arrows point at the GGO. Shortness of breath developed 3 days following this chest CT.

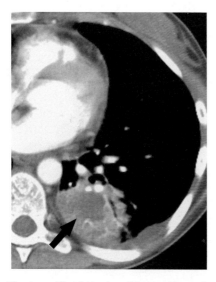

Fig. 19. *Aspergillus flavus* in a 26-year-old woman undergoing chemotherapy for relapsed acute lymphocytic leukemia following BMT with profound neutropenia and fever. Contrast-enhanced chest CT demonstrates a central region of lower attenuation (*arrow*) surrounded by an enhancing mass: the hypodense sign.

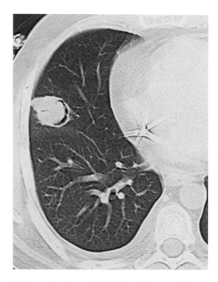

Fig. 20. Invasive aspergillosis in a 22-year-old man with acute myelogenous leukemia who presented with neutropenic fever 2 days following BMT. Chest CT 2 weeks after presentation and treatment initiation shows an eccentric cavitation in a right middle lobe nodule: the crescent sign.

than aspergillosis, but because both can be seen with other fungal infections, diagnosis of the exact fungal etiology requires diagnosis by culture or histology and cannot solely rely on CT appearances [50].

Candida pneumonia can be seen in severely immunocompromised patients but is a difficult diagnosis to establish because it is a common colonizer in this patient population, and is difficult to distinguish from the more common aspergillosis because most patients present with pulmonary nodules. These nodules are usually multiple, bilateral, with a lower lobe predominance, and range from 3 to 30 mm. Nodules as the sole CT finding are seen in less than a fifth of the patients, however, and are usually associated with other findings, such as GGO or consolidation. Consolidation is seen in two thirds of the patients and in half is the predominant finding. The consolidation is randomly distributed throughout both lungs in a segmental or subsegmental distribution [51]. The consolidation and GGO are caused by alveolar necrosis, proteinaceous exudate, and areas of exudative or proliferative phase of diffuse alveolar damage. The halo sign in candida pneumonia, like that seen in aspergillosis, is caused by localized candida inflammation with surrounding hemorrhage (Fig. 23). In a study comparing the imaging features of pulmonary invasive

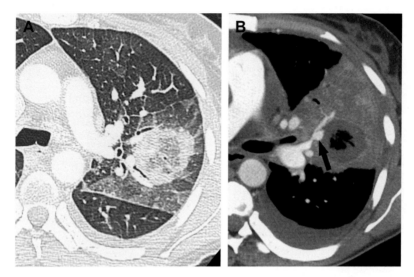

Fig. 21. Forty-nine-year-old woman with neutropenic fever following induction chemotherapy for acute myelogenous leukemia. (*A*) CT at the onset of shortness of breath shows a ring of soft tissue surrounding GGO within it: the reversed halo sign. Patient was treated for presumed Aspergillosis. (*B*) CT obtained 6 weeks following Fig. 21A shows interval development of a pseudoaneurysm (*arrow*) adjacent to some infarcted lung, which is embedded in left upper lobe consolidation. At lobectomy, the entire left upper lobe was infiltrated with mucormycosis.

aspergillosis with candidiasis, random nodules were more commonly seen with candidiasis, whereas centrilobular nodules were more common in aspergillosis but the prevalence of the halo sign, cavitation, and GGO was similar in both groups [52]. The most common fungal species in severely immunocompromised patients (aspergillus, mucor, fusarium, and candida) cannot reliably be distinguished by CT. Nonetheless, early CT imaging in those with suspected pulmonary fungal infection may be useful in management because of early detection of radiographically occult

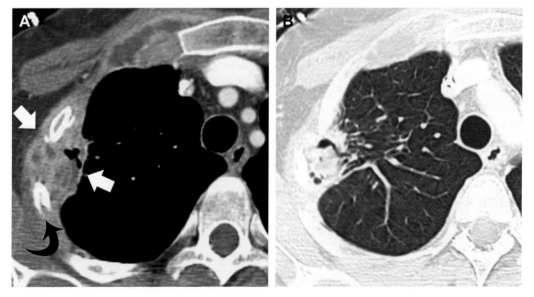

Fig. 22. Twenty-four-year-old woman after BMT with disseminated mucormycosis. (*A*) Contrast-enhanced chest CT shows invasion of a left upper lobe mass into the chest wall (*white arrows*) associated with rib destruction (*black arrow*). (*B*) Same patient demonstrates the crescent sign.

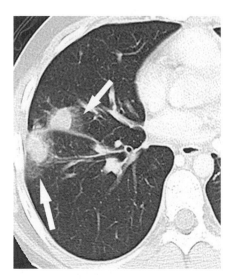

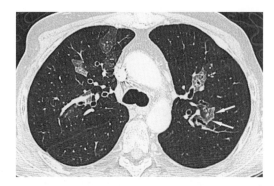

Fig. 24. *Pneumocystis jiroveci* pneumonia in a 53-year-old man after BMT for acute myelogenous leukemia. Contrast-enhanced chest CT shows central scattered GGO interspersed with normal lung parenchyma with interlobular septal thickening (*arrows*).

Fig. 23. Candida pneumonia in a neutropenic 11-year-old boy with metastatic osteosarcoma. Contrast-enhanced chest CT shows solid nodules with surrounding GGO (*arrows*): the halo sign.

pulmonary nodules, potentially allowing CT-guided bronchoscopic sampling, and early empiric antifungal treatment.

Pneumocystis jiroveci pneumonia ([PJP] previously known as *Pneumocystis carinii*), classified as a fungus, is rare in non-AIDS immunocompromised patients, compared with AIDS patients in which it is the most common opportunistic infection [53]. Abnormal chest radiographs usually with diffuse heterogenous pulmonary opacities with perihilar predominance were initially reported in 90% of patients with pneumocystis pneumonia [34]. The routine use of trimethoprim-sulfamethoxazole has decreased the incidence of this infection and increased the incidence of normal chest radiographs at presentation. The typical CT features include perihilar and scattered GGO interspersed with normal lung parenchyma, often with interlobular septal thickening (Fig. 24) [34]. These CT features differ from the typical CT features of other fungal infections but are similar to those seen with cytomegalovirus (CMV) pneumonia. Unfortunately, both CMV and pneumocystis pneumonia tend to occur at the same time after BMT, in the early phase, postengraftment period, and distinguishing between them radiographically is difficult. There are some CT features that are more commonly found in pneumocystis pneumonia compared with CMV: these include upper lobe predominance and a mosaic pattern with sharp demarcation, but distinction between the two is not done radiographically. When a severely immunocompromised patient with fever presents with these described CT features, however, treatment should first target CMV pneumonia because it is much more common than pneumocystis pneumonia in this patient population.

Viral infections

Viral pneumonias occur in up to 50% of immunocompromised non-AIDS patients and are a cause of serious respiratory illness in BMT and solid organ transplant patients. Of these infections, CMV is the most common, occurring in up to 55% of lung transplant recipients, and up to 35% of allogeneic BMT recipients [54]. CMV pneumonia on CT is bilateral and most patients have a combination of GGO or consolidation and pulmonary nodules. GGO or consolidation is seen in 90% of patients, whereas the nodules are seen in 59% (Fig. 25) [55]. Unlike fungal infections, in CMV pneumonia the nodules are all smaller than 1 cm. CT appearance of pure GGO can be seen in 3% to 30% of patients, but pure nodules are only seen in 9% of patients. CMV pneumonia cannot be distinguished radiographically from other respiratory viruses that also manifest with GGO, consolidation, and small nodules. Of these non-CMV pneumonias, respiratory syncytial virus is most common but other community acquired ones are also seen, such influenza A and B, parainfluenza, and adenovirus. Viral pneumonias occur at a similar time that pneumocystis pneumonia can be seen, yet tend to have a lower lobe predominance and pulmonary nodules [53].

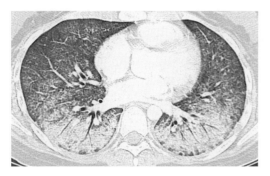

Fig. 25. Cytomegalovirus pneumonia in a 19-year-old woman receiving chemotherapy for relapsed acute lymphocytic leukemia. Contrast-enhanced chest CT shows diffuse air space disease, with both consolidation and GGO, with a lower lobe predominance.

Bacterial infections

Bacterial pneumonia can be nosocomial or community acquired. Outcome and radiographic appearance differ between the two. Nosocomial pneumonias in the solid organ transplant recipient are seen in the perioperative period, within the first month of transplantation. Gram-negative pathogens predominate but *Staphylococcus aureus* and even *Legionella* species are encountered [54]. In the BMT recipient, bacterial pneumonias are particularly prevalent during the pre-engraftment period of profound neutropenia, and most occur within 100 days of transplantation. In patients undergoing chemotherapy, bacterial pneumonia is seen when neutrophil counts are below 500 per milliliter, usually 1 week after chemotherapy. These pneumonias do not differ significantly from other nosocomial pneumonias and are of the bronchopneumonia type, ranging from focal peribronchial consolidation of one or more segments in a single lobe to involvement of multiple lobes. Some bacterial pathogens, such as legionella pneumonia, can involve an entire lobe. Others, pseudomonas or *S aureus*, can present with nodular or mass-like lesions. A normal chest radiograph is particularly common in the early phase of disease and in those patients with severe neutropenia. CT scanning may be useful in these cases. A special form of bacterial pulmonary infection, pyogenic airways disease, is now readily recognized by CT. It is usually caused by Streptococcus pneumonia and staphylococcus and more commonly seen in the BMT recipients. It results from bronchogenic dissemination of pyogenic bacteria and on CT can be seen as dilation and thickening of the bronchial walls, tree-in-bud

opacities, and some adjacent GGO or consolidation (Fig. 26). Interpretation should be cautious because mycobacterial infections commonly present with such airway manifestations and tree-in-bud opacities and even fungal pneumonias can show airway spread; the state of immunity should be kept in mind when interpreting these findings.

Mycobacterial infections

In developed countries *Mycobacterium tuberculosis* is uncommon after solid organ or bone marrow transplantation, although the risk in transplant recipients is 30 to 50 times higher than in the general population. Infection tends to occur late and is associated with chronic rejection or chronic graft-versus-host disease and is usually caused by reactivation of infection of the recipient or from the donor organ [54].

NTMB infections are more common than tuberculosis, usually from *Mycobacterium avium* complex infection. Diagnosis of pulmonary NTMB infection is often difficult because isolation of the organism from sputum or bronchoalveolar lavage fluid may represent airway colonization rather than infection and diagnosis is also based on the clinical presentation and the typical radiologic findings, which differ according to the immune status of the host. NTMB infection is uncommon in the severely immune compromised,

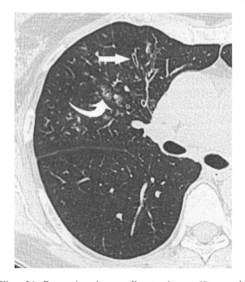

Fig. 26. Pyogenic airway disease in a 68-year-old woman with chronic lymphocytic pneumonia, fever, cough, and a normal chest radiograph. Non–contrast-enhanced chest CT shows bronchial wall thickening (*straight arrow*) and peribronchial GGO (*curved arrow*).

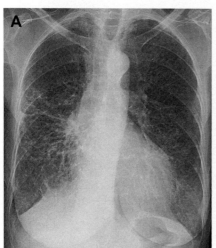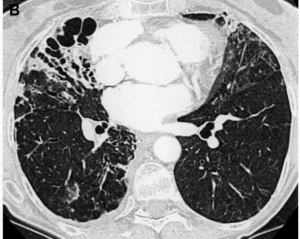

such as patients with lymphoproliferative disorders, transplant recipients, or those undergoing significant immunosuppressive therapy. When present it is usually disseminated and can be recovered from the blood, and is rarely isolated to the lung. When present, radiographic manifestations include mediastinal and hilar adenopathy, focal airspace disease, nodules, cavities, and diffuse interstitial opacities. The classic form of NTMB infection is seen in mildly immunosuppressed individuals, usually elderly white men with underlying lung disease, such as chronic obstructive lung disease or pulmonary fibrosis [56]. Chest radiographic findings are indistinguishable from reactivation tuberculosis and include apical opacities, biapical pleural thickening, and cavitation. CT findings demonstrate complex foci of high attenuation in the apices, cavities, and bronchiectasis in regions of most severe lung disease. Pleural thickening and small nodules (0.5–2 cm) are also common and can be found even in regions distant to the dominant focus of infection [56]. In elderly white women NTMB infection most often occurs in a bronchiectatic form. Chest radiographs show nodularity and linear opacities mainly in the middle lobe and lingula (Fig. 27). CT helps confirm that there is bronchiectasis in the middle lobe and lingula, associated with small peribronchial nodules, mucous plugging, and tree-in-bud opacities. Volume loss in these lobes and some pleural thickening adjacent to them and occasionally some mediastinal adenopathy may also be seen.

Patients with AIDS

Detection of infections in AIDS

The chest radiograph remains an important tool in assessing HIV-infected patients with respiratory symptoms, particularly if bacterial pneumonia is clinically suspected. When bacterial pneumonia is present the chest radiograph is commonly abnormal when the patient presents with acute onset of fever and productive cough [57–59]. Bacterial pneumonia is rarely the cause of an abnormal chest radiograph in the absence of symptoms [60].

In patients with AIDS, CT is superior to chest radiography in its sensitivity for parenchymal and airway abnormalities, its diagnostic accuracy, and its ability to evaluate thoracic complications [61,62]. CT imaging is especially useful in patients with respiratory symptoms with normal or nonspecific chest radiographs. Those patients suspected of having bacterial airway infections (see later), PJP, or tuberculosis may benefit most from CT [63]. Since the introduction of PJP prophylaxis, and highly active antiretroviral therapy (HAART), there has been a shift toward more subtle radiographic presentations of PJP [64,65]. The chest radiograph may be normal or near normal at initial presentation in 2% to 39% of patients with PJP [64,66,67]. Overall, high-resolution CT is more sensitive than chest radiography for detecting PJP, its accuracy in diagnosis ranging between 87% and 94% [61,62,68]. Among AIDS patients with

Fig. 27. *Mycobacterium avium* complex infection in an 80-year-old asymptomatic woman. (*A*) Frontal chest radiograph shows linear opacities mainly in the middle lobe and lingula. (*B*) CT shows that these linear opacities correspond to bronchiectasis in the middle lobe and lingula.

advanced immunosuppression and pulmonary tuberculosis, 10% to 20% also have a normal chest
radiograph [19,69,70]. In these cases CT frequently
demonstrates small nodules and mediastinal
lymphadenopathy [70].

Radiologic patterns

In patients with AIDS, focal or multifocal
consolidation in a segmental or lobar distribution
is often caused by bacterial pneumonias [57].
A combination of focal consolidation and history
of fever less than 1 week has a specificity of 94%
for bacterial pneumonia. Sensitivity is much less,
because about 50% of bacterial pneumonias are
associated with a radiographic pattern other
than focal consolidation [58,71,72]. For instance,
20% of bacterial pneumonias cause diffuse bilateral alveolar and interstitial infiltrates that mimic
PJP [67,73].

Nodules are a common finding on chest CT
performed in HIV-infected patients. Although
Hartman and colleagues [61] identified Kaposi's
sarcoma as the most common etiology for nodules
discovered on CT, other studies favor infectious
causes [74]. In one series of HIV-infected patients
undergoing chest CT, 36% had one or more pulmonary nodules. Bacterial pneumonia was the
most common etiology followed by tuberculosis
[75]. The same authors used the nodule size and
distribution on CT images to discriminate between infection and neoplastic etiologies. Nodules

measuring less than 1 cm and predominantly in
a centrilobular distribution are most likely caused
by infection [76].

Eighty-five percent of cavitary lung disease
seen on chest CT in patients with AIDS is caused
by bacterial infection [77]. *P aeruginosa* and *S aureus* are frequently among the causative pathogens, and mycobacterial coinfection is also
common [66,77,78]. Two opportunistic bacterial
pathogens, *Rhodococcus equi* and *Nocardia*, also
cause cavitating pneumonia in HIV-infected patients with advanced immune suppression
(Fig. 28). Both are acid fast and may cause pleural
effusions in addition to cavities. In HIV-infected
patients these organisms should be included with
mycobacterium in the differential diagnosis of
acid-fast pathogens that cause upper lobe–predominant cavitary disease and associated pleural
effusion.

CT evaluation of infection in patients with
AIDS occasionally reveals marked contrast enhancement and rapid contrast washout of lymph
node and soft tissue lesions. The broad differential
of such hypervascular lesions includes Kaposi's
sarcoma, Castleman's disease, and hypervascular
primary and metastatic neoplasms. In patients
with AIDS, bacillary angiomatosis, a systemic
infection by *Bartonella henselae* or *Bartonella
quintana*, can also cause markedly enhancing
lymph nodes [79]. This diagnosis should be considered in a nonhomosexual patient with findings

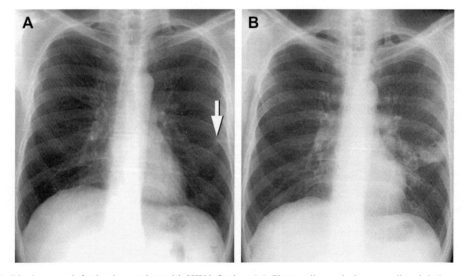

Fig. 28. Rhodococcus infection in a patient with HIV infection. (*A*) Chest radiograph shows small nodule (*arrow*) in the
left mid-lung. (*B*) Chest radiograph performed 6 weeks later demonstrates interval growth of the nodule, now beginning
to show signs of cavitation along its superior margin.

suggesting Kaposi's sarcoma. Biopsy may be required because bacillary angiomatosis is treatable, but when left untreated can be fatal.

Bacterial infection

Bacterial infections, including pyogenic airway disease and bacterial pneumonia, are the most common pulmonary infections diagnosed in HIV-infected individuals [57]. The risk of bacterial infection in HIV-infected individuals is affected by environmental exposures and CD4 lymphocyte counts. Risk is higher in patients with prior episode of PJP or a history of inhaled or intravenous drug abuse [71,80,81].

Mildly immunocompromised patients with CD4 counts lower than 500 cell/mm^3 are at an increased risk for developing bacterial pneumonia and the risk continues to increase as the CD4 count falls further. Prophylactic use of trimethoprim-sulfamethoxazole (Bactrim) for PJP (see later) provides some protection against bacterial infections. Nevertheless, despite a decline in the overall frequency of bacterial pneumonia in HIV-infected patients there has been an increase in the relative frequency of bacterial pneumonia compared with other infections in the chest [82,83].

Acute bronchitis is the most frequent infectious complication of AIDS in the lower respiratory tract, independent of the patient's immune status [71,73,82]. Airway diseases in AIDS patients are caused by bacterial agents, such as *Haemophilus influenzae, P aeruginosa, Streptococcus viridans,* and *S pneumoniae.* Abnormalities are typically absent or subtle on chest radiographs, but bronchial wall thickening and an interstitial or reticulonodular pattern may be detectable (Fig. 29) [71,82]. CT findings include bronchial dilatation and wall thickening and features of infectious bronchiolitis including tree-in-bud appearance of centrilobular nodular and branching opacities.

Bacterial pneumonia in HIV-infected patients differs from bacterial pneumonia in immunocompetent patients in four ways: (1) higher frequency of bacteremia, (2) unusual radiographic findings, (3) higher rate of pleural effusions, and (4) pneumonia caused by opportunistic bacteria [76]. Bacterial pneumonias in AIDS patients also tend to progress more rapidly and are more commonly complicated by cavities, abscess formation, and empyema [66].

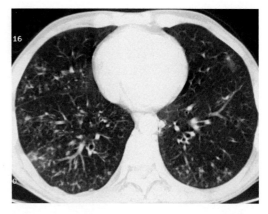

Fig. 29. Bacterial tracheobronchitis in an HIV-infected patient. CT shows centrilobular nodules; tree-in-bud opacities; and mild bronchiectasis, particularly in the left lower lobe.

Streptococcus pneumoniae and *H influenzae* are the most common etiologies for bacterial pneumonia in HIV-infected individuals [71,78,84]. *H influenzae* infection occurs less frequently overall, but is observed more commonly in patients with CD4 counts less than 100 cells/mm^3 [74]. Similar to HIV-seronegative patients, *S aureus* and *P aeruginosa* are the most frequent nosocomial pneumonias (Fig. 30) [60]. HIV-infected patients with severe immune suppression are susceptible to opportunistic bacterial infections (Table 2) [76,84].

Pneumocystis jiroveci pneumonia

PJP is a unicellular organism that behaves like a protozoan but is classified as a fungus [68,72]. PJP initially accounted for 65% of index diagnosis cases in AIDS, but has fallen to approximately 40% with the prophylactic use of trimethoprim-sulfamethoxazole and HAART [84]. Despite its decline in frequency, PJP remains the most common cause of life-threatening infection in AIDS patients [64,68]. Although PJP can occur at any level of immunosuppression, it typically occurs at CD4 counts below 200 cells/mm^3 [57,63,74].

The classic chest radiograph pattern in PJP is a bilateral perihilar or diffuse symmetric interstitial opacity, which may have a granular, reticular, or ground-glass texture (Fig. 31) [64,65]. Patients with a typical clinical presentation and these imaging findings are often empirically treated for PJP. If left untreated, the interstitial pattern can progress to parenchymal consolidation and ARDS. The typical high-resolution CT appearance of PJP consists of bilateral GGO that may

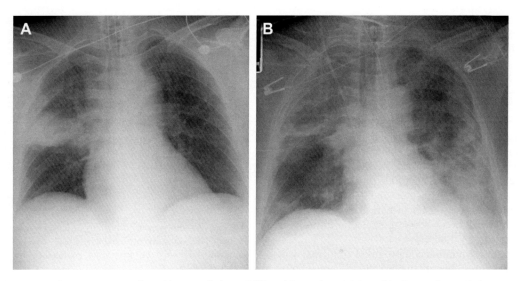

Fig. 30. Pseudomonas pneumonia and bacteremia in an HIV-positive patient. (*A*) Portable chest radiograph shows cavitating pneumonia in the right upper lobe with slight downward bowing of minor fissure. (*B*) Chest radiograph taken 4 days later shows development of extensive bilateral disease.

be geographic or patchy with a central perihilar predominance, sometimes interleaved by smooth interlobular septal thickening [61,65].

Cystic lung disease is now recognized as a common manifestation of PJP with a prevalence of 10% to 34% [59,64]. Cysts associated with PJP tend to be multiple and bilateral, of variable size and wall thickness, and are commonly associated with various amounts of GGO on CT. They can develop in any portion of the lung but have a predilection for the upper lobes and a subpleural location, the latter accounting for an increased incidence of pneumothoraces. A spontaneous pneumothorax in an AIDS patient is likely secondary to a ruptured subpleural cyst and virtually diagnostic of PJP (Fig. 32). Up to 35% of patients with cystic PJP develop a pneumothorax as opposed to 7% of patients with noncystic PJP [85].

Cysts may decrease in size or resolve after an acute episode of PJP, but CT scans frequently show residual cysts and fibrosis [86]. Some patients with PCP develop an atypical clinical presentation referred to as "chronic PJP," in which radiologic findings mirror a chronic inflammatory response associated with granulomatous inflammation and fibrosis. CT imaging demonstrates septal thickening, reticular opacities, architectural distortion, honeycombing, and traction bronchiectasis [65,87]. This combination of fibrosis and cysts may show predilection for the upper lobes, in which case it can be difficult to distinguish

PJP from tuberculosis. In the past, upper lobe predominance of radiologic abnormalities in PJP disease was attributed to the deposition of aerosolized pentamidine, but predominant upper lobe disease is now recognized in patients with PJP that have never used pentamidine.

Uncommon manifestations of PJP include pulmonary nodules, lobar consolidation, airway abnormalities, lymphadenopathy, and pleural effusions [59,64,65]. These findings are more commonly associated with other pathogens or neoplasm.

Mycobacterial infections

HIV-infected patients are at an increased risk of developing *M tuberculosis*, particularly those

Table 2
Bacterial pneumonia in patients infected by HIV

Radiologic finding	Immune suppression	Organism
Pneumonia	Mild > severe	Pneumococcus
Pneumonia	Severe > mild	*Haemophilus influenza*
Cavitary pneumonia	Mild to severe	Pseudomonas, Staphylococcus aureus
Cavitary pneumonia and effusion	Severe	Rhodococcus, Nocardia
Enhancing adenopathy	Severe	*Bartonella henselae, Bartonella quintana*

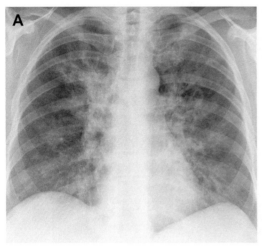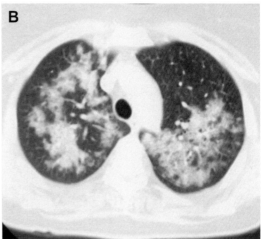

Fig. 31. *Pneumocystic jiroveci* pneumonia in a patient with HIV infection. (*A*) Chest radiograph demonstrates perihilar opacities that are most extensive in the upper lobes. (*B*) CT image from the same patient shows bilateral perihilar consolidation and GGO.

using intravenous drugs or living in regions where tuberculosis is endemic. *M tuberculosis* infection occurs in HIV-infected patients at all levels of immunosuppression, but the risk increases with decreasing CD4 counts as does the likelihood of progression to miliary or disseminated disease [22,32]. The risk of developing *M tuberculosis* is decreased by 70% to 90% by HAART therapy [88,89].

The radiographic appearance of pulmonary tuberculosis in HIV-infected patients is influenced

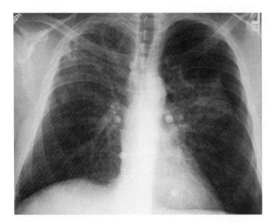

Fig. 32. Cystic *Pneumocystis carinii* pneumonia. Chest radiograph shows numerous thin-walled cysts, most evident in the upper lobes. Left-sided pneumothorax was a result of cyst rupture.

by the degree of immunosuppression [69,90,91]. In patients with CD4 counts greater than 200 cell/mm^3, the radiographic findings are similar to reactivation tuberculosis in immunocompetent patients. These include predominately upper lobe patchy consolidation, cavitation, nodular opacities, and evidence of bronchogenic spread. Involvement of the mid and lower lungs occurs more commonly in AIDS patients, possibly because of greater extent of bronchogenic spread [90]. High-resolution CT findings of endobronchial spread include bronchial wall thickening and bronchiolar disease (eg, centrilobular nodules).

In more severely immunocompromised patients (CD4 counts <200 cells/mm^3), the radiographic findings of tuberculosis resemble those typical of primary tuberculosis regardless of the mode (primary or reactivation) of infection. Radiographs show consolidation and lymphadenopathy, either alone or in combination (Fig. 33). A total of 60% to 75% of HIV-infected patients with pulmonary tuberculosis demonstrate enlarged lymph nodes on CT imaging, some of which demonstrate low-attenuation centers and peripheral rim enhancement following intravenous contrast [91]. This appearance, caused by necrotic lymphadenopathy, can also be seen in atypical mycobacterial and fungal infections (Fig. 34) [61]. Pleural effusions, when present, are often loculated and tend to be large [90]. With advanced HIV infection, the likelihood of

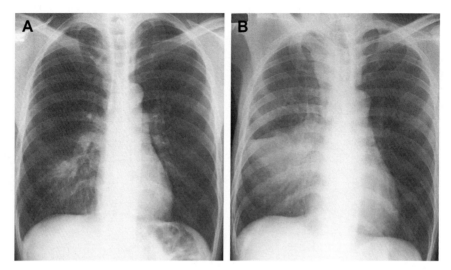

Fig. 33. Tuberculosis in an HIV-positive patient, primary tuberculosis pattern. (*A*) Frontal radiograph shows right hilar adenopathy and a right middle lobe parenchymal opacity. (*B*) Frontal radiograph taken 1 month after Fig. 33A, showing progressive right middle lobe consolidation. Effusions are commonly present in this pattern but are not seen on this radiograph.

disseminated tuberculosis increases. Seventy percent of patients with CD4 count less than 100 cells/mm^3 demonstrate extrathoracic disease and approximately one half of HIV-infected patients with extrathoracic involvement have a miliary pattern in the lungs [92].

NTMB is common among HIV-infected patients and is frequently disseminated at time of diagnosis. With improved survival among AIDS patients treated with HAART and PJP prophylaxis, NTMB disease is increasing in prevalence and for many patients disseminated NTMB is their first opportunistic infection [93]. A total of 96% of disseminated NTMB infections are caused by *Mycobacterium avium-intracellulare* complex. More than 95% occurring in patients with disseminated *M avium-intracellulare* have CD4 counts less than or equal to 50 cells/mm^3 [93]. The chest

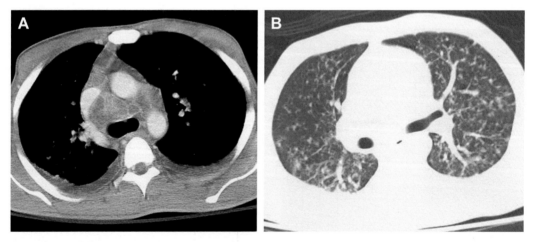

Fig. 34. Disseminated tuberculosis in an HIV-positive patient. (*A*) Contrast-enhanced CT image (mediastinal window settings) shows numerous enlarged low-attenuation mediastinal lymph nodes with peripheral enhancement. Similarly enlarged lymph nodes (not shown) were present in the abdomen. (*B*) CT section from the same patient (lung window settings) shows diffuse parenchymal nodules.

radiograph is frequently normal with disseminated *M avium-intracellulare* and localized pulmonary disease is less common than seen with disseminated *M tuberculosis*. When present, CT findings include multifocal patchy consolidation; ill-defined nodules, which may or may not cavitate; adenopathy; and findings of infectious bronchiolitis (Fig. 35) [63,66].

Patients being treated for tuberculosis or other infections who also receive HAART may develop transient worsening of clinical and radiographic findings as their cell-mediated immunity is partially restored [94]. This heightened inflammatory response has been referred to as "immune reconstitution inflammatory syndrome." This syndrome usually presents as a manifestation of an underlying mycobacterial (*M avium-intracellulare* or *M tuberculosis*) or viral infection but can manifest as sarcoid or other autoimmune disease [95,96]. Immune reconstitution inflammatory syndrome manifestations of *M tuberculosis* start within the first 2 months after initiating HAART, usually within 2 to 3 weeks. Patients may develop new or worsening lymphadenopathy, pulmonary infiltrates, and pleural effusions (Fig. 36). Although the radiologic findings are nonspecific, the temporal relationship to starting HAART is characteristic. To make this diagnosis, one must exclude new opportunistic infection, drug toxicity, noncompliance with antituberculous therapy, and multidrug-resistant tuberculosis [35,41].

Fungal infections

Cryptococcus neoformans, Histoplasma capsulatum, and *Coccidioides immitis* are three fungi that exploit the cell-mediated defects that are predominant in AIDS. These endemic mycoses cannot be killed effectively by nonimmune phagocytosis and require an effective cell-mediated immunity to prevent infection in a host [97]. In contrast, *Aspergillus* and *Mucor* species, which are killed by phagocytes, are less pathogenic in patients with AIDS. Overall, fungal infections are an uncommon cause of pulmonary infections in AIDS patients and when they do occur the patient is usually severely immunocompromised (CD4 counts < 100 cells/mm^3).

The most common cause of intrathoracic fungal infection complicating AIDS is *C neoformans*. The infection most commonly occurs in patients with CD4 counts below 200 cells/mm^3 and is usually systemic at time of presentation [98]. Chest imaging findings include reticular opacities; consolidation; single or multiple nodules (including miliary nodules); lymphadenopathy; and pleural effusions (Fig. 37) [57,98,99]. A shift from discrete nodules to more extensive pulmonary infiltration occurs with increasing immunosuppression.

The prevalence of histoplasmosis may exceed cryptococcosis in endemic regions, and this disease also frequently becomes disseminated in HIV-infected patients. At presentation a normal chest radiograph is seen in up to 50% of patients with disseminated disease but progresses to diffuse opacities concurrent with development of respiratory symptoms. High-resolution CT findings may include miliary nodules associated with disseminated disease, lymphadenopathy, and less commonly diffuse parenchymal consolidation. HIV-infected patients with coccidioidomycosis

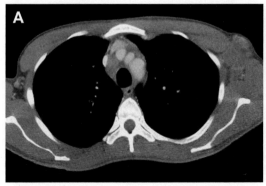 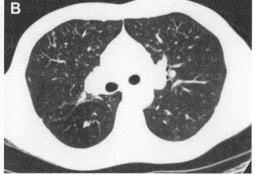

Fig. 35. Disseminated *Mycobacterium avium-intracellulare* in an HIV-positive patient. (*A*) CT section (mediastinal window settings) shows numerous enlarged low-attenuation lymph nodes in the left axilla and a single enlarged lymph node in the right paratracheal area. (*B*) CT section in lung windows shows scattered bilateral centrilobular nodules.

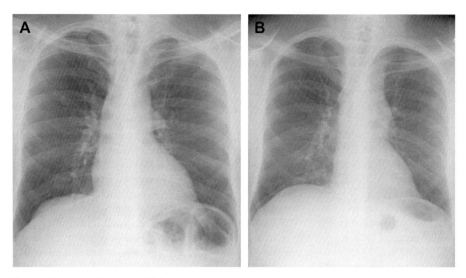

Fig. 36. Chest radiographs of patient with immune reconstitution syndrome. (*A*) Chest radiograph before the initiation of antiretroviral medications is normal. (*B*) Radiograph 2 months later shows widening of the mediastinal contours, particularly the left upper mediastinum, consistent with the development of mediastinal adenopathy.

usually present with a respiratory infection, a third of whom have meningitis. A normal chest radiograph is much less common than with histoplasmosis, but otherwise radiologic findings are similar [98,99].

Aspergillosis is uncommon in HIV-infected patients and most frequently occurs in advanced immunosuppression with CD4 counts frequently less than 50 cells/mm³. Most HIV-infected individuals who develop aspergillosis are also neutropenic secondary to advanced HIV infection,

antiretroviral therapy, or PJP prophylaxis, or have received corticosteroids [100]. The most common radiographic finding is thick-walled cavitary lesions (Fig. 38). Less common findings include single or multiple nodules, focal or diffuse consolidation, and pleural effusions [100,101]. The nodules may have a ground-glass halo surrounding them on high-resolution CT caused by local angioinvasion. Airway involvement by aspergillus occurs in HIV-infected patients with and without tissue invasion, the latter characterized by CT

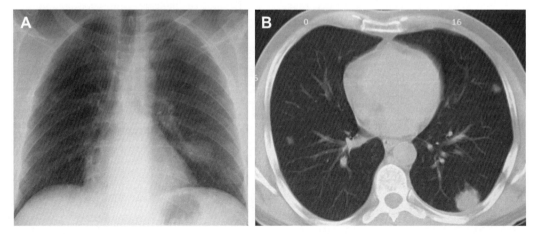

Fig. 37. HIV-positive patient with cryptococcus infection. (*A*) Chest radiograph shows mass in left lower lobe. (*B*) CT section reveals well-defined mass and other smaller nodules. Presence of discrete nodules is more common in HIV patients with lesser degrees of immunocompromise.

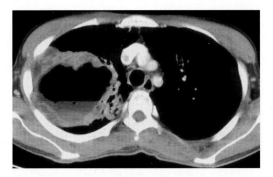

Fig. 38. CT of HIV-infected patient with invasive aspergillosis. CT section demonstrates thick-walled cavity occupying much of the right upper lobe.

findings ranging from subtle wall thickening and nodularity to airway obstruction with or without peribronchial opacities [63].

Viral infections

CMV is the most common viral pathogen of the lung in HIV-infected patients. CMV is frequently found incidentally in bronchoalveolar lavage fluid in AIDS patients with no associated pulmonary complications [102]. Although uncommon in AIDS patients, an increased occurrence of CMV pneumonia has been associated with use of systemic corticosteroids and prophylactic trimethoprim-sulfamethoxazole. Most patients with CMV pneumonia have disseminated disease and CD4 counts less than 100 cells/mm³. CT findings of CMV pneumonia include GGO, nodules, and alveolar consolidation [103]. Isolated airway disease can be caused by CMV, manifest as necrotizing tracheitis and bronchiolitis, the latter radiologically indistinguishable from other causes of infectious bronchiolitis.

Summary

Although basic chest radiography remains important in the assessment of infection, the use of CT continues to widen. Among hosts without immunocompromise, CT is most useful in assessing complications of infection, particularly pleural disease and the sequelae of lung necrosis. In non–immune-suppressed patients with micronodular opacities on chest radiograph, CT can also differentiate between airway-centered infection, such as mycoplasma, and blood-borne disseminated disease, such as miliary tuberculosis. Occasionally, CT demonstrates that parenchymal

opacities are caused by unsuspected noninfectious disease, such as pulmonary infarction.

CT should be used early in immune compromised patients to identify characteristic imaging findings early for improved prognosis; however, it should be interpreted with caution because imaging features of different pathogens overlap. General guidelines in severely immunocompromised patients are that the presence of large nodules and visualization of the halo sign are most suggestive of fungal infection [39]. Interpretation is improved when knowledge of the statistical likelihood of different pathogens after transplantation or last chemotherapy is taken into account. Diagnostic accuracy also depends on consideration of noninfectious posttransplantation complications (eg, bronchiolitis obliterans and cryptogenic organizing pneumonia).

The chest radiograph remains an important tool in assessing patients with AIDS and respiratory symptoms. CT has been shown to be especially useful, however, in patients with respiratory symptoms with normal or subtly abnormal chest radiograph. This is particularly true in the era of prophylactic trimethoprim-sulfamethoxazole and HAART, which has shifted the relative frequency of opportunistic infections in the HIV-infected patient population and made bacterial airway disease and atypical PJP infections more common. The patient's immune status (as referenced to CD4 lymphocyte count) remains the primary determinant of relative risk for specific thoracic infections and the radiographic appearance of pulmonary tuberculosis. Combined knowledge of the AIDS patient's presenting symptoms, immune status, and the imaging findings often shortens the differential diagnosis and yields a diagnosis with a higher level of confidence.

References

[1] Boersma WG, Daniels JM, Lowenbery A, et al. Reliability of radiographic findings and the relation to etiologic agents in community acquired pneumonia. Respir Med 2006;100(5):916–32.

[2] Heussel CP, Kauczor HU, Heussel G, et al. Early detection or pneumonia in febrile neutropenic patients: using thin section CT. Am J Roentgenol 1997;169(5):1347–53.

[3] Winer-Muram HT, Steiner RM, Gurney JW, et al. Ventilator-associated pneumonia in patients with adult respiratory distress syndrome: CT evaluation. Radiology 1998;208(1):193–9.

[4] Basi SK, Marrie TJ, Huang JQ, et al. Patients admitted to the hospital with suspected pneumonia

and normal chest radiographs: epidemiologic, microbiology and outcomes. Am J Med 2004;117(5):305–11.

[5] Hopstaken RM, Witbraad T, van Engelshoven JM, et al. Inter-observer variation in the interpretation of chest radiographs for pneumonia in community acquired lower respiratory tract infections. Clin Radiol 2004;59(8):743–52.

[6] Albaum MN, Hill LC, Murphy M, et al. Interobserver reliability of the chest radiograph inn community acquired pneumonia. Chest 1996;110(2):343–50.

[7] Winer-Muram HT, Rubin SA, Ellis JV, et al. Pneumonia and ARDS in patients receiving mechanical ventilation: diagnostic accuracy of chest radiography. Radiology 1993;188(2):479–85.

[8] Gattinoni L, Caironi P, Valenza F, et al. The role of CT-scan studies for the diagnosis and therapy of acute respiratory distress syndrome. Clin Chest Med 2006;27(4):559–70.

[9] Desai SR, Wells AU, Suntharalingam G, et al. Acute respiratory distress syndrome caused by pulmonary and extrapulmonary injury: a comparative CT study. Radiology 2001;218(3):689–93.

[10] Kearney SE, Davies CW, Davies RJ, et al. Computed tomography and ultrasound in parapneumonic effusions and empyema. Clin Radiol 2000;55(7):542–7.

[11] Tu CY, Hsu WH, Hsia TC, et al. Pleural effusions in febrile medical ICU patients: chest ultrasound study. Chest 2004;126(4):1274–80.

[12] Arenas-Jimenez J, Alonso-Charterina S, Sanchez-Paya J, et al. Evaluation of CT findings for diagnosis of pleural effusions. Eur Radiol 2000;10(4):681–90.

[13] Smolikov A, Smolyakova R, Riesenberg K, et al. Prevalence and clinical significance of pleural microbubbles in computed tomography of thoracic empyema. Clin Radiol 2006;61:513–9.

[14] Donnelly LF, Klosterman LA. Pneumonia in children: decreased parenchymal contrast enhancement–CT sign of intense illness and impending cavitary necrosis. Radiology 1997;215(3):817–20.

[15] Mody GN, Lau CL, Bhalla S, et al. Mycotic pulmonary artery pseudoaneurysm. J Thorac Imaging 2005;20(4):310–2.

[16] Hunt JP, Buechter KJ, Fakhry SM. Acinetobacter calcoaceticus pneumonia and the formation of pneumatoceles. J Trauma 2000;48(5):964–70.

[17] McGarry T, Giosa R, Rohman M, et al. Pneumatocele formation in adult pneumonia. Chest 1987;92(4):717–20.

[18] Stein DL, Haramati LB, Spindola-Franco H, et al. Intrathoracic lymphadenopathy in hospitalized patients with pneumococcal pneumonia. Chest 2005;127(4):1271–5.

[19] Leung AN. Pulmonary tuberculosis: the essentials. Radiology 1999;210(2):307–32.

[20] Choi YH, Kim SJ, Lee JY, et al. Scrub typhus: radiological and clinical findings. Clin Radiol 2000;55(2):140–4.

[21] Boroja M, Barrie JR, Raymond GS. Radiographic findings in 20 patients with hantavirus pulmonary syndrome correlated with clinical outcome. AJR Am J Roentgenol 2002;178(1):159–63.

[22] Rossi SE, Franquet T, Volpacchio M, et al. Tree in bud pattern at thin-section CT of the lungs: radiologic-pathologic overview. Radiographics 2005;25(3):789–801.

[23] Raoof S, Amchentsev A, Vlahos I, et al. Pictorial essay: multinodular disease. A high resolution CT scan diagnostic algorithm. Chest 2006;129(3):805–15.

[24] Shah RM, Miller W. Widespread ground glass opacity of the lung in consecutive patients undergoing CT: Does lobular distribution assist diagnosis? AJR Am J Roentgenol 2003;180(4):965–8.

[25] Shah RM, Friedman AC. CT angiogram sign: incidence and significance in lobar consolidations evaluated by contrast-enhanced CT. AJR Am J Roentgenol 1998;170(3):719–21.

[26] Revel M-P, Triki R, Chatellier G, et al. Is it possible to recognize pulmonary infarction on multisection CT images? Radiology 2007;244(3):875–82.

[27] Reittner P, Ward S, Heyneman L, et al. Pneumonia: high resolution CT findings in 114 patients. Eur Radiol 2003;13(3):515–21.

[28] Lee I, Kim TS, Yoon HK. *Mycoplasma pneumoniae* pneumonia: CT features in 16 patients. Eur Radiol 2006;16(3):719–25.

[29] Bramson RT, Griscom NT, Cleveland RH. Interpretation of chest radiographs in infants with cough and fever. Radiology 2005;236:22–9.

[30] Im JG, Itoh H, Shim YS, et al. Pulmonary tuberculosis: CT findings: early active disease and sequential change with anti-tuberculous therapy. Radiology 1993;186(3):656–60.

[31] Ors F, Deniz O, Bozlar U, et al. High resolution CT findings in patients with pulmonary tuberculosis: correlation with degree of smear positivity. J Thorac Imaging 2007;22(2):154–9.

[32] Martinez S, McAdams HP, Batchu CS. The many faces of pulmonary nontuberculous mycobacterial infection. AJR Am J Roentgenol 2007;189(1):177–86.

[33] Koh WJ, Lee KS, Kwon OJ, et al. Bilateral bronchiectasis and bronchiolitis at thin section CT: diagnostic implications in nontuberculous mycobacterial pulmonary infection. Radiology 2005;225(1):282–8.

[34] Primack SL, Muller NL. High-resolution computed tomography in acute diffuse lung disease in the immunocompromised patient. Radiol Clin North Am 1994;32(4):731–44.

[35] Caillot D, Casasnovas O, Bernard A, et al. Improved management of invasive pulmonary

aspergillosis in neutropenic patients using early thoracic computed tomographic scan and surgery. J Clin Oncol 1997;15:139–47.

[36] Ascioglu S, Rex JH, de Pauw B, et al. Defining opportunistic invasive fungal infections in immunocompromised patients with cancer and hematopoietic stem cell transplants: an international consensus. Clin Infect Dis 2002;34:7–14.

[37] Reichenberger F, Habicht J, Matt P, et al. Diagnostic yield of bronchoscopy in histologically proven invasive pulmonary aspergillosis. Bone Marrow Transplant 1999;24:1195–9.

[38] Subira M, Martino R, Rovira M, et al. Clinical applicability of the new EORTC/MSG classification for invasive pulmonary aspergillosis in patients with hematological malignancies and autopsy-confirmed invasive aspergillosis. Ann Hematol 2003; 82:80–2.

[39] Escuissato DL, Gasparetto EL, Marchiori E, et al. Pulmonary infections after bone marrow transplantation: high-resolution CT findings in 111 patients. AJR Am J Roentgenol 2005;185:608–15.

[40] Franquet T, Gimenez A, Hidalgo A. Imaging of opportunistic fungal infections in immunocompromised patient. Eur J Radiol 2004;51:130–8.

[41] Connolly JE Jr, McAdams HP, Erasmus JJ, et al. Opportunistic fungal pneumonia. J Thorac Imaging 1999;14:51–62.

[42] Erasmus JJ, McAdams HP, Tapson VF, et al. Radiologic issues in lung transplantation for end-stage pulmonary disease. AJR Am J Roentgenol 1997; 169:69–78.

[43] Kontoyiannis DP, Bodey GP. Invasive aspergillosis in 2002: an update. Eur J Clin Microbiol Infect Dis 2002;21:161–72.

[44] Logan PM, Primack SL, Miller RR, et al. Invasive aspergillosis of the airways: radiographic, CT, and pathologic findings. Radiology 1994;193:383–8.

[45] Greene RE, Schlamm HT, Oestmann JW, et al. Imaging findings in acute invasive pulmonary aspergillosis: clinical significance of the halo sign. Clin Infect Dis 2007;44:373–9.

[46] Primack SL, Hartman TE, Lee KS, et al. Pulmonary nodules and the CT halo sign. Radiology 1994;190:513–5.

[47] Kuhlman JE, Fishman EK, Siegelman SS. Invasive pulmonary aspergillosis in acute leukemia: characteristic findings on CT, the CT halo sign, and the role of CT in early diagnosis. Radiology 1985; 157:611–4.

[48] Lionakis MS, Kontoyiannis DP. Fusarium infections in critically ill patients. Semin Respir Crit Care Med 2004;25:159–69.

[49] McAdams HP, Rosado de Christenson M, Strollo DC, et al. Pulmonary mucormycosis: radiologic findings in 32 cases. AJR Am J Roentgenol 1997; 168:1541–8.

[50] Chamilos G, Marom EM, Lewis RE, et al. Predictors of pulmonary zygomycosis versus invasive

pulmonary aspergillosis in patients with cancer. Clin Infect Dis 2005;41:60–6.

[51] Franquet T, Muller NL, Lee KS, et al. Pulmonary candidiasis after hematopoietic stem cell transplantation: thin-section CT findings. Radiology 2005; 236:332–7.

[52] Althoff Souza C, Muller NL, Marchiori E, et al. Pulmonary invasive aspergillosis and candidiasis in immunocompromised patients: a comparative study of the high-resolution CT findings. J Thorac Imaging 2006;21:184–9.

[53] Vogel MN, Brodoefel H, Hierl T, et al. Differences and similarities of cytomegalovirus and pneumocystis pneumonia in HIV-negative immunocompromised patients: thin-section CT-morphology in the early phase of the disease. Br J Radiol 2007; 80(995):516–23.

[54] Kotloff RM, Ahya VN, Crawford SW. Pulmonary complications of solid organ and hematopoietic stem cell transplantation. Am J Respir Crit Care Med 2004;170:22–48.

[55] Franquet T, Lee KS, Muller NL. Thin-section CT findings in 32 immunocompromised patients with cytomegalovirus pneumonia who do not have AIDS. AJR Am J Roentgenol 2003;181: 1059–63.

[56] Miller WT Jr. Spectrum of pulmonary nontuberculous mycobacterial infection. Radiology 1994;191: 343–50.

[57] Boiselle PM, Aviram G, Fishman JE. Update on lung disease in AIDS. Semin Roentgenol 2002;37: 54–71.

[58] Selwyn PA, Pumerantz AS, Durante A, et al. Clinical predictors of *Pneumocystis carinii* pneumonia, bacterial pneumonia, and tuberculosis in hospitalized patients with HIV infection. AIDS 1998;12: 885–93.

[59] Boiselle PM, Tocino I, Hooley RJ, et al. Chest radiograph diagnosis of *Pnemocystis carinii* pneumonia, bacterial pneumonia and pulmonary tuberculosis in HIV-positive patients: accuracy, distinguishing features, and mimics. J Thorac Imaging 1997;12:47–53.

[60] Gold JA, Rom WA, Harkin TJ. Significance of abnormal chest radiograph findings in patients with HIV-1 infection without respiratory symptoms. Chest 2002;121:395–408.

[61] Hartman TE, Primack SL, Muller NL, et al. Diagnosis of thoracic complications in AIDS: Accuracy of CT. AJR Am J Roentgenol 1994; 162:547–53.

[62] Kang EY, Staples CA, McGuinness G, et al. Detection and differential diagnosis of pulmonary infections and tumors in patients with AIDS: value of chest radiography versus CT. AJR Am J Roentgenol 1996;166:15–9.

[63] McGuiness G, Gruden JF, Bhalla M, et al. AIDS-related airway disease. AJR Am J Roentgenol 1997;168:67–77.

[64] Kuhlman JE. Pneumocystic infections: the radiologist's perspective. Radiology 1996;198:623–35.

[65] Boiselle PM, Crans CA, Kaplan MA. The changing face of *Pneumocystis carinii* pneumonia in AIDs patients. AJR Am J Roentgenol 1999;172:1301–9.

[66] Maki DD. Pulmonary infections in HIV/AIDS. Semin Roentgenology 2000;35:124–39.

[67] Opravil M, Marinecek B, Fuchs W, et al. Shortcomings of chest radiography in detecting *Pneumocystis carinii* pneumonia. J Acquir Immune Defic Syndr 1994;7:39–45.

[68] Gruden JF, Huang L, Turner J, et al. High-resolution CT in the evaluation of clinically suspected *Pneumocystis carinii* pneumonia in AIDS patients with normal, equivocal, or nonspecific radiographic findings. AJR Am J Roentgenol 1997;169:967–75.

[69] Greenberg SD, Frager D, Suster B, et al. Active pulmonary tuberculosis in patients with AIDS; spectrum of radiographic findings (including a normal appearance). Radiology 1994;193:115–9.

[70] Leung AN, Braumer MN, Gamsu G, et al. Pulmonary tuberculosis: comparison of CT findings in HIV-seropositive and HIV-seronegative patients. Radiology 1996;198:687–91.

[71] Hirschtick RE, Glassroth J, Jordan MC, et al. Bacterial pneumonia in persons infected with the human immunodeficiency virus. N Engl J Med 1995; 333:845–51.

[72] Amorosa JK, Nahass RG, Nosher JL, et al. Radiologic distinction of pyogenic pulmonary infection from *Pneumocystis carinii* pneumonia in AIDS patients. Radiology 1990;175:721–4.

[73] Cordero E, Pachon J, Rivero A, et al. *Haemophilus influenzae* pneumonia in human immunodeficiency virus–infected patients. Clin Infect Dis 2000;30: 461–5.

[74] Martinez-Marcos FJ, Viciana P, Canas E, et al. Etiology of solitary pulmonary nodules in patients with human immunodeficiency virus infection. Clin Infect Dis 1997;24:908–13.

[75] Jasmer RM, Edinburgh KJ, Thompson A, et al. Clinical and radiographic predictors of pulmonary nodules in HIV-infected patients. Chest 2000;117: 1023–30.

[76] Edinburgh KJ, Jasmer RM, Huang L. Multiple pulmonary nodules in AIDS: usefulness of CT in distinguishing among potential causes. Radiology 2000;214:427–32.

[77] Aviram G, Fishman JE, Sagar M. Cavitary lung disease in AIDS: etiologies and correlation with immune status. AIDS Patient Care STDS 2001;15: 353–61.

[78] Mayaud C, Parrot A, Cadranel J. Pyogenic bacterial lower respiratory infection in human immunodeficiency virus-infected patients. Eur Respir J 2002;36:28–39.

[79] Moore EH, Russel LA, Klein JS, et al. Bacillary angiomatosis in patients with AIDS; multiorgan imaging findings. Radiology 1995;197:67–72.

[80] Caiaffa WT, Vlahov D, Graham NM, et al. Drug smoking, *Pneumocystis carinii* pneumonia, and immunosuppression increase risk of bacterial pneumonia in human immunodeficiency virus–seropositive injection drug users. Am J Respir Crit Care Med 1994;150:1493–500.

[81] Afessa B, Green G. Bacterial pneumonia in hospitalized patients with HIV infection. Chest 2000; 117:1017–22.

[82] Verghese A, Al-Samman M, Nabhan D, et al. Bacterial bronchitis and bronchiectasis in human immunodeficiency virus infection. Arch Intern Med 1994;154:2086–91.

[83] Wolff AJ, O'Donnell AE. Pulmonary manifestations of HIV infection in the era of highly active antiviral therapy. Chest 2001;120:1888–93.

[84] Brecher CW, Aviram G, Boiselle PM. CT and radiography of bacterial respiratory infections in AIDS patients. AJR Am J Roentgenol 2003;180: 1203–9.

[85] Chow C, Templeton PA, White CS. Lung cysts associated with *Pneumocystis carinii* pneumonia: radiographic characteristics, natural history and complications. AJR Am J Roentgenol 1993;161: 527–31.

[86] Wassermann K, Pothoff G,, Kirn E, et al. Chronic *Pneumocystis carinii* pneumonia in AIDS. Chest 1993;104:667–72.

[87] Jones BE, Young SM, Antoniskis D, et al. Relationship of the manifestations of tuberculosis to CD4 cell counts in patients with human immunodeficiency virus infection. Am Rev Respir Dis 1993; 148:1292–7.

[88] Garardi E, Antonucci G, Vanacore P,, et al. Tuberculosis in HIV-infected persons in the context of wide availability of highly active antiretroviral therapy. Eur Respir J 2004;24:11–7.

[89] Geng E, Kreiswirth B, Burzynski J, et al. Clinical and radiographic correlates to primary and reactivation tuberculosis: a molecular epidemiology study. JAMA 2005;293:2740–5.

[90] Saurborn D, Fishman JE, Boiselle PM. The imaging spectrum of pulmonary tuberculosis in AIDS. J Thorac Imaging 2002;17:28–33.

[91] Laissy JP, Cadi M, Boudiaf ZE, et al. Pulmonary tuberculosis: computed tomography and high-resolution computed tomography patterns in patients who are either HIV-negative or HIV-seropositive. J Thorac Imaging 1998;13:58–64.

[92] Hill AR, Somasundaram P,, Brustein S, et al. Disseminated tuberculosis in the acquired immunodeficiency syndrome. Am Rev Respir Dis 1991;144: 1164–70.

[93] Chin DP, Hopewell PC. Mycobacterial complications of HIV infection. Clin Chest Med 1996;17: 697–711.

[94] Fishman JE, Saraf-Lavi E, Narita M, et al. Pulmonary tuberculosis in AIDS patients: transient chest radiographic worsening after initiation of

antiretroviral therapy. AJR Am J Roentgenol 2000;174:43–9.

[95] French MA, Price P, Stone SF. Immune restoration disease after antiretroviral therapy. AIDS 2004;18: 1615–25.

[96] Wittram C, Fogg J, Farber H. Immune restoration syndrome manifested by pulmonary sarcoidosis. AJR Am J Roentgenol 2001;177:1427.

[97] Schaffner A, Davis CE, Schaffner T, et al. In vitro susceptibility to killing by neurophil granulocytes discriminates between primary pathogenicity and opportunism. J Clin Invest 1986;78:511–24.

[98] Davies SF, Sarosi GA. Fungal pulmonary complications. Clin Chest Med 1996;17:725–44.

[99] Marchiori E, Muller NL, Souza AS, et al. Pulmonary disease in patients with AIDS: high-resolution CT and pathologic findings. AJR Am J Roentgenol 2005;184:757–64.

[100] Mylonakis E, Barlam TF, Flanigan T, et al. Pulmonary aspergillosis and invasive disease in AIDS; review of 342 cases. Chest 1998;114:251–62.

[101] Staples CA, Kang EY, Wright JL, et al. Invasive pulmonary aspergillosis in AIDS: radiographic, CT, and pathologic findings. Radiology 1995;196: 409–14.

[102] Uberti-Foppa C, Lillo F, Terreni MR, et al. Cytomegalovirus pneumonia in AIDS patients: value of cytomegalovirus culture from BAL fluid and correlation with lung disease. Chest 1998;113:919–23.

[103] McGuinness G. Changing trends in the pulmonary manifestations of AIDS. Radiol Clin North Am 1997;35:1029–82.

**ELSEVIER
SAUNDERS**

Clin Chest Med 29 (2008) 107–116

**CLINICS
IN CHEST
MEDICINE**

Imaging of Pulmonary Thromboembolism

Meltem Gulsun Akpinar, MD[a,b,*], Lawrence R. Goodman, MD, FACR[a]

[a]*Department of Radiology, Medical College of Wisconsin, 9200 W. Wisconsin Avenue, Milwaukee, WI 53226-3596, USA*
[b]*Department of Radiology, Hacettepe University, Sihhiye, Ankara, 06100, Turkey*

Pulmonary thromboembolism (PE) is the third most common cardiovascular disease after myocardial infarction and stroke [1]. It is also one of the most controversial disorders, with ongoing debate as to the best approach for diagnosis and the best means of treatment.

PE is not a single entity. Approximately 90% of all pulmonary thromboemboli originate from deep veins of lower extremities [2]. Together, deep venous thrombosis (DVT) and pulmonary embolism constitute venous thromboembolism. The older literature states that when untreated, PE is fatal in 30% of patients. With better imaging able to diagnose smaller pulmonary thromboemboli, it is likely that 10% is a more realistic rate [3].

Fatality rates fall to 2% to 10% with proper diagnosis and treatment with anticoagulants [4–7]. Nevertheless, anticoagulant therapy has serious risks, including hemorrhage. Therefore, false-positive diagnosis must be kept to a minimum. Because clinical symptoms and laboratory findings of PE are nonspecific and seldom provide definitive diagnosis, the diagnosis relies on imaging methods. Chest radiography, ventilation/perfusion (V/Q) scan, venous Doppler ultrasound of the lower extremities, and pulmonary angiography have been used frequently. Chest radiographic findings are nonspecific and V/Q scans are often not definitive. Pulmonary angiography, still considered the "gold standard," is invasive, time consuming, and underutilized.

With the introduction of helical CT in the early 1990s, direct visualization of PE became possible. Advances in CT technology have made CT pulmonary angiography (CTA) the most frequently used

diagnostic method for PE in recent years [8]. MRI also provides direct imaging of PE; however, its value in large patient populations has not been tested and its use in critically ill patients is somewhat limited.

Chest radiography

Chest radiography is the first-line imaging method in the evaluation of PE. The most commonly seen findings of PE on chest radiographs are atelectasis, small pulmonary opacities, and pleural effusion [9,10]. Hampton's hump is a peripheral wedge-shaped, pleural-based parenchymal density representing a pulmonary infarct. This pleural-based parenchymal density may also be seen in other diseases such as pneumonia and septic pulmonary emboli. Westermark's sign refers to reduction in size of occluded pulmonary arteries. It is sometimes difficult to recognize this sign unless the patient has comparison films (Fig. 1A, B). This finding is also nonspecific and may be seen in emphysema or old infections. Another sign is the enlargement of a major arterial trunk at the hilum. None of these three signs is seen frequently.

The chest radiographic signs of PE are all nonspecific [11]. Patients who have PE often have normal chest radiographs. Further investigation with other imaging methods is mandatory. The role of the chest radiograph in evaluation of PE is to rule out other disease processes such as pneumothorax or pneumonia, which can mimic symptoms of PE, and to guide V/Q scanning.

Ventilation/perfusion scanning

PE is recognized as one or several perfusion defects on perfusion scans (Fig. 2). Because there

* Corresponding author.
E-mail address: meltemgulsun@hotmail.com (M. Gulsun Akpinar).

0272-5231/08/$ - see front matter © 2008 Elsevier Inc. All rights reserved.
doi:10.1016/j.ccm.2007.11.003

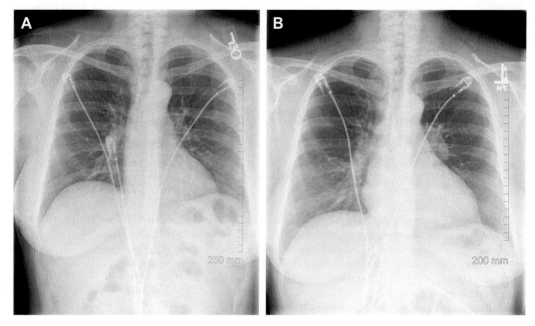

Fig. 1. Forty-five-year-old woman. Figs. 1–4 and 6 are from the same patient. (*A*) Initial chest radiograph from prior admission was normal. (*B*) Subsequent chest radiograph demonstrates reduced size of segmental and subsegmental pulmonary arteries in both upper lobes and the left lower lobe (Westermark's sign). The central pulmonary arteries are slightly increased in size.

are many causes of perfusion defects other than PE, such as obstructive airway disease, pneumonia, atelectasis, edema, and vasculitis, ventilation scans have been added to the perfusion scan to increase the specificity. Perfusion defects with normal ventilation strongly suggest PE.

V/Q scans are interpreted as negative, low, intermediate, and high probability. A normal V/Q scan essentially excludes the diagnosis of PE, and a high probability V/Q scan has a 96% positive predictive value in high-risk patients according to the Prospective Investigation of Pulmonary Embolism Diagnosis (PIOPED) data [12]. It is unfortunate that most of the V/Q scans (60%–70%) are interpreted as low or intermediate probability and are nondiagnostic [12–14]. When the chest radiograph is normal, however, as many as 80% to 90% of studies are definitive [15].

Pulmonary arteriography

On invasive pulmonary arteriography, emboli are seen as complete obstruction, intraluminal filling defects, or a decrease in flow rate [16]. For many years, pulmonary arteriography has been accepted as the gold standard and the most sensitive and specific method available for diagnosis of

PE. Pulmonary arteriography, however, is invasive, expensive, time-consuming, may not be readily available, and has complications. Accurate statistics for morbidity and mortality are difficult to obtain. In recent studies, the morbidity of pulmonary arteriography has been shown to be 1% and mortality was absent [17]. Many clinicians still have the exaggerated perception that pulmonary arteriography has moderate to high morbidity and mortality. There is no generally accepted indication for pulmonary arteriography, although it has been recommended as part of the workup for patients who have nondiagnostic scintigraphy. After the introduction of CTA, the role of conventional pulmonary arteriography has been questioned further. It is used significantly less frequently. Many investigators now question whether pulmonary arteriography should remain the gold standard [18,19].

Transesophageal echocardiography

Central pulmonary emboli are directly visualized with transesophageal echocardiography. Peripheral emboli are not imaged. Right ventricular overload can also be evaluated, which is important in assessment of the patient's

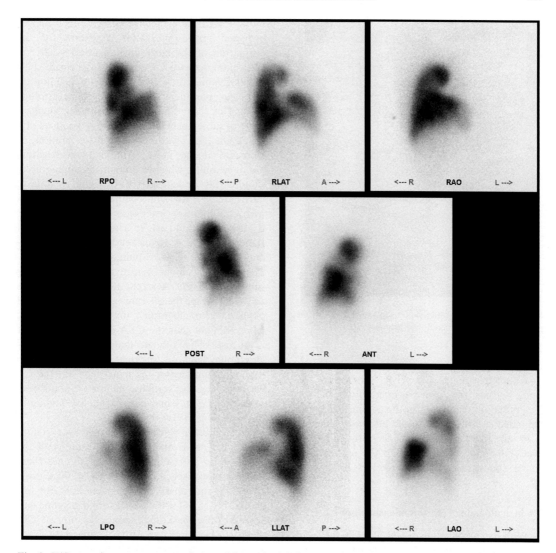

Fig. 2. V/Q scan demonstrates no perfusion of the entire left lung and multiple segmental perfusion defects predominantly in the upper lobe of the right lung.

cardiopulmonary status and prognosis. Transesophageal echocardiography may not be available at all centers. Its primary role is in patients who have suspected massive emboli and are too unstable to move elsewhere for imaging.

Doppler ultrasonography

Lower-extremity venous Doppler ultrasonography is widely available and easily obtained for patients who have symptoms of DVT. It is noninvasive and inexpensive. DVT is seen as partial or complete filling defects in the veins, with lack of compressibility of the vessel (Fig. 3). Doppler ultrasonography has high sensitivity and specificity (95% and 96%, respectively) [20]; however, this is true only for the popliteal, femoral, and saphenous veins. Its sensitivity is much lower for calf vein, and evaluation of the inferior vena cava and iliac veins is often not possible with ultrasound, depending on patient factors [21]. Another drawback of Doppler ultrasound is its insensitivity in the detection of nonocclusive thrombi [22–24].

Contrast venography

Contrast venography is still considered the most reliable test and gold standard in diagnosis

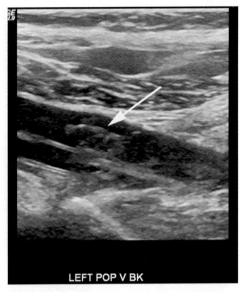

Fig. 3. Doppler ultrasonography shows DVT in the left popliteal vein as an incomplete filling defect (*arrow*).

of DVT [25]. Contrast venography has the ability to completely image the pelvic, thigh, and calf veins; however, it is invasive, operator dependent, uses radiation, and requires the administration of iodinated contrast material. In addition, phlebitis is an infrequent complication. Since the introduction of Doppler ultrasound and CT venography, contrast venography has been used less frequently.

CT in acute pulmonary thromboembolism

With the introduction of helical CT in the early 1990s, acquisition of a volume data set in a single breath hold (18–30 seconds) at optimal contrast enhancement became possible. The first study comparing CTA with pulmonary arteriography was published in 1992 and reported 100% sensitivity and 96% specificity for the diagnosis of PE [26]. In a subsequent study using electron-beam CT, Teigen and colleagues [27] reported similar results of high sensitivity (95%) and specificity (80%) for spiral CT. These results, however, were for central pulmonary emboli only. Later studies evaluating central and subsegmental arteries demonstrated lower sensitivity and specificity [28].

Advances in CT technology, with the introduction of faster scanners and multidetector row CT, enabled acquisition of thinner slices in a shorter time period, decreasing respiratory-

motion artifacts. Higher-quality thinner images provided improved spatial resolution for the evaluation of the subsegmental arteries [29–33]. With multidetector CT scanning, the entire chest can be scanned in 4 to 8 seconds, depending on technical parameters and the CT technology used. This technology enabled routine visualization of subsegmental arteries on a good-quality CT angiogram without respiratory motion or increased image noise. Although investigators are questioning whether pulmonary angiography should still be considered the gold standard, most studies are still comparing CTA results with a pulmonary arteriography gold standard. By using thrombi casts in a pig model as a gold standard, Baile and colleagues [18] compared 1-mm-thin CTA slices to pulmonary angiography. They found similar sensitivities for detecting subsegmental PE. A recent PIOPED II analysis showed that in the 20 cases in which CTA and pulmonary angiography disagreed, an expert panel thought that the CTA diagnosis was right in 14 cases. They thought that the pulmonary angiographic diagnosis was right in two cases. In the four remaining cases, the panel felt that the CT was true negative initially, but that emboli were subsequently present when pulmonary angiography was done [19].

Interobserver variability of CTA is significantly dependent on the technical quality of the examination [34]. With the use of thinner slices and increased speed provided by multidetector row CTs, interobserver agreement has also improved [31,35,36]. PIOPED II found a kappa statistic for CT of 0.73 (95% confidence interval [CI]: 0.68%–78%) compared with a kappa statistic for angiography of 0.66 (95% CI: 0.48%–59%).

CTA enables direct visualization of PE. Acute PE can be seen as a complete, a central partial, or an eccentric partial filling defect (Fig. 4A, B). A central partial filling defect presents as "polo mint sign" or "railway track sign" when perpendicular or parallel to the long axis of the vessel, respectively. With complete filling defects, vessels may be enlarged compared with those of the same generation. Indirect signs of acute PE include wedge-shaped peripheral opacities, representing pulmonary infarcts. Atelectasis and pleural effusion are nonspecific findings of acute PE.

How sensitive and specific is CTA? How reliable is CT in excluding important pulmonary emboli? If CT is negative, how often do patients return with embolic problems in the next few months if they are untreated? There is a range of

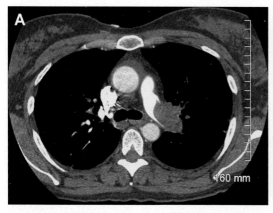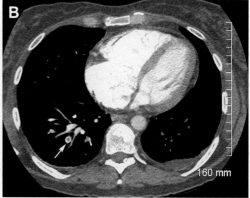

Fig. 4. (*A*) CTA demonstrates acute PE in the left main pulmonary artery as a complete filling defect; the vessel is enlarged. (*B*) At the level of ventricles, a central partial filling defect of the acute PE (*arrow*) is seen in the right lower lobe posterobasal segmental artery (Polo mint sign). Right ventricle and right atrium are moderately dilated, suggesting right heart strain.

sensitivities and specificities reported in the literature. Recently, PIOPED II reported a sensitivity and a specificity of 83% and 96%, respectively, whereas others have reported sensitivities of 90% or greater [35,37,38]. With current-generation scanners, the latter is probably a better estimate.

Numerous studies have been performed over the last 10 years that have followed-up CT patients who did not have evidence of PE and were not treated for pulmonary embolus. Quiroz and colleagues [39] reviewed 15 studies that had at least a 3-month follow-up. A total of 3500 patients were evaluated. The negative predictive value for CT was 99.1% (95% CI: 98.7%–99.5%). The negative likelihood ratio was 0.07 (95% CI: 0.05%–0.11%). There did not appear to be a significant difference in risk of subsequent PE using a single-slice versus a multislice detector. These studies support the view that a good-quality CT angiogram without pulmonary emboli justifies withholding treatment without further imaging. PIOPED II cautioned, however, that if the preclinical probability (Wells score) was high, then a negative CT angiogram may not always be reliable. Unless the CT is absolutely pristine and normal, additional imaging of the legs or lungs is warranted. Likewise, a positive CT and low clinical evaluation may require further evaluation when PEs are confined to small vessels.

Stein [3] tried to reconcile the discrepancy between the relatively high number of undetected pulmonary emboli (false negatives) in the PIOPED II study with the very low number of subsequent pulmonary emboli found on 3-month follow-up. His statistical argument was based on PIOPED data. The authors included data from other studies and broadened the argument:

1. Assume 10% to 17% of PE are missed (CT false negative).
2. Assume 5% to 10% of patients who have small PE (presumably the ones missed on CT) have subsequent PE if untreated. (These estimates are based on PE recurrence in patients who were not anticoagulated after a low-probability V/Q scan).
3. Five percent to 10% of 10% to 17% equals 0.5% to 1.7%, which is approximately the 99.1% sensitivity calculated by Quiroz and colleagues [39].

The strongest argument against treating every small embolus comes indirectly from the outcome studies. If CTA is approximately 90% sensitive, and 10% of patients who have emboli—presumably small emboli—go undetected and untreated, then mortality and morbidity from pulmonary emboli in the next few months should be high. Quiroz and colleagues [39] showed that this mortality and morbidity is approximately 1%, which suggests that most difficult-to-diagnose (presumably small) emboli do not lead to unfavorable clinical outcomes.

Still to be determined is whether every patient who has a small pulmonary embolus needs treatment. There is a growing body of literature that suggests that patients who have small emboli, no evidence of DVT, and good cardiopulmonary reserve may do better without anticoagulation than with anticoagulation [40–42].

CT in chronic pulmonary thromboembolism

Chronic PE is seen on CT as an eccentric filling defect contiguous with the vessel wall, reduced diameter of pulmonary arteries, vascular bands, and webs (Fig. 5). Calcification within the clot is the most specific finding of chronic PE. Indirect findings include enlarged main pulmonary arteries secondary to pulmonary arterial hypertension, prominent collateral bronchial arteries, and mosaic perfusion of the lung. Small subpleural scars are nonspecific but commonly seen findings of chronic PE on CT [43]. Perfusion scanning often shows multiple perfusion defects.

It is important to consider the diagnosis of chronic thromboembolic disease in all patients presenting with unexplained pulmonary hypertension. In young patients who have suspected primary pulmonary hypertension, V/Q scanning is often an appropriate test to exclude thromboembolic pulmonary hypertension. In older individuals or those who have underlying lung disease, however, CTA is probably more specific because of the high frequency of indeterminate perfusion defects in this population. Although a proportion of cases of chronic thromboembolism may be missed on CTA [44,45], the presence of central thrombus on CTA is a useful predictor of the likelihood of improvement following thromboendarterectomy [46,47].

CT venography

In 1998, Loud and colleagues [48] described the use of combined CTA and indirect CT venography of the lower extremities. Indirect CT venography was obtained without additional contrast administration. Three minutes after administration of intravenous contrast material for CTA, contiguous or sequential images were obtained through the pelvis and lower extremities. Acute DVT was visualized directly as a complete or partial filling defect within the vessel (Fig. 6). Acute thrombi may completely obstruct vessel lumen, and the veins are enlarged. There is also perivenous stranding and mural enhancement. In chronic DVT, veins are smaller compared with the accompanying arteries, and the most specific finding is calcification of the vein.

CT venography is routinely used after CTA in some institutions; however, there is considerable radiation to the pelvis, which is important, especially in young patients. At the authors' institution, patients younger than 40 years who do not have symptoms of DVT do not undergo CT venography. Pelvic radiation can be reduced further by using one 5-mm image every 2 cm rather than performing continuous imaging, and by scanning from the acetabulum rather than from the iliac crest because DVT isolated to the iliac veins is very rare [49].

Radiation exposure from CTA is lower than from pulmonary angiography, but CTA is associated with a higher radiation burden than V/Q scanning. Reducing the dose by using appropriate technical parameters and dose modulation

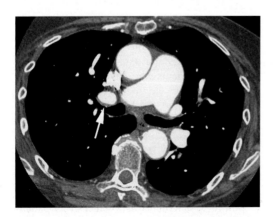

Fig. 5. Chronic PE in the right upper lobe pulmonary artery (*arrow*) is seen as an eccentric filling defect. Main pulmonary artery is moderately dilated.

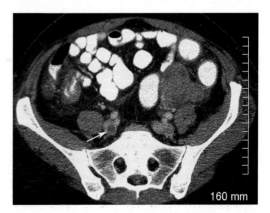

Fig. 6. Acute DVT in right common iliac vein is visualized as a near-complete filling defect (*arrow*). There is also a filling defect in left common iliac vein.

programs becomes especially important in patients followed-up with repeat CT angiograms.

Allergic reactions to iodinated contrast material, renal failure, and severe heart failure are contraindications to CTA. The use of gadolinium chelates instead of iodinated contrast medium in CTA has been reported and is promising for those who have allergic reactions to CT contrast media. The use of gadolinium in renal failure patients is debatable because of its potential to induce nephrogenic systemic fibrosis [50].

Indeterminate CT angiograms usually result from respiratory artifacts or inadequate opacification of pulmonary arteries and from increased image noise in obese patients. The prevalence of indeterminate CTA examinations has been reported to be 2% to 13% [35,36,42]. This prevalence is much less than that of V/Q scanning and is similar to that of pulmonary angiography.

Because CTA is widely available and readily accessible, it is considered the first-line modality in evaluation of PE in most institutions, rather than V/Q scanning. CTA is a rapid procedure. It provides alternative diagnoses responsible for symptoms of the patients, which cannot be determined by other diagnostic tests for PE. It is also cost-effective in the diagnostic workup of PE, although its cost varies among countries and even institutions. The severity of the pulmonary embolism can also be assessed with CTA by the evaluation of right ventricle dilatation, suggesting right ventricular failure [51].

Magnetic resonance angiography

Lack of radiation and iodinated contrast material administration are major advantages of MRI over CT. Currently, high-resolution magnetic resonance angiography (MRA) images can be obtained with gradient echo techniques during a single breath hold and using intravenous gadolinium by performing dynamic imaging. Like CT, deep veins of the pelvis and lower extremities can be evaluated with magnetic resonance venography (MRV) as a combined approach with MRA. MRV has very high sensitivity and specificity for pelvic venous imaging and DVT [52–54]. Emboli are directly visualized as filling defects in MRA and MRV, as in CT and pulmonary arteriography. Although MRI is noninvasive, the length of examinations and limited patient access to critically ill, dyspneic, and monitored patients are disadvantages. It is also expensive and operator and reader dependent.

Several investigators compared MRA with pulmonary arteriography [55–57]. Sensitivities of MRA ranged between 48% and 100%. Following intravenous administration of gadolinium and using very short echo times, pulmonary perfusion can also be visualized. Kluge and colleagues [58] evaluated the diagnostic accuracy of three MRI techniques (real-time MRI, MRA, and MR perfusion imaging) and compared them with 16-multidetector row CT to assess acute PE to the subsegmental level. They found the combined MR protocol to be reliable and sensitive compared with 16-multidetector row CT in the diagnosis of PE. MR perfusion imaging was sensitive for the detection of PE, whereas real-time MRI and MRA were specific.

Recently, the use of gadolinium in renal failure patients has been shown to cause nephrogenic systemic fibrosis, suggesting that allergy to iodinated contrast is the only current indication for MRI [50].

Diagnostic algorithm

PIOPED II has recently emphasized the value of objective pretest probability scoring (eg, Wells score) and the use of D-dimer in eliminating the need for imaging in a significant number of outpatients [59]. This step should be the first in patient triage, before imaging is considered.

Imaging of PE begins with the chest radiograph. It is helpful to rule out other disease processes that can mimic symptoms of PE. When the chest radiograph is normal, patients are usually evaluated with V/Q scan to take advantage of its low radiation and high negative predictive value. When the chest radiograph is not normal or the V/Q scan is inconclusive, the patient undergoes CTA.

Patients who have symptoms of DVT alone undergo Doppler venous ultrasonography of lower extremities. At the authors' institution, CT venography is routinely obtained after CTA in patients older than 40 years. Pulmonary arteriography is reserved for patients who have inconclusive CTA. Patients who have iodine allergy or are pregnant may be referred to MRI.

The optimal imaging evaluation of pregnant patients for PE is controversial. Although V/Q scan has a lower effective dose of radiation to the mother compared with CTA, the reverse is true for the fetus. Normally, a V/Q scan is preferred as first-line imaging after a normal chest radiograph to rule out PE, especially in young patients, but in pregnant patients, CTA is preferred to V/Q scan because it gives less radiation to the fetus. Imaging starts with lower-etremity ultrasound. When DVT is detected, the lungs are not imaged.

Summary

Introduction of helical and multidetector row CT technology has changed the algorithm of PE imaging. With multidetector row CTs, thinner images can be obtained in a shorter time, greatly increasing the diagnostic yield. CT can also provide alternative diagnoses that cannot be made by other methods, and CT venography can provide evaluation for DVT as part of the same examination.

Acknowledgments

The authors wish to thank Sylvia Bartz for her help in preparing this manuscript.

References

[1] Goldhaber SZ. Pulmonary embolism. Lancet 2004; 363(9417):1295–305.

[2] Byrne JJ, O'Neil EE. Fatal pulmonary emboli: a study of 130 autopsy-proven fatal pulmonary emboli. Am J Surg 1952;83:47–54.

[3] Stein PD. Outcome studies of pulmonary embolism versus accuracy. Case fatality rate and population mortality rate from pulmonary embolism and deep venous thrombosis. p. 355–6. 2nd edition. In: Stein PD, editor. Pulmonary embolism. Malden (MA): Blackwell Publishing; 2007. p. 19–23.

[4] Goldhaber SZ, Elliott CG. Acute pulmonary embolism: part I: epidemiology, pathophysiology, and diagnosis. Circulation 2003;108(22):2726–9.

[5] Dalen JE, Alpert JS. Natural history of pulmonary embolism. Prog Cardiovasc Dis 1975;17(4):259–70.

[6] Carson JL, Kelley MA, Duff A, et al. The clinical course of pulmonary embolism. N Engl J Med 1992;326(19):1240–5.

[7] Matsumoto AH, Tegtmeyer CJ. Contemporary diagnostic approaches to acute pulmonary emboli. Radiol Clin North Am 1995;33(1):167–83.

[8] Stein PD, Kayali F, Olson RE. Trends in the use of diagnostic imaging in patients hospitalized with acute pulmonary embolism. Am J Cardiol 2004; 93(10):1316–7.

[9] Worsley DF, Alavi A, Aronchick JM, et al. Chest radiographic findings in patients with acute pulmonary embolism: observations from the PIOPED Study. Radiology 1993;189(1):133–6.

[10] Buckner CB, Walker CW, Purnell GL. Pulmonary embolism: chest radiographic abnormalities. J Thorac Imaging 1989;4(4):23–7.

[11] Greenspan RH, Ravin CE, Polansky SM, et al. Accuracy of the chest radiograph in diagnosis of pulmonary embolism. Invest Radiol 1982;17(6): 539–43.

[12] PIOPED investigators. Value of the ventilation/perfusion scan in acute pulmonary embolism: results of the prospective investigation of pulmonary embolism diagnosis (PIOPED). JAMA 1990;263:2753–9.

[13] Goodman LR, Lipchik RJ. Diagnosis of acute pulmonary embolism: time for a new approach. Radiology 1996;199:25–7.

[14] van Beek EJ, Brouwers EM, Song B, et al. Lung scintigraphy and helical computed tomography for the diagnosis of pulmonary embolism: a meta-analysis. Clin Appl Thromb Hemost 2001;7(2):87–92.

[15] Forbes KPN, Reid JH, Murchison JT. Do preliminary chest X-ray findings define the optimum role of pulmonary scintigraphy in suspected pulmonary embolism? Clin Radiol 2001;56:397–400.

[16] Wittram C, Kalra MK, Maher MM, et al. Acute and chronic pulmonary emboli: angiography-CT correlation. AJR Am J Roentgenol 2006;186:S421–9.

[17] Johnson MS. Current strategies for the diagnosis of pulmonary embolus. J Vasc Interv Radiol 2002; 13(1):13–23.

[18] Baile EM, King GG, Muller NL, et al. Spiral computed tomography is comparable to angiography for the diagnosis of pulmonary embolism. Am J Respir Crit Care Med 2000;161(3 Pt 1):1010–5.

[19] Wittram C, Waltman AC, Shepard J-AO, et al. Discordance between CT and angiography in the PIOPED II study. Radiology 2007;244(3):883–9.

[20] Weinmann EE, Salzmann EW. Deep-vein thrombosis. N Engl J Med 1994;331:1630–41.

[21] Kearon C, Julian JA, Math M, et al. Noninvasive diagnosis of deep venous thrombosis. Ann Intern Med 1998;128(8):663–77.

[22] Cronan JJ. Venous thromboembolic disease: the role of US. Radiology 1993;186:619–30.

[23] Davidson BL, Elliot C, Lensing AW. Low accuracy of color Doppler ultrasound in the detection of proximal leg vein thrombosis in asymptomatic high-risk patients: the RD Heparin Arthroplasty Group. Ann Intern Med 1992;117:735–8.

[24] Jongbloets LM, Lensing AW, Koopman MM, et al. Limitations of compression ultrasound for the detection of symptomless postoperative deep vein thrombosis. Lancet 1994;343(8906):1142–4.

[25] Bettmann MA. Venography. In: Baum S, editor. Abrams' angiography. vol 2. Boston: Little, Brown and Company; 1997. p. 1743–54.

[26] Remy-Jardin M, Remy J, Wattinne L, et al. Central pulmonary thromboembolism: diagnosis with spiral volumetric CT with the single-breath-hold technique—comparison with pulmonary angiography. Radiology 1992;185(2):381–7.

[27] Teigen CL, Maus TP, Sheedy PF 2nd, et al. Pulmonary embolism: diagnosis with electron-beam CT. Radiology 1993;188(3):839–45.

[28] Goodman LR, Curtin JJ, Mewissen MW, et al. Detection of pulmonary embolism in patients with unresolved clinical and scintigraphic diagnosis: helical CT versus angiography. AJR Am J Roentgenol 1995;164(6):1369–74.

[29] Remy-Jardin M, Baghaie F, Bonnel F, et al. Thoracic helical CT: influence of subsecond scan time and thin collimation on evaluation of peripheral pulmonary arteries. Eur Radiol 2000;10(8):1297–303.

[30] Ghaye B, Szapiro D, Mastora I, et al. Peripheral pulmonary arteries: how far in the lung does multidetector row spiral CT allow analysis? Radiology 2001;219(3):629–36.

[31] Schoepf UJ, Holzknecht N, Helmberger TK, et al. Subsegmental pulmonary emboli: improved detection with thin-collimation multi-detector row spiral CT. Radiology 2002;222(2):483–90.

[32] Raptopoulos V, Boiselle PM. Multi-detector row spiral CT pulmonary angiography: comparison with single-detector row spiral CT. Radiology 2001;221:606–13.

[33] Perrier A, Roy P-M, Sanchez O, et al. Multidetector-row computed tomography in suspected pulmonary embolism. N Engl J Med 2005;352(17):1760–8.

[34] Herold CJ, Remy-Jardin M, Grenier PA, et al. Prospective evaluation of pulmonary embolism: initial results of the European multicenter trial (ESTIPEP) [abstract]. Radiology 1998;209(P):299.

[35] Coche E, Verschuren F, Keyeux A, et al. Diagnosis of acute pulmonary embolism in outpatients: comparison of thin-collimation mutlidetector row spiral CT and planar ventilation-perfusion scintigraphy. Radiology 2003;229:757–65.

[36] Brunot S, Corneloup O, Latrabe V, et al. Reproducibility of multi-detector spiral computed tomography in detection of sub-segmental acute pulmonary embolism. Eur Radiol 2005;15:2057–63.

[37] Blachere H, Latrabe V, Montaudon M, et al. Pulmonary embolism revealed on helical CT angiography: comparison with ventilation-perfusion radionuclide lung scanning. AJR Am J Roentgenol 2000;174(4):1041–7.

[38] Qanadli SD, Hajjam ME, Mesurolle B, et al. Pulmonary embolism detection: prospective evaluation of dual-section helical CT versus selective pulmonary arteriography in 157 patients. Radiology 2000;217(2):447–55.

[39] Quiroz R, Kucher N, Zou KH, et al. Clinical validity of a negative computed tomography scan in patients with suspected pulmonary embolism: a systematic review. JAMA 2005;293(16):2012–7.

[40] Goodman LR. Small pulmonary emboli: what do we know? Radiology 2005;234(3):654–8.

[41] Engelke C, Rummeny EJ, Marten K. Pulmonary embolism at multi-detector row CT of chest: one-year survival of treated and untreated patients. Radiology 2006;239(2):563–75.

[42] Eyer BA, Goodman LR, Washington L. Clinicians' response to radiologists' reports of isolated subsegmental pulmonary embolism or inconclusive interpretation of pulmonary embolism using MDCT. AJR Am J Roentgenol 2005;184(2):623–8.

[43] Wittram C, Maher MM, Yoo AJ, et al. CT angiography of pulmonary embolism: diagnostic criteria and causes of misdiagnosis. Radiographics 2004; 24(5):1219–38.

[44] Bergin CJ, Sirlin C, Deutsch R, et al. Predictors of patient response to pulmonary thromboendarterectomy. AJR Am J Roentgenol 2000;174:509–15.

[45] Tunariu N, Gibbs SJ, Win Z, et al. Ventilation-perfusion scintigraphy is more sensitive than multidetector CTPA in detecting chronic thromboembolic pulmonary disease as a treatable cause of pulmonary hypertension. J Nucl Med 2007;48:680–4.

[46] Bergin CJ, Sirlin CB, Hauschildt JP, et al. Chronic thromboembolism: diagnosis with helical CT and MR imaging with angiographic and surgical correlation. Radiology 1997;204:695–702.

[47] Oikonomou A, Dennie CJ, Muller NL, et al. Chronic thromboembolic pulmonary arterial hypertension: correlation of postoperative results of thromboendarterectomy with preoperative helical contrast-enhanced computed tomography. J Thorac Imaging 2004;19:67–73.

[48] Loud PA, Grossman ZD, Klippenstein DL, et al. Combined CT venography and pulmonary angiography: a new diagnostic technique for suspected thromboembolic disease. AJR Am J Roentgenol 1998;170:951–4.

[49] Goodman LR, Stein PD, Beemath A, et al. CT venography: continuous helical images versus reformatted discontinuous images using PIOPED II data. AJR Am J Roentgenol 2007;189:1–7.

[50] Broome DR, Girguis MS, Baron PW, et al. Gadodiamide-associated nephrogenic systemic fibrosis: why radiologists should be concerned. AJR Am J Roentgenol 2007;88:586–92.

[51] Reid JH, Murchison JT. Acute right ventricular dilatation: a new helical CT sign of massive pulmonary embolism. Clin Radiol 1998;53:694–8.

[52] Laissy JP, Cinqualbre A, Loshkajian A, et al. Assessment of deep venous thrombosis in the lower limbs and pelvis: MR venography versus duplex Doppler sonography. AJR Am J Roentgenol 1996; 67:971–5.

[53] Spritzer CE, Norconk JJ, Sostman HD, et al. Detection of deep venous thrombosis by magnetic resonance imaging. Chest 1993;104:54–60.

[54] Dupas B, El Kouri D, de Faucal P, et al. Angiomagnetic resonance imaging of iliofemorocaval venous thrombosis. Lancet 1995;346:17–9.

[55] Meaney JF, Weg JG, Chenevert TL, et al. Diagnosis of pulmonary embolism with magnetic resonance angiography. N Engl J Med 1997;336:1422–7.

[56] Gupta A, Frazer CK, Ferguson JM, et al. Acute pulmonary embolism: diagnosis with MR angiography. Radiology 1999;210:353–9.

[57] Hurst DR, Kazerooni EA, Stafford-Johnson D, et al. Diagnosis of pulmonary embolism: comparison of CT angiography and MR angiography in canines. J Vasc Interv Radiol 1999;10:309–18.

[58] Kluge A, Luboldt W, Bachmann G. Acute pulmonary embolism to the subsegmental level: diagnostic accuracy of three MRI techniques compared with 16-MDCT. AJR Am J Roentgenol 2006;187:W7–14.

[59] Stein PD, Woodard PK, Weg JG, et al. Diagnostic pathways in acute pulmonary embolism: recommendations of the PIOPED II investigators. Radiology 2007;242(1):15–21.

ELSEVIER SAUNDERS

Clin Chest Med 29 (2008) 117–131

CLINICS IN CHEST MEDICINE

Imaging of Occupational and Environmental Lung Diseases

Masanori Akira, MD, PhD

Department of Radiology, Kinki Cuo Chest Medical Center, 1180 Nagasone-cho, Kita-ku, Sakai City, Osaka 591-8555, Japan

Imaging techniques for occupational lung disease

The chest radiograph has for many years been a pivotal investigation for detection and characterization of occupational lung disease. The International Labor Organization (ILO) system of International Classification of Radiographs of Pneumoconiosis, originally developed for epidemiologic studies of occupational lung disease, may also assist in clinical interpretation of the disease [1]. The ILO classification system has been extensively validated by comparison with duration and intensity of dust exposure, pathologic extent of disease, and outcome; however, it is clear that CT is more sensitive than chest radiography in the detection of pleuroparenchymal abnormalities in pneumoconiosis. In particular, high-resolution CT (HRCT) is a more sensitive diagnostic tool to demonstrate lesions of pneumoconiosis. In addition, HRCT is useful in achieving more accurate categorization of the parenchymal changes in pneumoconiosis [2,3]. The optimal technique for detection of pneumoconiosis likely includes a combination of conventional thick-section CT and thin-section HRCT. Thin sections are important because some early centrilobular lesions of pneumoconiosis with relatively low attenuation values may not be detected by using thick sections: conversely, if thin sections alone are used, the relatively low profusion of nodules on each individual thin CT slice may preclude recognition. Thus, conventional CT and HRCT techniques should be used in combination for the early detection of micronodules in pneumoconiosis [4]. With modern spiral CT acquisitions, the use of maximum-intensity projection

techniques may facilitate identification of micronodules [5,6]. Similarly, in workers who have asbestos exposure, noncontiguous HRCT imaging is insufficient to exclude the presence of pleural plaques because minimal pleural plaques located in the skipped area are not included in HRCT [7]. In these individuals, it is preferable to conduct a spiral scan with the patient in the supine position for detecting pleural plaques, tumors, and other possible pathologies, followed by HRCT imaging with the patient prone for the early diagnosis of lung and pleural disease.

Although MRI is not useful for the detection of pneumoconiosis or pleural plaques, it has been reported to be superior to CT in selected patients who have potentially resectable mesothelioma [8]. T2-weighted MRI can allow discrimination between pleural plaques and malignant mesothelioma.

There is some preliminary evidence that positron emission tomography (PET) with fluorodeoxyglucose (FDG) might be useful in demonstrating parenchymal fibrotic changes in idiopathic pulmonary fibrosis (IPF) [9,10]. This technique, however, has not yet been applied to pneumoconioses. PET imaging may be useful in distinguishing benign from malignant asbestos-related pleural disease. PET in conjunction with CT scanning has improved diagnosis and staging in pleural mesothelioma [11,12].

Silicosis

Silicosis is a fibrotic disease of the lungs caused by inhalation of crystalline silicon dioxide (silica), and usually occurs after many years of exposure. It is rare for the chest radiograph to become abnormal before 20 years of exposure. Silicosis is

E-mail address: akira@kch.hosp.go.jp

characterized on the chest radiograph and chest CT by the presence of small, discrete nodules that are usually 2 to 5 mm in diameter but may range from 1 to 10 mm, found mainly in the upper and posterior lung zones (Fig. 1) [13,14]. These nodules tend to coalesce and form massive fibrotic lesions. Confluence of nodules along the pleura may result in pseudoplaques. Progressive massive fibrosis (PMF) is seen as irregularly shaped masses, most frequently in the apical and posterior segments of the upper and lower lobes, with peripheral parenchymal distortion (Fig. 2). Cavitation can occur from ischemic necrosis or accompanying tuberculosis. PMF in the upper zones of the lung may be mistaken for bronchogenic carcinoma and vice versa. PMF, however, is typically bilateral and often symmetric. PMF lesions may uncommonly be calcified. The lateral interface of the mass typically parallels the lateral chest wall. In addition, the natural history of the lesion on serial imaging is useful in the differential diagnosis between PMF and lung cancer or tuberculosis: PMF tends to be much more slowly progressive than these other entities. When serial images are not available, MRI may be useful for differentiating PMF from lung cancer. On MRI, lung cancer appears as a high-signal-intensity lesion on T2-weighted images, whereas the PMF is characterized on MRI by signal isointensity on T1-weighted images and hypointensity on T2-weighted images [15]. With PET, PMF often shows significantly increased FDG uptake and may therefore be confused with lung cancer [13].

Egg-shell calcifications in hilar and mediastinal lymph nodes are occasionally seen in silicosis. A similar egg-shell pattern of nodal calcification may be seen in sarcoidosis and chronic beryllium disease (CBD). There is no doubt that diffuse interstitial fibrosis occurs in silica and coal workers, but it is unknown whether this is related to silica or coal dust inhalation. About 10% to 20% of pneumoconioses show evidence of diffuse interstitial fibrosis similar to interstitial pneumonia, both radiologically and pathologically, in addition to typical pneumoconiotic lesions [16–18]. Various pleural abnormalities can also occur in silicosis, especially in advanced disease. Pleural effusion is found in 11% at chest radiography and CT, and pleural thickening is found in 58% at CT [19].

Accelerated silicosis follows shorter, heavier exposure (usually 4–10 years). Its imaging manifestations are generally similar to those of chronic silicosis. Acute silicosis follows intense exposure to fine dust of high silica content for periods measured in months. Radiologic and pathologic findings of acute silicosis are similar to those of pulmonary alveolar proteinosis [13,14].

In patients who have simple silicosis, it has been shown that reduced levels of lung function

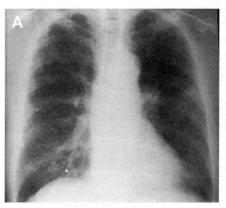 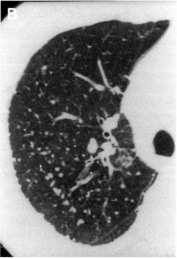

Fig. 1. Silicosis. (*A*) Chest radiograph shows multiple small nodules in both lungs, predominantly in the upper and middle zones. Many of the nodules appear to be calcified. (*B*) HRCT scan shows well-defined multiple small nodules with a perilymphatic (centrilobular and subpleural) distribution.

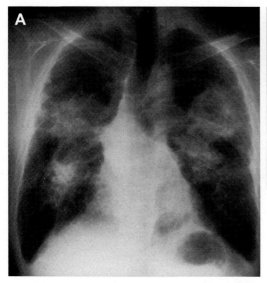
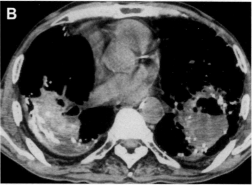

Fig. 2. Complicated silicosis. (*A*) Chest radiograph shows bilateral lung masses with distortion of adjacent lung and hyperexpansion of the lower lobes. The lateral margins of the masses are parallel to the chest wall. Peripheral cicatricial emphysema is evident, and there is a cavity in the left upper lung mass. (*B*) CT image viewed at mediastinal window settings depicts bilateral cavitating conglomerate masses with calcification. There is marked associated pleural thickening.

correlated with superimposed emphysema rather than nodular profusion [14]. Several articles have suggested that silicosis is a risk factor for emphysema, even in nonsmokers [20–22]. Recently, Arakawa and colleagues [23] reported that the extent of air trapping expressed by paired inspiratory and expiratory thin-section CT scans was the best CT index in the assessment of obstructive derangement in workers exposed to silica dust.

Coal worker's pneumoconiosis

The inhalation of coal mine dust may lead to the development of coal worker's pneumoconiosis (CWP); silicosis may also develop, depending on the silica content of the coal. The characteristic lesion of CWP is the collection of closely packed, dust-laden macrophages around the respiratory bronchiole, containing little collagen (coal dust macules). These lesions are usually associated with dilatation of respiratory bronchioles—so-called "focal emphysema." Another type of lesion is the fibrotic nodule. PMF may also occur in CWP: the imaging appearance of PMF in CWP is similar to that in silicosis; however, PMF of CWP is histopathologically distinguished from a silicotic conglomeration by the excess of black dust and by

the absence of individually identifiable silicotic nodules with their distinctive whorled pattern in the aggregate [14].

According to the ILO 1980 International Classification of Radiographs of Pneumoconiosis, small rounded opacities smaller than 1.5 mm in diameter are classified as p, those between 1.5 and 3 mm as q, and those between 3 and 10 mm as r. PMF or large opacities are defined radiologically as lesions of 1 cm or greater in longest diameter. The HRCT appearance in patients who have radiographic type p pneumoconiosis, including CWP, is characterized by minute branching lines or ill-defined punctate opacities, usually in a centrilobular location (Fig. 3). Micronodules can be seen in the subpleural areas, and confluence of subpleural nodules may simulate pleural plaques, referred to as pseudoplaques. Small nonperipheral areas of low attenuation with a central dot are sometimes seen, and they correspond to focal emphysema [2]. Opacities of the q and r types are characterized by sharply demarcated, rounded nodules or contracted nodules. Several investigators [24,25] have reported that coal workers who have p type opacities have a lower transfer factor and a more compliant lung than those who have q or r type opacities. This may be related to the development of focal emphysema.

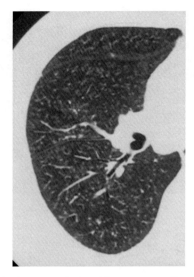

Fig. 3. Pneumoconiosis with p-type small nodules. HRCT scan shows multiple small nodules throughout the lung. They are located around the end of broncho-vascular branches and separated from the pulmonary vein or the pleura at a distance of about 2 to 3 mm, suggesting that the lesions exist in the centrilobular region.

Mixed-dust pneumoconiosis

Mixed-dust pneumoconiosis is defined as pneumoconiosis caused by concomitant exposure to silica and to less fibrogenic dusts such as iron, silicates, and carbon. Generally, as the proportion of silica increases, the number of silicotic nodules increases in proportion to the mixed-dust nodules.

Typical occupations associated with the diagnosis of mixed-dust pneumoconiosis include metal miners, quarry workers, foundry workers, pottery and ceramics workers, and stonemasons. Microscopically, the mixed-dust fibrotic nodule is characterized by a stellate shape and has a central hyalinized collagenous zone surrounded by linearly and radially arranged collagen fibers admixed with dust-containing macrophages. The radiologic findings of mixed-dust pneumoconiosis include a mixture of small rounded and irregular opacities [14]. Honeycombing and emphysematous spaces are also seen (Fig. 4).

Asbestos-related disorders

Pleuropulmonary changes related to asbestos dust exposure include asbestosis, pleural plaques, benign pleural effusion, diffuse pleural thickening, round atelectasis, lung cancer, and mesothelioma. Except for benign pleural effusion, asbestos-related pleuropulmonary complications usually occur after 20 or more years of exposure.

Pleural plaque is a localized thickening of the parietal pleura. Pleural plaques usually develop 20 years after asbestos exposure and serve only as a marker for such exposure. They occur most commonly on the middle part of the diaphragm, on the posterolateral chest wall between the seventh and 10th ribs, or on the lateral chest wall between the sixth and ninth ribs [26]. Unlike diffuse pleural thickening, no impairment of lung

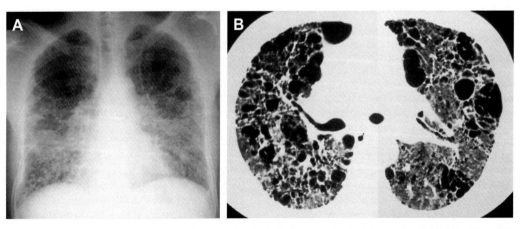

Fig. 4. Images obtained in a 60-year-old man who had pathologically proved mixed-dust pneumoconiosis. Chest radiograph shows a coarse reticulonodular pattern with middle and lower zonal predominance. (A) There is upper-lobe emphysema. (B) HRCT scan shows multiple cysts and bullae, traction bronchiectasis, and areas of ground-glass attenuation with intralobular interstitial thickening. Autopsy showed diffuse interstitial fibrosis with mixed-dust nodules and no silicotic nodules.

function is associated with pleural plaques. On the chest radiograph, pleural plaques must be differentiated from normal anatomic shadows, particularly extrapleural fat. Extrapleural fat may be radiographically differentiated from pleural plaque by its smooth, wavy margin and by the fact that it usually extends all the way to the lung apices. Chest radiographs have a low sensitivity for plaque detection, particularly for noncalcified pleural plaques. The percentage of pleural plaques detected on chest roentgenograms is variable, ranging from 8.3% to 40.3% depending on the detection criteria and population [27]. CT can demonstrate plaques along the mediastinum, paravertebral areas, and diaphragm, which are difficult to assess by conventional radiography (Fig. 5). CT is almost twice as sensitive as chest radiography for detecting pleural plaques. CT can readily distinguish pleural plaques from extrapleural fat.

Diffuse pleural thickening involves the visceral pleura and is frequently the result of prior asbestos-related exudative effusions. The definition of diffuse pleural thickening varies. In the United Kingdom, the plain radiographic criteria used for diffuse pleural thickening are the following: it may be unilateral or bilateral; it must cover at least 25% of the total chest wall on a chest radiograph (50% if unilateral); and it must extend to a thickness of at least 5 mm in at least one site on the chest radiograph [28]. McLoud and colleagues [29] defined diffuse pleural thickening as

a smooth uninterrupted pleural density extending over at least one fourth of the chest wall, with or without obliteration of the costophrenic angle. On CT scans, Lynch and colleagues defined diffuse pleural thickening as a continuous sheet of pleural thickening more than 5 cm wide, more than 8 cm in craniocaudal extent, and more than 3 mm thick (Fig. 6). Like benign asbestos-related pleural effusion, diffuse pleural thickening is less specific than pleural plaques but can be attributed to asbestos exposure when other causes are excluded.

Rounded atelectasis occurs when an area of visceral pleural fibrosis invaginates into the parenchyma and causes the underlying lung to become atelectatic. Rounded atelectasis appears as a masslike lesion that often mimics a pulmonary neoplasm. The most helpful features in the diagnosis of rounded atelectasis with CT are the following: contiguity to areas of diffuse pleural thickening; a lentiform or wedge-shaped outline; a characteristic "comet tail" of vessels and bronchi sweeping into the margins of the mass; and evidence of volume loss in the affected lobe, often with hyperlucency of the adjacent lung (Fig. 7) [30]. The appearance of rounded atelectasis on MRI is described as a lesion with signal intensity similar to that of the liver on T1-weighted images, with bronchovascular bundles curving into the pleural-based mass. MRI shows curved low signal lines or a distinct curvilinear nonenhanced area contiguous to the thickened visceral pleura in the atelectatic lung tissue, probably corresponding to enfolded visceral pleura [31].

Asbestosis is defined as diffuse interstitial fibrosis of the lung because of exposure to asbestos dust. The common HRCT findings include interstitial lines (intralobular interstitial

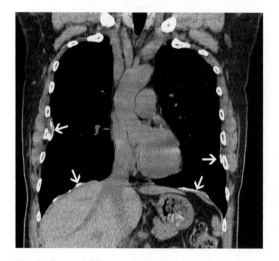

Fig. 5. Coronal CT scan obtained with mediastinal window settings shows pleural plaques on the lateral chest walls and diaphragm (*arrows*).

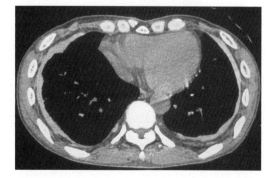

Fig. 6. CT scan of an asbestos-exposed person shows bilateral circumferential diffuse pleural thickening, slightly hyperdense relative to the chest wall muscles.

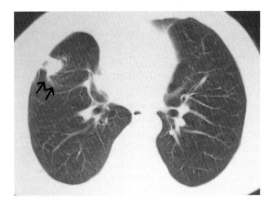

Fig. 7. Rounded atelectasis. CT scan shows a peripheral mass that abuts thickened pleura, with comet tail distortion of the vascular structures (*arrows*).

thickening and interlobular septal thickening), subpleural curvilinear lines, subpleural dotlike opacities, pleura-based nodular irregularities, parenchymal bands, patchy areas of ground-glass attenuation, traction bronchiectasis, and honeycombing (Figs. 8 and 9). Based on HRCT–pathologic correlation, subpleural curvilinear lines have been shown to represent peribronchiolar fibrotic thickening combined with flattening and collapse

of the alveoli caused by fibrosis. The intralobular interstitial thickening is pathologically caused by peribronchiolar fibrosis, with subsequent involvement of the alveolar ducts [14].

The earliest findings in asbestosis on HRCT have been shown to be subpleural dotlike opacities connected with the most peripheral branch of the pulmonary artery (Fig. 10). Paired serial CT images have revealed that these subpleural dotlike opacities and branching lines increased in number over time and that the confluence of dots created pleura-based nodular irregularities and subpleural curvilinear lines [32]. CT scans obtained in a prone position are important for distinguishing between gravity-related physiologic phenomena and mild fibrosis.

Asbestosis and IPF (ie, usual interstitial pneumonia; UIP) have similar radiographic manifestations apart from pleural diseases. Copley and colleagues [33] reported that the thin-section CT pattern of asbestosis closely resembled that of biopsy-proved UIP and differed markedly from that of biopsy-proved nonspecific interstitial pneumonia (NSIP). They reported that the asbestosis cases, as compared with the NSIP cases, were characterized by higher coarseness scores and a lower proportion of ground-glass opacification,

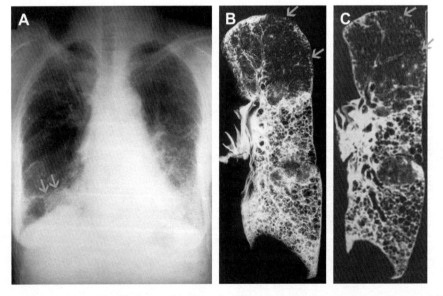

Fig. 8. Images from a woman who died at age 75 years after 31 years in the asbestos textile industry and 25 years of exposure. (*A*) Chest radiograph obtained 1 month before death shows diffuse, small, irregular opacities. This patient also had primary squamous cell carcinoma in the right lower lobe (*arrowheads*). Postmortem low-kilovoltage radiograph (*B*) and HRCT scan (*C*) of the inflated and fixed left lung show honeycombing in the lower two thirds of the lung. Subpleural nodular opacities are also seen (*arrows*). (*From* Akira M, et al. Asbestosis: high-resolution CT-pathologic correlation. Radiology 1990;176:390; with permission.)

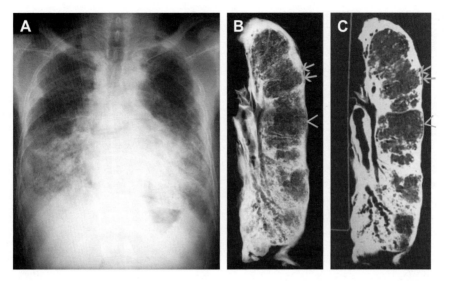

Fig. 9. Images from man who died at age 56 years after 42 years in the asbestos textile industry and 22 years of exposure. (*A*) Chest radiograph obtained 1 month before death shows coarse reticular opacities, predominantly in the lower lung zones; "shaggy heart"; and extensive bilateral pleural thickening. Postmortem low-kilovoltage radiograph (*B*) and HRCT scan (*C*) of the inflated and fixed left lung show diffuse pleural thickening and pleural-based opacities extending along the bronchovascular sheath. Subpleural curvilinear line (*arrows*) and subpleural nodular opacities (*arrowhead*) are also seen. (*From* Akira M, et al. Asbestosis: high-resolution CT-pathologic correlation. Radiology 1990;176:393; with permission.)

whereas coarseness scores and proportions of ground-glass opacification did not differ significantly between the UIP and asbestosis groups. In early disease, it may be possible to discern the effects of fibrosis on the subpleural secondary pulmonary lobule, with asbestosis having initially centrilobular densities due to the deposition of

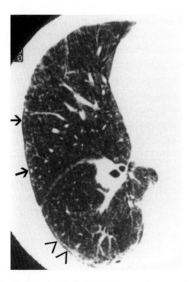

Fig. 10. Early asbestosis. HRCT scan shows subpleural dots (*arrows*) and subpleural curvilinear line (*arrowheads*).

fibers by way of airways, whereas immunologically mediated IPF is more widespread, resulting in traction effects on the bronchioles. In one study, a combination of subpleural dots, subpleural lines, and parenchymal bands was found in 35% of 80 patents who had asbestosis, whereas this combination was found in 1% of 80 patients who had IPF; a combination of subpleural dots, subpleural lines, parenchymal bands, and mosaic perfusion was found in 21% of the 80 patients who had asbestosis but in none of the 80 patients who had IPF [34].

The relationship between asbestos exposure and malignant mesothelioma has been established. Malignant pleural mesothelioma may manifest as unilateral pleural effusion, diffuse pleural thickening, or both on the plain chest radiograph. CT plays a key role in the diagnosis of mesothelioma and is likely to be the initial study for determining resectability in most cases. CT can be used to assist diagnosis by a guiding percutaneous needle biopsy. The CT findings of rindlike pleural involvement, mediastinal pleural involvement, pleural nodularity, and pleural thickness greater than 1 cm are independent findings for the differentiation of malignant pleural diseases from benign pleural disease (Fig. 11) [35].

124   AKIRA

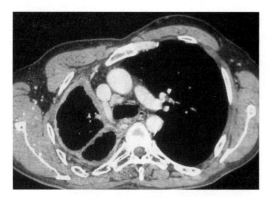

Fig. 11. CT scan obtained with mediastinal window settings in a patient who had malignant pleural mesothelioma shows circumferential pleural thickening with mediastinal involvement (pleural rind), ipsilateral volume loss due to encasement of the lung, and extension along the major fissure.

MRI is superior to CT in identifying local invasion by mesothelioma into the diaphragm, endothoracic fascia, or chest wall [36]. Although malignant pleural mesothelioma staging with CT and multiplanar reformatting has not been studied extensively, volumetric CT technique can improve the visualization of tumor extent, especially in regions such as the diaphragm that may be difficult to assess with axial imaging (Fig. 12).

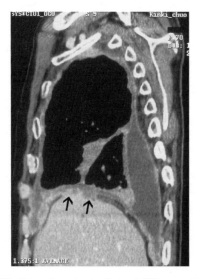

Fig. 12. Coronal contrast-enhanced CT scan obtained with mediastinal window settings in a patient who had malignant pleural mesothelioma shows invasion of the diaphragmatic muscle (*arrows*).

Talcosis

Talc is a hydrated magnesium silicate used in the manufacture of leather, rubber, paper, textiles, and ceramic tiles. It is usually incorporated into such products with other elements such as iron and nickel and is often found in association with minerals such as quartz, mica, kaolin, and asbestos. Talcosis can produce several radiographic appearances: a nodular pattern resembling silicosis or mixed-dust fibrosis, including, in some cases, large opacities; a diffuse interstitial pattern, simulating asbestosis; or a combination of nodular and linear patterns [37].

HRCT findings in patients who have pulmonary talcosis caused by the inhalation of talc consist of small centrilobular and subpleural nodules, conglomerated masses containing focal areas of high attenuation, septal lines, subpleural lines, ground-glass opacities, and lobular low-attenuation areas (Fig. 13) [38]. Pleural plaques and enlarged lymph nodes containing focal areas of high attenuation may also be seen [38]. The HRCT findings in patients who have pulmonary talcosis resulting from chronic intravenous drug abuse include diffuse small nodules, perihilar conglomerate masses with areas of high attenuation, ground-glass opacities, and lower-lobe panacinar emphysema [39,40].

Berylliosis

Beryllium disease is a multisystem disorder caused by exposure to dust, fumes, or aerosols of beryllium metal or its salts. There are two types of lung injury related to beryllium exposure: an acute chemical pneumonitis (acute berylliosis) and a chronic granulomatous disease (CBD). Acute berylliosis is rare today because of industrial control measures. CBD develops in up to 16% of exposed workers, depending on individual genetic susceptibility and the extent and type of exposure.

The radiographic and CT appearances of CBD are similar to those of sarcoidosis. Mediastinal and hilar lymphadenopathy is less common in CBD. On CT, enlarged lymph nodes are detected in the pulmonary hila in 32% of patients who have CBD, and in the mediastinum in 25% of patients. The most common CT abnormalities are parenchymal nodules and septal lines (Fig. 14). The nodules are often distributed along the bronchovascular bundles or interlobular septa, similar to the distribution seen in sarcoidosis [41].

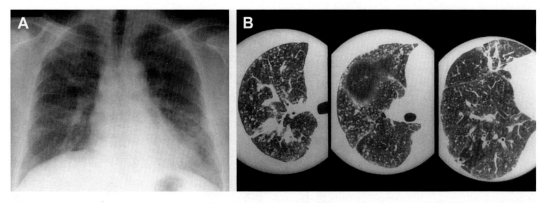

Fig. 13. Talc pneumoconiosis. (*A*) Chest radiograph shows fine nodular and irregular opacities diffusely distributed throughout both lungs and confluent opacities. (*B*) Right upper lung, middle lung, and lower lung. HRCT scan shows fine nodular opacities, mainly distributed in a centrilobular location, with confluent peribronchovascular nodules in the right upper lung.

Hard-metal lung disease

Hard metal is an alloy of tungsten carbide in a matrix of cobalt to which small amounts of titanium, nickel chromium, niobium, vanadium, titanium, or molybdenum may be added. Respiratory effects produced by exposure to hard metal include asthmatic reactions, bronchiolitis, hypersensitivity pneumonitis (HP) or alveolitis, and pulmonary fibrosis [42]. Cobalt is generally considered the main cause of hard-metal lung disease. Hard-metal lung disease is a rare form of occupational lung disease, and the existence of a possible genetic susceptibility has been suggested [43]. The most characteristic pathologic finding in hard-

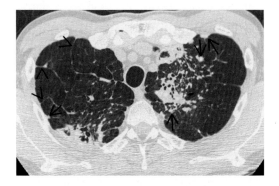

Fig. 14. CBD related to exposure to beryllium at a ceramics factory. CT scan through the upper lobes demonstrates bilateral conglomerate masses (subpleural on the right and peribronchovascular on the left) associated with marked architectural distortion, septal thickening (*arrowheads*), and peribronchovascular and subpleural nodularity (*arrows*). Findings are indistinguishable from those of sarcoidosis.

metal lung disease is the presence of "bizarre" or "cannibalistic" multinucleated giant cells in the interstitium and alveolar lumen [44].

The radiologic appearance of hard-metal interstitial lung disease may be variable and may mimic sarcoidosis, NSIP, and UIP [45]. HRCT findings consist of bilateral ground-glass opacities or consolidation in panlobular or multilobular form, extensive reticular opacities, and traction bronchiectasis (Fig. 15). Honeycombing may be seen. The findings of panlobular and multilobular ground-glass opacities or consolidation correspond histopathologically to areas of interstitial thickening caused by inflammatory cell infiltration and intra-alveolar accumulation of macrophages and multinucleated giant cells. The findings of parenchymal distortion, traction bronchiectasis, reticulation, or a combination of these correspond histopathologically to areas of interstitial fibrosis [44,46]. The HRCT findings in early stages of hard-metal interstitial lung disease are characterized by fine nodular opacities and areas of ground-glass attenuation without traction bronchiectasis, mainly in the lower lobes (Fig. 16).

Aluminum pneumoconiosis

Exposure to aluminum, alumina, and pot-room fumes has been associated with diffuse interstitial fibrosis [47]. Diffuse interstitial fibrosis attributable to aluminum exposure is usually most severe in the upper lung zones, although it may be diffuse. Desquamative interstitial pneumonia, granulomatous lung reaction, and pulmonary alveolar proteinosis develop after exposure to fumes from aluminum welding, have also been described [48].

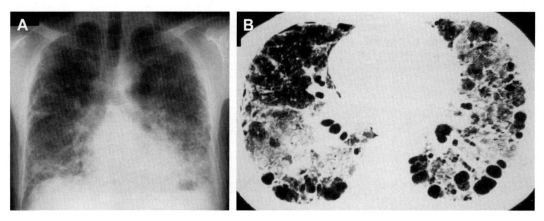

Fig. 15. Giant cell interstitial pneumonitis in a patent who had a history of exposure to hard metal for 5 years. (*A*) Chest radiograph shows coarse reticular opacity with peripheral patchy areas of dense opacity, predominantly in the lower lung zones. (*B*) HRCT scan reveals air space consolidation and ground-glass attenuation with traction bronchiectasis. Multiple cysts are seen.

The radiologic appearances of aluminum pneumoconiosis may be variable and may mimic silicosis, sarcoidosis, NSIP, and UIP. They include nodular, reticular, and upper-lung fibrosis patterns, and so on [44]. The nodular pattern consists of well-defined nodules 2 to 5 mm in diameter (identical to those of silicosis) or ill-defined centrilobular nodules diffusely distributed throughout both lungs. In the reticular pattern, HRCT findings are similar to those of UIP, and honeycombing may be seen. The distribution may be upper-lung predominant or diffuse, and such a distribution is distinct from that of IPF or asbestosis. There may be conglomeration with shrinkage in both upper lungs. Ground-glass opacities, with traction bronchiectasis mimicking NSIP, are also seen (Fig. 17). Increased density of mediastinal lymph nodes may be seen [49].

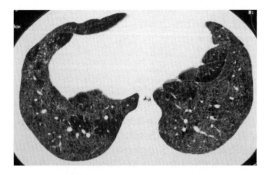

Fig. 16. Hard-metal lung disease. HRCT scan shows diffuse small, ill-defined nodules with ground-glass opacity. Appearances in this case are similar to those of HP.

The HRCT findings in the early stages of aluminosis are characterized by small rounded and ill-defined centrilobular opacities mainly in the upper lobes, and the opacities cannot be assessed using chest radiography [50].

Welder's lung

Exposure to welding fumes is known to be a risk factor for chronic respiratory disorders such as pneumoconiosis, chronic bronchitis, and lung cancer [51]. The principal component of the inhaled dust is iron oxide. Diffuse pulmonary fibrosis has often been attributed to inhalation of agents other than iron oxide, such as silica or asbestos, during welding. Some experimental studies, however, suggest that a large amount of iron or welding fume may also be able to produce nodular fibrosis [52].

The typical HRCT findings in arc welder's siderosis are diffusely distributed ill-defined centrilobular micronodules and fine branching lines mimicking HP (Fig. 18). In some welders, a honeycomb pattern and ground-glass opacities are also found [44,53]. Conglomerated masses with areas of high attenuation are rarely seen. The masses with areas of high attenuation correspond histologically to organizing pneumonia with siderosis (Fig. 19) [44].

Hypersensitivity pneumonitis

HP is an immunologic disorder characterized by granulomatous interstitial pneumonia associated with exposure to occupational or environmental

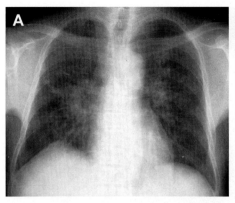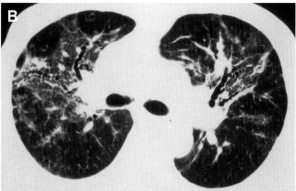

Fig. 17. Aluminum pneumoconiosis. (*A*) Chest radiograph shows fine nodular, reticular, and ground-glass opacities more pronounced in the upper and middle lung zones. (*B*) HRCT scan shows areas of peribronchovascular ground-glass attenuation with architectural distortion and traction bronchiectasis.

antigens. A unique form of HP, summer-type HP, in which signs and symptoms appear in summer and subside spontaneously in midautumn, is seen in Japan. HP has recently been described in patients exposed primarily to aerosolized *Mycobacterium avium-intracellulare* complex, and called "hot-tub lung" [54].

HRCT findings in acute HP typically consist of diffuse ground-glass opacity or airspace consolidation. HRCT findings in subacute HP are characterized by small centrilobular nodular opacities and patchy ground-glass opacities showing a mosaic pattern. Expiratory CT scans are useful for detecting air trapping, which may suggest the diagnosis in combination with other features [14]. Chronic HP (CHP) may show features similar to those of subacute HP but may also be associated with irregular fibrotic opacities, traction bronchiectasis, and honeycombing (Fig. 20). Unlike IPF, the fibrosis of CHP is often

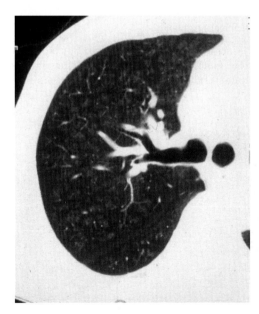

Fig. 18. HRCT scan of welder's siderosis. Ill-defined centrilobular nodules and branching opacities diffusely distribute throughout the lung, mimicking those of HP.

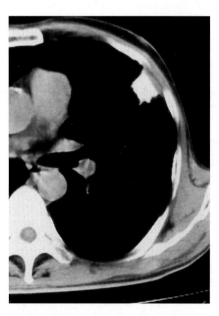

Fig. 19. Organizing pneumonia with welder's siderosis. CT scan at mediastinal windows (level, 30 H; width, 300 H) shows pulmonary mass with high-attenuation material. The transbronchial biopsy specimen from the mass showed organization with siderosis.

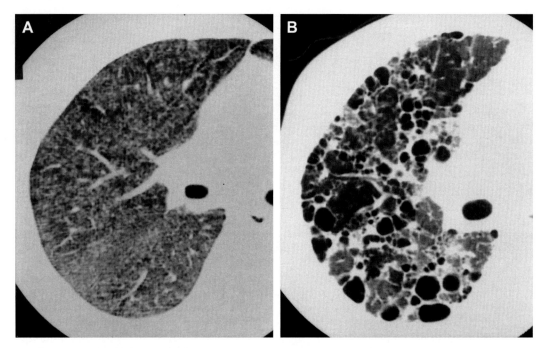

Fig. 20. Initial (*A*) and follow-up (*B*) HRCT scans in a 39-year-old woman with who had repeated episodes of summer-type HP for several years. (*A*) Centrilobular nodules and patchy areas of ground-glass attenuation are diffusely distributed in the lung. (*B*) Follow-up scan obtained 6 years later demonstrates progression of parenchymal changes, forming honeycomb cysts, traction bronchiectasis, bullae, and multilobular areas of low attenuation.

situated predominantly in the upper or middle lung zones or it shows no zonal predominance. The presence of centrilobular nodules on HRCT helps distinguish CHP from IPF. Lobular areas of low attenuation or a mosaic pattern representing air trapping is common in CHP and uncommon in IPF. Thin-walled cysts of 3 to 25 mm in diameter can be seen in patients who have CHP;

however, some cases of CHP may have findings identical to those of UIP [55].

Chemical pneumonitis

Chemical pneumonitis is caused by exposure to toxic fumes of gases such as sulfur dioxide, ammonia, chlorine, phosgene, oxides of nitrogen,

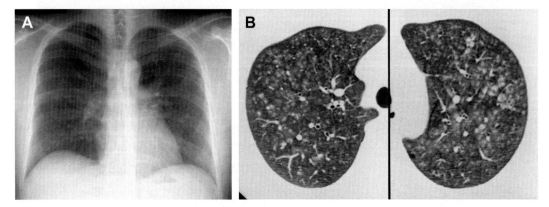

Fig. 21. Images from man who was exposed to chlorine gas. (*A*) Chest radiograph shows patchy areas of consolidation and ground-glass opacity in both lungs. (*B*) HRCT scan shows centrilobular nodular areas of ground-glass attenuation diffusely distributed throughout the lungs.

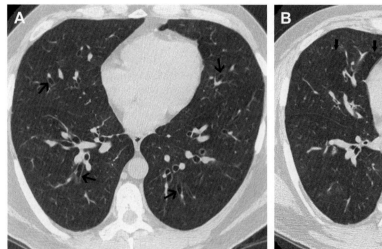
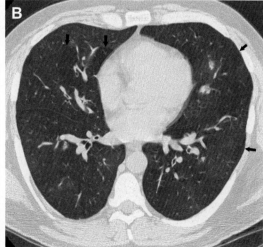

Fig. 22. Flavor workers' lung in a 41-year-old man who had bronchiolitis obliterans related to exposure to diacetyl in flavor manufacturing. (*A*) Inspiratory CT shows widespread cylindric bronchiectasis (*arrows*). (*B*) Expiratory CT shows patchy air trapping (*arrows*). Findings are consistent with severe bronchiolitis obliterans. (*Courtesy of* David A. Lynch, MD, PhD, Denver, CO)

and ozone. Silo filler's disease is an acute lung injury caused by inhalation of nitrogen dioxide in or near an agricultural silo. Highly soluble gases such as ammonia, sulfur dioxide, and hydrochloric acid are absorbed in the upper respiratory tract and result in upper airway irritation. Death may occur as a result of laryngeal edema. A large exposure may result in pulmonary edema. A less soluble gas such as nitrogen dioxide is not removed in the upper passages and reaches the more peripheral areas of the respiratory tree to cause pulmonary edema (Fig. 21) [14]. These patients recover with few pulmonary sequelae. Bronchiolitis obliterans or bronchiectasis has developed in several survivors. An asthmalike condition can arise after a single inhalation of miscellaneous irritant agents, and the condition is known as reactive airways dysfunction syndrome [56].

Newer occupational lung diseases

With evolving occupational exposures, CT has been of assistance in the detection and characterization of novel exposure-related conditions such as flock worker's lung and flavor worker's lung (Fig. 22). Flock worker's lung, related to inhalation of tiny nylon fibers, is characterized by ground-glass abnormality and centrilobular nodularity [57]. Flavor worker's lung, occurring in workers exposed to the flavoring agent diacetyl,

is characterized by mosaic attenuation with expiratory air trapping [58].

Summary

The chest radiograph is the basic tool for identifying occupational and environmental lung diseases; however, its sensitivity and specificity for the diagnosis of occupational and environmental lung diseases are low. HRCT is the optimal method of recognizing parenchymal abnormalities in occupational and environmental disease. MRI and FDG-PET can be useful for the diagnosis and staging of malignancy. With the exception of pleural plaques, the CT findings of occupational and environmental lung diseases are nonspecific. Therefore, correlation of imaging features with history of exposure, other clinical features, and sometimes pathology is needed for the diagnosis of pneumoconiosis.

References

[1] Guidelines for the use of ILO international classification of radiographs of pneumoconiosis, revised edition. Occupational Safety and Health Series no. 22. Geneva, Switzerland: International Labor Organization; 1980.
[2] Akira M, Higashihara T, Yokoyama K, et al. Radiographic type p pneumoconiosis: thin-section CT. Radiology 1898;171:117–23.

[3] Remy-Jardin M, Remy J, Farre I, et al. Computed tomographic evaluation of silicosis and coal worker's pneumoconiosis. Radiol Clin North Am 1992;30:1155–75.

[4] Gevenois PA, Pichot E, Dargent F, et al. Low grade coal worker's pneumoconiosis: comparison of CT and chest radiography. Acta Radiol 1994;35:351–6.

[5] Remy-Jardin M, Remy J, Artaud D, et al. Diffuse infiltrative lung disease: clinical value of sliding-thin-slab maximum intensity projection CT scans in the detection of mild micronodular patterns. Radiology 1996;200:333–9.

[6] Beigelman-Aubry C, Hill C, Guibal A, et al. Multi-detector row CT and postprocessing techniques in the assessment of diffuse lung disease. Radiographics 2005;25:1639–52.

[7] Gevenois PA, De Vuyst P, Dedeire S, et al. Conventional and high-resolution CT in asymptomatic asbestos-exposed workers. Acta Radiol 1994;35:226–9.

[8] Weber M-A, Bock M, Plathow C, et al. Asbestos-related pleural disease: value of dedicated magnetic resonance imaging techniques. Invest Radiol 2004;39:554–64.

[9] Meissner HH, Soo Hoo GW, Khonsary SA, et al. Idiopathic pulmonary fibrosis: evaluation with positron emission tomography. Respiration 2006;73:197–202.

[10] Misumi S, Lynch DA. Idiopathic pulmonary fibrosis/usual interstitial pneumonia: imaging diagnosis, spectrum of abnormalities, and temporal progression. Proc Am Thorac Soc 2006;3:307–14.

[11] Benard F, Sterman D, Smith RJ, et al. Metabolic imaging of malignant pleural mesothelioma with fluorodeoxyglucose positron emission tomography. Chest 1998;114:713–22.

[12] Benard F, Sterman D, Smith RJ, et al. Prognostic value of FDG PET imaging in malignant pleural mesothelioma. J Nucl Med 1999;40:1241–5.

[13] Kim K-II, Kim CW, Lee MK, et al. Imaging of occupational lung disease. Radiographics 2001;21:1371–91.

[14] Akira M. High-resolution CT in the evaluation of occupational and environmental disease. Radiol Clin North Am 2002;40:43–59.

[15] Matsumoto S, Mori H, Miyake H, et al. MRI signal characteristics of progressive massive fibrosis in silicosis. Clin Radiol 1998;53:510–4.

[16] Katabami M, Dosaka-Akita H, Honma K, et al. Pneumoconiosis-related lung cancers: preferential occurrence from diffuse interstitial fibrosis-type pneumoconiosis. Am J Respir Crit Care Med 2000;162:295–300.

[17] Honma K, Chiyotani K. Diffuse interstitial fibrosis in nonasbestos pneumoconiosis—a pathological study. Respiration 1993;60:120–6.

[18] Arakawa H, Johkoh T, Honma K, et al. Chronic interstitial pneumonia in silicosis and mix-dust pneumoconiosis: its prevalence and comparison of CT findings with idiopathic pulmonary fibrosis. Chest 2007;131:1870–6.

[19] Arakawa H, Honma K, Saito Y, et al. Pleural disease in silicosis: pleural thickening, effusion, and invagination. Radiology 2005;236:685–93.

[20] Begin R, Filion R, Ostiguy G. Emphysema in silica- and asbestos-exposed workers seeking compensation. A CT scan study. Chest 1995;108:647–55.

[21] Cowie RL, Hay M, Thomas RG. Association of silicosis, lung dysfunction, and emphysema in gold miners. Thorax 1993;48:746–9.

[22] Hnizdo E, Sluis CG, Baskind E, et al. Emphysema and airway obstruction in non-smoking South African gold miners with long exposure to silica dust. Occup Environ Med 1994;51:557–63.

[23] Arakawa H, Gevenois PA, Saito Y, et al. Silicosis: expiratory thin-section CT assessment of airway obstruction. Radiology 2005;236:1059–66.

[24] Cockcroft A, Berry G, Cotes JE, et al. Shape of small opacities and lung function in coalworkers. Thorax 1982;37:765–9.

[25] Hankinson JL, Palmes ED, Lapp NL. Pulmonary air space size in coal miners. Am Rev Respir Dis 1979;119:391–7.

[26] Rosenstock L, Hudson LD. The pleural manifestations of asbestos exposure. Occup Med 1987;2(2):383–407.

[27] Gefter WB, Conant EF. Issues and controversies in the plain-film diagnosis of asbestos-related disorders in the chest. J Thorac Imaging 1988;3(4):11–28.

[28] Report by the Industrial Injuries Advisory Council in accordance with Section 171 of the Social Security Administration Act 1992:asbestos related diseases. London: Her Majesty's Stationery Office; 1996.

[29] McLoud TC, Woods BO, Carrington CB, et al. Diffuse pleural thickening in the asbestos-exposed population. AJR Am J Roentgenol 1985;144:9–18.

[30] Lynch DA, Gamsu G, Aberle DR. Conventional and high-resolution computed tomography in the diagnosis of asbestos-related diseases. RadioGraphics 1989;9:523–51.

[31] Verschakelen JA, Demaerel P, Coolen J, et al. Rounded atelectasis of the lung: MR appearance. AJR Am J Roentgenol 1989;152:965–6.

[32] Akira M, Yokoyama K, Yamamoto S, et al. Early asbestosis: evaluation with high-resolution CT. Radiology 1991;178:409–16.

[33] Copley SJ, Wells AU, Sivakumaran P, et al. Asbestosis and idiopathic pulmonary fibrosis: comparison of thin-section CT features. Radiology 2003;229:731–6.

[34] Akira M, Yamamoto S, Inoue Y, et al. High-resolution CT of asbestosis and idiopathic pulmonary fibrosis. AJR Am J Roentgenol 2003;181:163–9.

[35] Leung AN, Müller NL, Miller RR. CT in differential diagnosis of diffuse pleural disease. AJR Am J Roentgenol 1990;154:487–92.

[36] Heelan RT, Rusch VW, Begg CB, et al. Staging of malignant pleural mesothelioma: comparison of

CT and MR imaging. AJR Am J Roentgenol 1999; 172:1039–47.

[37] Jones RN, Weill H, Parkes WR. Disease related to non-asbestos silicates. In: Parkes WR, editor. Occupational lung disorders. 3rd edition. London: Butterworths; 1994. p. 536–70.

[38] Akira M, Kozuka T, Yamamoto S, et al. Inhalational talc pneumoconiosis: radiographic and computed tomographic findings in 14 patients. AJR Am J Roentgenol 2007;188:326–33.

[39] Padley SPG, Adler BD, Staples CA, et al. Pulmonary talcosis: CT findings in three cases. Radiology 1993;186:125–7.

[40] Ward S, Heyneman LE, Reittner P, et al. Talcosis associated with IV abuse of oral medications: CT findings. AJR Am J Roentgenol 2000;174:789–93.

[41] Lynch DA. Beryllium-related diseases. In: Gevenois PA, De Vyust P, editors. Imaging of occupational and environmental disorders of the chest (Medical Radiology, Diagnostic Imaging and Radiation Oncology). Berlin: Springer-Verlag; 2006. p. 249–56.

[42] Nemery B, Verbeken EK, Demedts M. Giant cell interstitial pneumonia (hard metal lung disease, cobalt lung). Semin Respir Crit Care Med 2001;22:435–48.

[43] Verougstraete V, Mallants A, Buchet J-P, et al. Lung function changes in workers exposed to cobalt compounds. A 13-year follow-up. Am J Respir Crit Care Med 2004;170:162–6.

[44] Akira M. Uncommon pneumoconioses: CT and pathologic findings. Radiology 1995;197:403–9.

[45] Gotway MB, Golden JA, Warnock M, et al. Hard metal interstitial lung disease: high-resolution computed tomography appearance. J Thorac Imaging 2002;17:314–8.

[46] Choi JW, Lee KS, Chung MP, et al. Giant cell interstitial pneumonia: high-resolution CT and pathologic findings in four adult patients. AJR Am J Roentgenol 2005;184:268–72.

[47] Maier LA. Clinical approach to chronic beryllium disease and other nonpneumoconiotic interstitial lung diseases. J Thorac Imaging 2002;17:273–84.

[48] Nemery B. Metal toxicity and the respiratory tract. Eur Respir J 1990;3:202–19.

[49] Vahlensieck M, Overlack A, Müller K-M. Computed tomographic high-attenuation mediastinal lymph nodes after aluminum exposition. Eur Radiol 2000;10:1945–6.

[50] Kraus T, Schaller KH, Angerer J, et al. Aluminosis—detection of an almost forgotten disease with HRCT. J Occup Med Toxicol 2006;1:4–12.

[51] Sferlazza SJ, Beckett WS. The respiratory health of welders. State of the art. Am Rev Respir Dis 1991; 143:1134–48.

[52] Sung JH, Choi B-G, Maeng S-H, et al. Recovery from welding-fume-exposure-induced lung fibrosis and pulmonary function changes in Sprague Dawley rats. Toxicol Sci 2004;82:608–13.

[53] Yoshii C, Matsuyama T, Takazawa A, et al. Welder's pneumoconiosis: diagnostic usefulness of high-resolution computed tomography and ferritin determinations in bronchoalveolar lavage fluid. Intern Med 2002;41:1111–7.

[54] Embil J, Warren P, Yakrus M, et al. Pulmonary illness associated with exposure to mycobacterium-avium complex in hot tub water: hypersensitivity pneumonitis or infection? Chest 1997;111:813–6.

[55] Lynch DA, Newell JD, Logan PM, et al. Can CT distinguish hypersensitivity pneumonitis from idiopathic pulmonary fibrosis? AJR Am J Roentgenol 1995;165:807–11.

[56] Rabinowitz PM, Siegel MD. Acute inhalational injury. Clin Chest Med 2002;23:707–15.

[57] Weiland DA, Lynch DA, Jensen SP, et al. Thin-section CT findings in flock worker's lung, a work-related interstitial lung disease. Radiology 2003; 227:222–31.

[58] Akpinar-Elci M, Travis WD, Lynch DA, et al. Bronchiolitis obliterans syndrome in popcorn production plant workers. Eur Respir J 2004;24: 298–302.

CLINICS
IN CHEST
MEDICINE

Clin Chest Med 29 (2008) 133–147

Imaging of Idiopathic Interstitial Pneumonias

Takeshi Johkoh, MD, PhD

Department of Radiology, Kinki Central Hospital of Mutual Aid Association of Public School Teachers,
Kurumazuka 3-1, Itami, Hyogo 664-8533, Japan

Idiopathic interstitial pneumonias are a heterogeneous group of diseases characterized histologically by inflammation and fibrosis of the parenchymal interstitial tissue. Their cause is unknown, and some degree of airspace disease commonly accompanies the interstitial abnormality in all these conditions. Idiopathic interstitial pneumonias are classified into acute interstitial pneumonia (AIP), cryptogenic organizing pneumonia (COP), nonspecific interstitial pneumonia (NSIP), usual interstitial pneumonia (UIP), desquamative interstitial pneumonia (DIP), respiratory bronchiolitis–associated interstitial lung disease (RB-ILD), and lymphoid interstitial pneumonia (LIP) [1]. In this article, the imaging findings of each idiopathic interstitial pneumonia are described, paying special attention to the characteristic CT findings.

Acute interstitial pneumonia

AIP is a rapidly progressive and histologically distinct form of interstitial pneumonia. Clinically, respiratory failure develops over days or a week. Its pathologic finding is described as diffuse alveolar damage (DAD) that is indistinguishable from the histologic pattern found in acute respiratory distress syndrome (ARDS) [2]. In early disease, histologic abnormalities consist of alveolar wall thickening by edema fluid and inflammatory cells, alveolar airspace filling by proteinaceous exudates, and hyaline membranes on the surface of transitional airways (Fig. 1). Fibroblastic tissue increases in amount as the disease progresses and is eventually transformed into mature collagen.

The pathologic appearance of DAD can be separated into acute exudative, subacute proliferative or organized, and chronic fibrotic phases.

Typical radiologic findings consist of bilateral airspace consolidation and ground-glass opacity [3]. The appearance rapidly changes and the extent of abnormalities increases within a few days. This rapid evolution is an important feature for the diagnosis of AIP. Typical CT or high-resolution CT (HRCT) findings of this condition include extensive areas of ground-glass attenuation and patchy areas of airspace consolidation (see Fig. 1; Fig. 2) [3–5]. Other common findings are architectural distortion, traction bronchiectasis, thickening of bronchovascular bundles, and thickening of interlobular septa. No zonal predominance is found.

The extent of ground-glass attenuation and traction bronchiectasis increases as disease evolves and fibrosis develops [4,5]. Ichikado and colleagues [6] established a scoring system that calculates the amount of ground-glass attenuation and the extent of traction bronchiectasis and found that it is a reliable predictor of prognosis of AIP. Ichikado and colleagues [4] correlated the HRCT and histologic findings in 14 patients who had pathologically proved AIP. Areas of ground-glass attenuation and consolidation without traction bronchiectasis were present in the exudative or early proliferative phases, whereas traction bronchiectasis was seen in the late proliferative and fibrotic phases (see Figs. 1 and 2). Honeycombing is seen in a small number of patients and correlates with the presence of interstitial fibrosis, alveolar destruction, and dilatation of distal airspace [4,5].

Tomiyama and colleagues [7] compared thin-section CT findings from 25 patients who had

E-mail address: johkoh@sahs.med.osaka-u.ac.jp

0272-5231/08/$ - see front matter © 2008 Elsevier Inc. All rights reserved.
doi:10.1016/j.ccm.2007.11.006

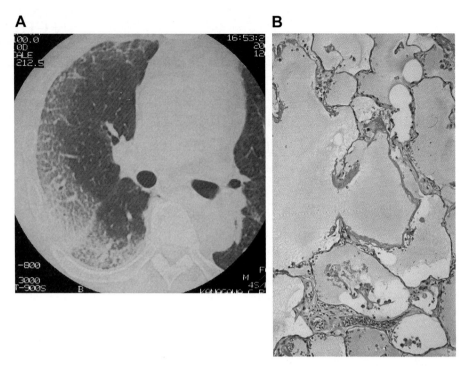

Fig. 1. AIP. (*A*) HRCT shows diffuse ground-glass attenuation in the peripheral lung zone. Note that signs of architectural distortion such as traction bronchiectasis are not seen. (*B*) A photomicrograph demonstrates hyaline membranes along alveolar duct and alveolar filling by exudates. This patient is in the exudative phase of AIP (hemotoxiline-eosine, original magnification ×10).

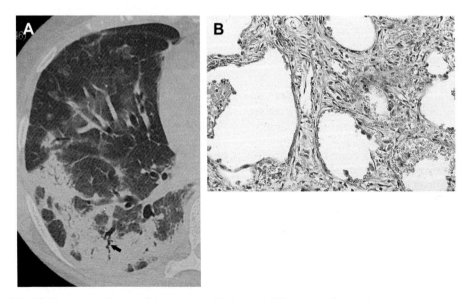

Fig. 2. AIP. (*A*) Nonsegmental areas of airspace consolidation and diffuse areas of ground-glass attenuation are seen on HRCT. Airspace consolidation in the dependent lung is accompanied by traction bronchiectasis (*arrow*) and loss of volume. (*B*) Photomicrograph demonstrating organizing DAD (hemotoxiline-eosine, original magnification ×10).

ARDS with those from 25 patients who had AIP. Patients who had AIP had a greater prevalence of honeycombing and were more likely to have a symmetric bilateral distribution than patients who had ARDS. The high prevalence of honeycombing may be due to some cases of AIP being superimposed on previously unrecognized UIP.

Cryptogenic organizing pneumonia

COP is a clinicopathologic entity described by Davison and colleagues [8] and was previously called bronchiolitis obliterans organizing pneumonia (BOOP) [9]. Although the term *BOOP* is still commonly used, the term *COP* is preferred because it conveys the essential features of the

syndrome as described in the following text and avoids confusion with airway disease [1].

COP is pathologically characterized by the presence of fibroblastic tissue within alveolar airspace and the lumina of respiratory bronchioles and alveolar ducts and by a variable degree of fibrosis and chronic inflammation of the parenchymal interstitium (Fig. 3) [8,9]. Katzenstein and Myers [10] claimed that COP should be excluded from idiopathic interstitial pneumonias because parenchymal interstitial abnormalities are not prominent. The author, however, believes that COP should be included in the classification of idiopathic interstitial pneumonias because of its idiopathic nature and its tendency on occasion to be confused with other forms of idiopathic

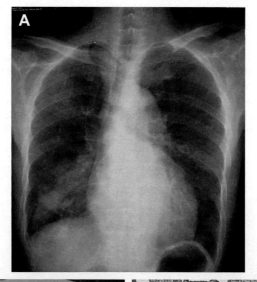

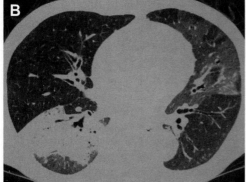
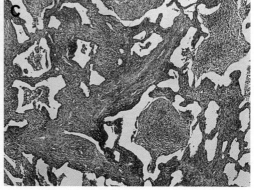

Fig. 3. COP. (*A*) Chest radiograph shows consolidation in the right lower lung. Ground-glass opacity is seen in right upper and left middle lung. (*B*) An area of airspace consolidation is seen in right lower lobe on HRCT. Ground-glass attenuation is present in the left lung. (*C*) Photomicrograph from the area of airspace consolidation shows diffuse intraluminal organizing pneumonia (hemotoxiline-eosine, original magnification ×10).

interstitial pneumonias. Patients who have idiopathic COP typically present with a 1- to 6-month history of nonproductive cough; low-grade fever, malaise, and shortness of breath [9].

The most common radiographic findings are bilateral or unilateral airspace consolidation (see Fig. 3) [8,9,11]. Irregular linear opacities may be present, but they are seldom a major feature. Sometimes, large nodular opacities (> 1 cm) are seen. The distribution is usually patchy. In some patients, the consolidation has a peripheral and subpleural distribution similar to that seen in chronic eosinophilic pneumonia [11,12].

Typical CT findings also consist of unilateral or bilateral areas of airspace consolidation (see Fig. 3) [13–15]. Subpleural distribution, peribronchial distribution, or both are seen in almost 60% of cases (see Fig. 3) [15]. Areas of ground-glass attenuation are also common. Thirty percent to 50% of cases show small, ill-defined nodules, and they are more common in immune-compromised patients than in immune-competent patients [15]. Air bronchiolograms with traction bronchiectasis may be seen in patients who have extensive consolidation, and are usually restricted to these areas. Large nodules or masslike areas of consolidation are occasionally seen (Fig. 4) [16].

These nodules sometimes show irregular borders or spiculation, mimicking adenocarcinoma. Sometimes, COP shows unique findings such as the reversed halo sign (Fig. 5) [17] and perilobular pattern (Fig. 6) [18]. Reversed halo sign is defined as central ground-glass opacity surrounded by more dense airspace consolidation of crescentic and ring shapes. This sign is seen in 19% of patients who have COP [17]. The perilobular region comprises the structures bordering secondary pulmonary lobules, such as interlobular septa, pleura, pulmonary veins, large bronchus, and large pulmonary arteries [19,20]. Perilobular pattern is defined as predominant distribution of airspace consolidation at the periphery of the secondary pulmonary lobule. In one report, 57% of patients who had COP had this finding [18].

The areas of airspace consolidation on CT correspond histologically to the regions of lung parenchyma that show accumulation of organizing exudate (intraluminal organization) (see Fig. 3) [13,21]. Areas of ground-glass attenuation correlate with areas of alveolar septal inflammation and minimal intraluminal organization (see Fig. 4) [21]. Accumulation of organizing exudate in the perilobular alveoli contributes to reversed halo sign and perilobular pattern [17,18,20].

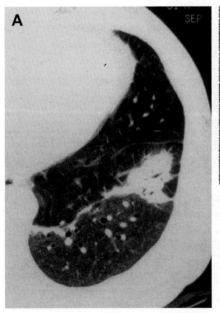
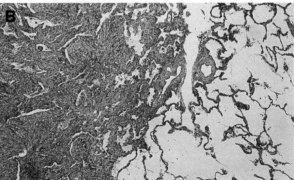

Fig. 4. COP. (*A*) A nodule with irregular border is seen in the left lower lobe on HRCT. Ground-glass abnormality is also present. (*B*) The nodule on CT histologically corresponds to intraluminal organization and airspace consolidation (hemotoxiline-eosine, original magnification ×10). The ground-glass attenuation correlates with alveolar septal inflammation.

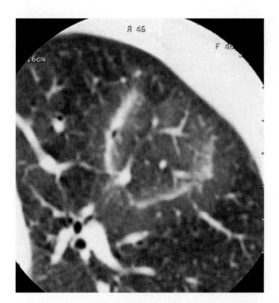

Fig. 5. COP. HRCT demonstrates a central ground-glass opacity surrounded by a ring-shaped area of more dense airspace consolidation, representing the reversed halo sign. (*Courtesy of* Dr. Masahiko Kusumoto, National Cancer Center, Tokyo, Japan).

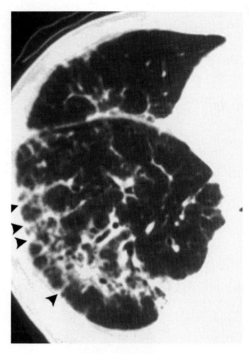

Fig. 6. COP. Linear areas of airspace consolidation are distributed along perilobular structures on HRCT (*arrowheads*). This finding is called a perilobular pattern.

Nonspecific interstitial pneumonia

Lung biopsy samples from some patients who have idiopathic interstitial disease do not fit into any well-defined histologic patterns of idiopathic interstitial pneumonia. The recognition of such diseases led to proposals of the term *nonspecific interstitial pneumonia* by Katzenstein and Fiorelli [22]. NSIP is characterized histologically by interstitial inflammation and fibrosis without specific features that allow a diagnosis of other idiopathic interstitial pneumonias [10,22]. It is therefore largely a diagnosis of exclusion.

Katzenstein and Fiorelli [22] divided NSIP into three major subgroups based on the amount of inflammation and fibrosis in the lung biopsies: group I primarily involves interstitial inflammation (Fig. 7); group II involves inflammation and fibrosis (Fig. 8); and group III primarily involves fibrosis (Fig. 9). The prognosis of NSIP correlates with differences in the dominant pathology—whether a cellular or fibrotic pattern of NSIP is present and dominates [22–25]. At the cellular end of the spectrum, the NSIP pattern consists primary of mild to moderate interstitial chronic inflammation, usually with lymphocytes and a few plasma cells [10,22,25]. The lung typically is uniformly involved, but the distribution of the lesions is often patchy. At

the fibrotic end of the spectrum, the NSIP pattern consists of dense or loose interstitial fibrosis in varying degrees, and the connective tissue is temporally homogeneous [22–25]. In some cases, the pattern of fibrosis is patchy in distribution, causing remodeling of the lung architecture [24].

The radiographic findings consist mainly of ground-glass opacity or airspace consolidation involving predominantly the lower lung zone (see Fig. 7). A reticular pattern or a combination of reticular and ground-glass pattern is also seen [26]. Loss of volume is commonly seen (see Fig. 7).

The most common CT manifestations consist of patchy or confluent areas of ground-glass attenuation, often with lower or peribronchiolar predominance, patchy areas of airspace consolidation, and intralobular reticulation (see Figs. 7–9) [26,27]. Loss of volume and traction bronchiectasis, indicating architectural distortion, are commonly seen on CT (see Figs. 8 and 9) [27]. Although honeycombing may be present, it tends to be mild. Johkoh and colleagues [27] correlated CT findings with pathologic subgroups in 55 patients. The extent of traction bronchiectasis and intralobular reticulation at thin-section CT correlated with increased fibrosis in NSIP.

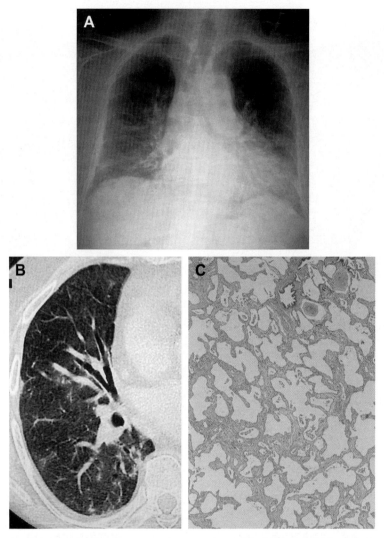

Fig. 7. NSIP Group I. (*A*) Chest radiograph shows ground-glass opacities in both lower lungs. (*B*) HRCT demonstrates peribronchovascular ground-glass attenuation in the right lower lung. Note that traction bronchiectasis is not seen. (*C*) Pure alveolar septal inflammation is the only finding on photomicrograph (hemotoxiline-eosine, original magnification ×10).

One report compared HRCT with the pathologic findings in NSIP [28]. The areas of ground-glass attenuation corresponded histologically to alveolar septal thickening by inflammatory cells and fibrous tissue (see Fig. 7), whereas the areas of consolidation were related to intraluminal organization or foci of honeycombing in which the cystic spaces were filled with mucus (see Figs. 8 and 9). Recently, Manganas and colleagues [29] suggested that the cases that had airspace consolidation should be excluded from NSIP and diagnosed as COP because airspace consolidation often corresponded to intraluminal organization.

Tsubamoto and colleagues [30] evaluated whether the subtypes of NSIP could be differentiated from other idiopathic interstitial pneumonias on the basis of findings on HRCT. Group I NSIP was misdiagnosed as AIP, as DIP or RB-ILD, and as LIP in 8.3% of patients. Group II NSIP was misdiagnosed as COP in 10% of patients, as LIP in 6.7%, as AIP in 3.3%, and as DIP or RB-ILD in 3.3%, respectively. Group III NSIP was misdiagnosed as UIP in 6.7% of patients, as COP in 6.7%, and as DIP or RB-ILD in 3.3%. In most patients, NSIP can be distinguished from other idiopathic interstitial pneumonias based on

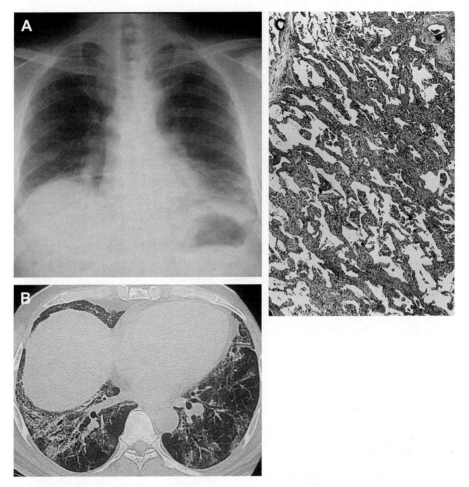

Fig. 8. NSIP Group II. (*A*) Chest radiograph shows ground-glass opacities and loss of volume in both lower lungs. (*B*) Areas of ground-glass attenuation and reticular abnormality along bronchi and bronchioles are seen on HRCT. Traction bronchiectasis is also seen. (*C*) In addition to alveolar septal inflammation, photomicrograph shows fibrosis in alveolar septa and lumens (hemotoxiline-eosine, original magnification ×10).

the findings on HRCT. Only a small percentage of patients who had predominantly fibrotic NSIP (group 1, 2, 3 NSIP) showed overlap with the HRCT findings of UIP.

Usual interstitial pneumonia

UIP is the most common type of interstitial pneumonia and corresponds to the clinical diagnosis of idiopathic pulmonary fibrosis (IPF). IPF occurs most commonly in patients aged 50 to 70 years [1,10]. Its prognosis is poor, with a mean survival of approximately 4 years from the onset of symptoms [10,31]. Periods of rapid decline are sometimes recognized, and this rapidly progressive phase is called acute exacerbation [32].

The important histologic findings consist of architectural distortion, fibrosis (often with honeycombing), scattered fibroblastic foci, patchy distribution, and involvement of the periphery of the lobule [10,25]. It has a heterogeneous appearance at low magnification, with alternating areas of normal lung, interstitial inflammation, fibrosis, and honeycombing change ("spatial heterogeneity") (Fig. 10). This admixture of normal tissue, new inflammation, and old fibrosis is also referred to as "temporal heterogeneity." The histologic changes affect the peripheral subpleural parenchyma most severely. In patients who have acute exacerbation, the pathologic findings are a combination of UIP and DAD or organizing pneumonia (Fig. 11) [32].

140 JOHKOH

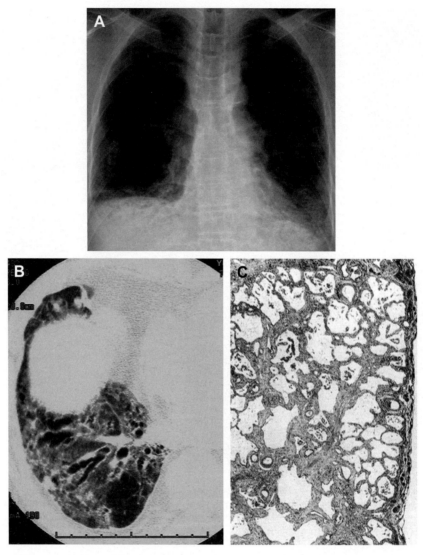

Fig. 9. NSIP Group III. (*A*) Chest radiograph shows ground-glass opacity, fine reticular abnormality, and loss of volume in both lower lungs. (*B*) HRCT shows ground-glass attenuation and fine reticular abnormality along bronchi and bronchioles. Traction bronchiectasis is widespread. (*C*) Pure alveolar septal fibrosis is widely distributed on micrograph (hemotoxiline-eosine, original magnification ×10).

The radiographic findings of UIP consist of bilateral irregular linear opacities, causing a reticular pattern (see Fig. 10) [33,34]. A predominance of lower lung zones and loss of lung volume is commonly seen. The reticular pattern is initially fine, becoming coarser as fibrosis progresses. The end stage of UIP shows diffuse honeycombing.

The characteristic CT findings consist of intralobular reticular opacities and honeycombing distributing mainly in the subpleural regions and lung bases (see Fig. 10) [1,35]. The bronchioles and bronchi in areas of fibrosis are often dilated and tortuous (traction bronchiolectasis and bronchiectasis) As is seen histologically, parenchymal involvement is typically patchy on CT, with areas of normal and markedly abnormal lung often present in the same lobe, and sometimes even in the same lobule. Honeycombing is seen on CT in most cases and typically involves the subpleural regions and lung bases [35,36]. Honeycombing on CT is defined as clustered cystic airspaces usually

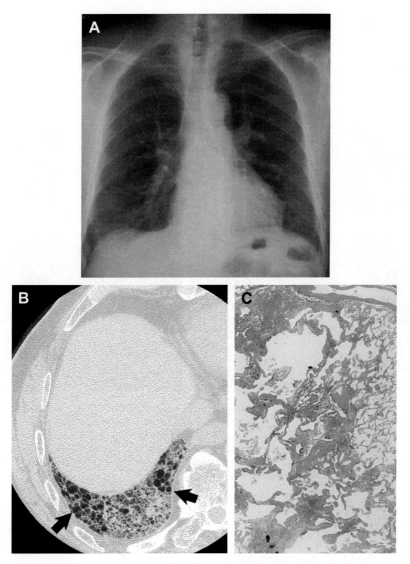

Fig. 10. UIP. (*A*) Chest radiograph shows ground-glass opacity, reticular abnormality, and loss of volume in both lower lungs. (*B*) Honeycombing (*arrows*), ground-glass attenuation, and reticular abnormality are seen in the same area on HRCT. This appearance corresponds to pathologic temporal heterogeneity. (*C*) Photomicrograph has a heterogeneous appearance at low magnification, with alternating areas of normal lung, interstitial inflammation, fibrosis, and honeycombing change ("spatial and temporal heterogeneity") (hemotoxiline-eosine, original magnification ×10).

measuring 2 to 10 mm in diameter and having well-defined walls (see Fig. 8). The cysts typically share walls and usually occur in several layers. The presence of predominantly subpleural and basal reticulation and honeycombing on CT is practically diagnostic of UIP. This combination had a positive predictive value of 96% in the diagnosis of IPF [37]. Irregular thickening of interlobular septa and patchy areas of ground-

glass attenuation are commonly seen but are less conspicuous than intralobular reticular opacity and honeycombing [35,36].

The intralobular reticular opacities reflect the presence of periacinar septal fibrosis [38]. Irregular thickening of interlobular septa reflects the presence of fibrosis in the periphery of the secondary pulmonary lobules [20,39,40]. Areas of ground-glass attenuation correspond to alveolar

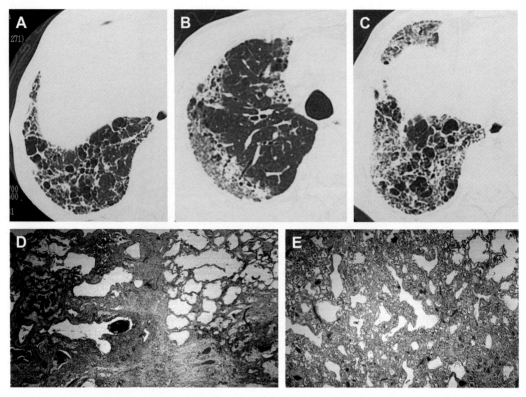

Fig. 11. Acute exacerbation of UIP. (*A*) HRCT through the right lower lung before onset of acute exacerbation shows typical findings of UIP including honeycombing, reticular opacities, and peripheral predominance. (*B*, *C*) At onset of acute exacerbation, diffuse nonsegmental areas of ground-glass attenuation are seen on CT, superimposed on background of reticular abnormality and honeycombing. (*D*) One pathologic specimen shows typical findings of UIP including spatial heterogeneity (hemotoxiline-eosine, original magnification ×10). (*E*) Another specimen demonstrates organizing DAD (hemotoxiline-eosine, original magnification ×10).

septal inflammation or to fibrosis below the resolution of HRCT [41]. Ground-glass attenuation should be considered to represent inflammation only when there are no associated CT findings of fibrosis such as intralobular reticular opacities, honeycombing, and traction bronchiectasis in the same area [42].

The CT findings of acute exacerbation consist of extensive multifocal, diffuse, or peripheral ground-glass attenuation superimposed on a background of chronic fibrosis (see Fig. 11) [43,44]. A retrospective review of 17 cases of acute exacerbation of IPF identified three HRCT patterns of increasing opacification: peripheral (n = 6), multifocal (n = 6), and diffuse (n = 5). All cases were bilateral. On biopsy, the peripheral pattern of abnormality on CT was associated with the presence of active fibroblastic foci and had good prognosis, whereas the multifocal and diffuse patterns

were associated with more typical features of acute DAD superimposed on UIP and had poor prognosis [43].

Using univariate and multivariate analyses, Sumikawa and colleagues [45] retrospectively analyzed CT findings of chronic idiopathic interstitial pneumonias to determine which findings were most helpful for distinguishing idiopathic interstitial pneumonia (especially NSIP) from UIP. Multivariate logistic regression analysis showed that the independent findings distinguishing UIP from cellular NSIP were the extent of honeycombing and the most proximal bronchus with traction bronchiectasis (odds ratios, 5.16 and 0.37, respectively); the finding that distinguished UIP from fibrotic NSIP was the extent of honeycombing (odds ratio, 2.10). Thus, the most useful finding when differentiating UIP from NSIP is the extent of honeycombing [45].

Desquamative interstitial pneumonia

DIP is an uncommon form of idiopathic interstitial pneumonia that occurs most frequently in patients between 40 and 50 years old [33]. Approximately 90% of patients are cigarette smokers [33,46]. DIP is more common in men than in women by a ratio of 2:1. The prognosis of DIP is generally good. Most patients improve with smoking cessation and corticosteroids [33]. The overall survival rate is about 70% after 10 years [10,33].

A characteristic pathologic finding of DIP is the presence of numerous macrophages within alveolar airspaces (Fig. 12) [10,33]. This involvement is typically uniform in severity within affected lobes. Interstitial inflammation and fibrosis are usually mild but may be moderate to severe.

On chest radiography, ground-glass opacity is commonly seen in the lower lung zones [33]. Peripheral predominance is sometimes found.

Areas of ground-glass attenuation are present on CT in all cases (see Fig. 12) [46]. DIP has a lower zone distribution in most cases and a peripheral distribution in almost 60% of cases. Irregular linear opacities and intralobular reticular opacities are frequent but limited in extent and usually confined to the lungs. Cysts and emphysematous changes are also seen, presumably due to accompanying emphysema (Fig. 13). Honeycombing is uncommon.

Areas of ground-glass attenuation are due to a combination of diffuse filling of alveolar airspaces by macrophages and diffuse mild septal fibrosis [47]. Irregular linear opacities and intralobular reticular opacities are presumed to correlate with alveolar septal fibrosis.

Respiratory bronchiolitis–interstitial lung disease

Respiratory bronchiolitis (RB) is a common incidental finding in cigarette smokers and is also

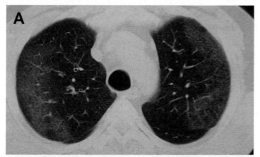
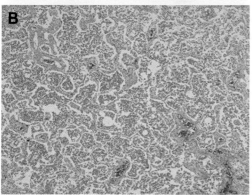

Fig. 12. DIP. (*A*) Homogeneous areas of ground-glass attenuation show nonsegmental and subpleural distribution on HRCT. (*B*) Photomicrograph shows the presence of numerous macrophages within alveolar airspaces (hemotoxiline-eosine, original magnification ×10).

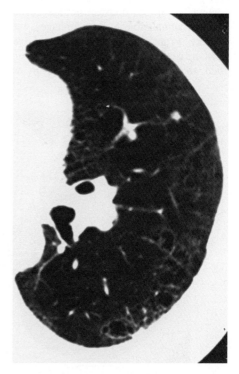

Fig. 13. DIP. In addition to areas of ground-glass attenuation, paraseptal emphysema and numerous cysts are seen on HRCT.

called "smoker's bronchiolitis" [48,49]. It is characterized histologically by the presence of macrophages within respiratory bronchioles and adjacent alveoli (Fig. 14) [48,49]. RB by itself is not associated with any symptoms [1]; however, a small percentage of patients have more extensive disease that looks like interstitial lung disease (ILD) [1,48,49]. This condition (RB-ILD) occurs most frequently in patients between 30 and 40 years old [50,51].

There is some overlap between the histologic findings of RB-ILD and those of DIP. Histologically, RB-ILD has a bronchiolocentric distribution, whereas DIP is diffuse [1]. In addition, some patients who have DIP are never-smokers [52]; therefore, although RB-ILD and DIP may represent different parts of a spectrum [53], they are currently considered separate entities [1,52].

Almost 30% of patients who have RB-ILD have a normal chest radiograph, whereas ground-glass shadows or mild reticular shadows can be seen on chest radiographs of the remaining 70% [54,55].

The most common CT findings consist of centrilobular nodules (see Fig. 11), areas with ground-glass attenuation, and bronchial wall thickening [53,55]. Centrilobular nodules correlate with the accumulation of macrophages within respiratory bronchioles and adjacent alveoli, whereas areas with ground-glass attenuation correspond to macophage accumulation in wide areas of alveolar ducts and alveoli (see Fig. 14) [55]. The abnormalities can involve all lobes but tend to have an upper-lobe predominance. Smoking-related centrilobular emphysema is commonly present.

Lymphoid interstitial pneumonia

LIP is a clinicopathologic term [56,57]. Its histologic characteristic is polyclonal proliferation of lymphoid cells with diffuse infiltration of the pulmonary interstitium. LIP is female predominant. The average age of patients is 50 years. Clinical symptoms include dyspnea, cough, and chest pain [56,57].

The American Thoracic Society/European Respiratory Society 2002 consensus report defined LIP as an interstitial pneumonia [1] because its clinical and radiologic presentation enters the differential diagnosis of diffuse lung disease and, histologically, its pattern is unequivocally that of an interstitial pneumonia. In this definition, the term *LIP* is limited to conditions with extensive alveolar septal lymphocytic infiltration based on the concept that LIP is one of the interstitial pneumonias [2].

Characteristic CT findings of LIP diagnosed by recent criteria have been unclear. The author has seen some cases of LIP with lower-lobe predominant ground-glass attenuation (Fig. 15). Honeycombing and cysts were also seen on CT (see

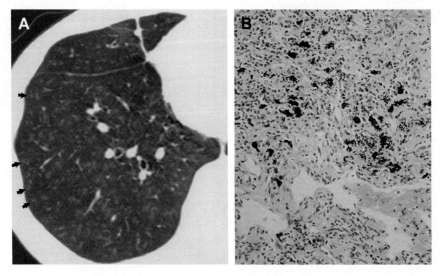

Fig. 14. RB-ILD. (*A*) Diffuse centrilobular ground-glass opacities are seen on CT (*arrows*). (*B*) Photomicrograph demonstrates macrophages within respiratory bronchioles and adjacent alveoli (hemotoxiline-eosine, original magnification ×10).

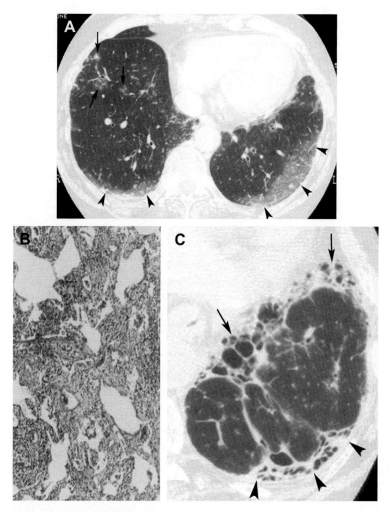

Fig. 15. LIP. (*A*) Areas of ground-glass attenuation (*arrowheads*) show nonsegmental and subpleural distribution on HRCT. Centrilobular and peribronchovascular ground-glass opacities (*arrows*) are also seen. (*B*) Photomicrograph demonstrates extensive alveolar septal infiltration by lymphoid cells (hemotoxiline-eosine, original magnification ×10). (*C*) Two years later, the areas of subpleural ground-glass attenuation have evolved into cysts (*arrows*) or honey-combing (*arrowheads*).

Fig. 15). Further investigations are necessary to clarify the characteristic imaging findings of LIP.

Recognizing and understanding the characteristic imaging findings of idiopathic interstitial pneumonias requires substantial experience. It is hoped that this review article will be a useful tool for the daily clinical practice of general chest physicians and radiologists.

References

[1] American Thoracic Society/European Respiratory Society. International Multidisciplinary Consensus Classification of the idiopahtic interstitial pneumonias. Am J Respir Crit Care Med 2002;165: 277–304.

[2] Katzenstein AL, Myers JL, Mazur MT. Acute interstitial pneumonia. A clinicopathologic, ultrastructural, and cell kinetic study. Am J Surg Pathol 1986;10:256–67.

[3] Primack SL, Hartman TE, Ikezoe J, et al. Acute interstitial pneumonia: radiographic and CT findings in nine patients. Radiology 1993;188:817–20.

[4] Ichikado K, Johkoh T, Ikezoe J, et al. Acute interstitial pneumonia: high-resolution CT findings correlated with pathology. AJR Am J Roentgenol 1997; 168:333–8.

[5] Johkoh T, Müller NL, Taniguchi H, et al. Acute interstitial pneumonia: thin-section CT findings in 36 patients. Radiology 1999;211:859–63.

[6] Ichikado K, Suga M, Muranaka H, et al. Prediction of prognosis for acute respiratory distress syndrome with thin-section CT: validation in 44 cases. Radiology 2006;238:321–9.

[7] Tomiyama N, Müller NL, Johkoh T, et al. Acute respiratory distress syndrome and acute interstitial pneumonia: comparison of thin-section CT findings. J Comput Assist Tomogr 2001;25:28–33.

[8] Davison AG, Heard BE, McAllister WAC, et al. Cryptogenic organizing pneumonias. Q J Med 1983;207:382–94.

[9] Epler GR, Colby TV, McLoud TC, et al. Bronchiolitis obliterans organizing pneumonia. N Engl J Med 1985;312:152–8.

[10] Katzenstein AL, Myers JL. Idiopathic pulmonary fibrosis: clinical relevance of pathological classification. Am J Respir Crit Care Med 1998;157: 1301–15.

[11] Müller NL, Guerry-Force ML, Staples CA, et al. Differential diagnosis of bronchiolitis obliterans with organizing pneumonia and usual interstitial pneumonia: clinical functional, and radiologic findings. Radiology 1987;162:151–6.

[12] Bartter T, Irwin RS, Nash G, et al. Idioapthic bronchiolitis obliterans organizing pneumonia with peripheral infiltrates on chest radiogram. Arch Intern Med 1989;149:273–9.

[13] Müller NL, Staples CA, Miller RR. Bronchiolitis obliterans organizing pneumonia. CT features in 14 patiensts. AJR Am J Roentgenol 1990;154:983–7.

[14] Bouchardy LM, Kuhiman JE, Ball WC, et al. CT findings in bronchiolitis obliterans organizing pneumonia (BOOP) with radiographic, clinical, and histologic correlation. J Comput Assist Tomogr 1993;17:352–7.

[15] Lee KS, Kullnig P, Hartman TE, et al. Cryptogenic organizing pneumonia: CT features in 43 patients. AJR Am J Roentgenol 1994;162:569–74.

[16] Akira M, Yamamoto S, Sakatani M. Bronchiolitis obliterans organizing pneumonia manifesting as multiple large nodules or masses. AJR Am J Roentgenol 1998;170:291–5.

[17] Kim SJ, Lee KS, Ryu YH, et al. Reversed halo sign on high-resolution CT of cryptogenic organizing: diagnostic implications. AJR Am J Roentgenol 2003;180:1251–4.

[18] Ujita M, Renzonl EA, Veeraraghaven S, et al. Organizing pneumonia: perilobular pattern at thin-section CT. Radiology 2004;232:757–61.

[19] Murata K, Khan A, Herman PG. Pulmonary parenchymal disease: evaluation with high-resolution CT. Radiology 1989;170:629–35.

[20] Johkoh T, Müller NL, Ichikado K, et al. Perilobular pulmonary opacities: high-resolution CT findings and pathologic correlation. J Thorac Imaging 1999;14:172–7.

[21] Nishimura K, Itoh H. High-resolution computed tomographic features of bronchiolitis obliterans organizing pneumonia. Chest 1992;102:26S–31S.

[22] Katzenstein AL, Fiorelli RF. Nonspecific interstitial pneumonia/fibrosis. Histologic features and clinical significance. Am J Surg Pathol 1994;18:136–47.

[23] Bjoraker JA, Ryu JH, Edwin MK, et al. Prognostic siginificance of histologic subsets in idiopathic pulmonary fibrosis. Am J Respir Crit Care Med 1998;157:99–103.

[24] Nagai S, Kitaichi M, Itoh H, et al. Idiopathic nonspecific interstitial pneumonia/fibrosis: comparison with idiopathic pulmonary fibrosis and BOOP. Eur Respir J 1998;12:1010–9.

[25] Travis WD, Matsui K, Moss JE, et al. Idiopathic nonspecific interstitial pneumonia: prognostic significance of cellular and fibrosis patterns. Survival comparison with usual interstitial pneumonia and desquamative interstitial pneumonia. Am J Surg Pathol 2000;24:19–33.

[26] Park JS, Lee KS, Kim JS, et al. Nonspecific interstitial pneumonia with fibrosis: radiographic and CT findings in seven patients. Radiology 1995;195:645–8.

[27] Johkoh T, Müller NL, Colby TV, et al. Nonspecific interstitial pneumonia: correlation between thin-section CT findings and pathologic subgroups in 55 patients. Radiology 2002;225:199–204.

[28] Kim TS, Lee KS, Chung MP, et al. Nonspecific interstitial pneumonia with fibrosis: high-resolution CT and pathologic findings. AJR Am J Roentgenol 1998;171:1645–50.

[29] Manganas H, Desai S, Hansell DM, et al. Organizing pneumonia with or without fibrosis: computed tomography prognostic determinants. Am J Respir Crit Care Med 2007;175:A150.

[30] Tsubamoto M, Müller NL, Johkoh T, et al. Pathologic subgroups of nonspecific interstitial pneumonia: differential diagnosis from other idiopathic interstitial pneumonias on high-resolution computed tomography. J Comput Assist Tomogr 2005;29:793–800.

[31] American Thoracic Society. Idiopathic pulmonary fibrosis: diagnosis and treatment. International consensus statement. American Thoracic Society (ATS) and the European Respiratory Society (ERS). Am J Respir Crit Care Med 2000;161:646–64.

[32] Kondo Y, Taniguchi H, Kawabata Y, et al. Acute exacerbation in idiopathic pulmonary fibrosis. Analysis of clinical and pathologic findings in three cases. Chest 1993;103:1808–12.

[33] Carrington CB, Gaensler EA, Coute RE, et al. Natural history and treated course of usual and desquamative interstitial pneumonia. N Engl J Med 1978;298:801–9.

[34] Grenier P, Chevret S, Beigelman C, et al. Chronic diffuse infiltrative lung disease: determination of the diagnostic value of clinical data, chest radiography, and CT with Bayesian analysis. Radiology 1994;191:383–90.

[35] Müller NL, Colby TV. Idiopathic interstitial pneumonia: high-resolution CT and histologic findings. Radiographics 1997;17:1016–22.

[36] Nishimura K, Kitaichi M, Izumi T, et al. Usual interstitial pneumonia: histologic correlation with high-resolution CT. Radiology 1992;182:337–42.

[37] Hunninghake G, Zimmerman M, Schwartz T, et al. Utility of lung biopsy for the diagnosis of idiopathic pulmonary fibrosis. Am J Respir Crit Care Med 2001;164:193–6.

[38] Johkoh T, Itoh H, Müller NL, et al. Crazy-paving appearance at thin-section CT: spectrum of disease and pathologic findings. Radiology 1999;211: 155–60.

[39] Webb WR, Stein MG, Finkbeiner WE, et al. Normal and disease isolated lungs: high-resolution CT. Radiology 1988;166:81–7.

[40] Kang EY, Grenier P, Laurent F, et al. Interlobular septal thickening: patterns at high-resolution computed tomography. J Thorac Imaging 1996;11: 260–4.

[41] Leung AN, Miller RR, Müller NL. Parenchymal opacification in chronic infiltrative lung diseases: CT-pathologic correlation. Radiology 1993;188: 209–14.

[42] Remy-Jardin M, Giraud F, Remy J, et al. Importance of ground glass attenuation in chronic diffuse infiltrative lung disease: pathologic-CT correlation. Radiology 1993;189:693–8.

[43] Akira M, Hamada H, Sakatani M, et al. CT findings during phase of accelerated deterioration in patients who have idiopathic pulmonary fibrosis. AJR Am J Roentgenol 1997;168:79–83.

[44] Collard HR, Moore BB, Flaherty KR, et al. Pulmonary perspective: acute exacerbations of idiopathic pulmonary fibrosis. Am J Respir Crit Care Med 2007;176:636–43.

[45] Sumikawa H, Johkoh T, Ichikado K, et al. Usual interstitial pneumonia and chronic idiopathic interstitial pneumonia: analysis of CT appearance in 92 patients. Radiology 2006;241:258–66.

[46] Hartman TE, Primack SL, Swensen SJ, et al. Desquamtive interstitial pneumonia: thin-section CT findings in 22 patients. Radiology 1993;187: 787–90.

[47] Akira M, Yamamoto S, Hara H, et al. Serial computed tomographic evaluation in desquamative interstitial pneumonia. Thorax 1997;52:333–7.

[48] Colby TV. Bronchiolitis: pathologic considerations. Am J Clin Pathol 1998;109:101–9.

[49] Müller NL, Miller RR. Diseases of the bronchioles: CT and histopathologic findings. Radiology 1995; 196:3–12.

[50] Myers JL, Veal CF, Shin MS, et al. Respiratory bronchiolitis causing interstitial lung disease: a clinicopathologic study of six cases. Am Rev Respir Dis 1987;135:880–4.

[51] King TE. Respiratory bronchiolitis-associated interstitial lung disease. Clin Chest Med 1993;14: 693–8.

[52] Craig PJ, Wells AU, Doffman S, et al. Desquamative interstitial pneumonia, respiratory bronchiolitis and their relationship to smoking. Histopathology 2004; 45:275–82.

[53] Heyneman LE, Ward S, Lynch DA, et al. Respiratory bronchiolitis, respiratory bronchiolitis-interstitial lung disease, and desquamative interstitial pneumonia: different entities or part of the spectrum of the same disease process? AJR Am J Roentgenol 1999;173:1617–22.

[54] Yousem SA, Colby TV, Gaenseler EA. Respiratory bronchiolitis-associated interstitial lung disease and its relationship to desquamative interstitial pneumonia. Mayo Clin Proc 1989;64:1373–80.

[55] Prak J, Brown KK, Tuder R, et al. Respiratory bronchiolitis-associated interstitial lung disease: radiologic features with clinical and pathologic correlation. J Comput Assist Tomogr 2002;26: 13–20.

[56] Nicholson AG, Wotherspoon AC, Diss TC, et al. Reactive pulmonary lymphoid disorders. Histopathology 1995;19:357–63.

[57] Koss MN, Hochholzer L, Langloss JM, et al. Lymphoid interstitial pneumonitis: clinicopathologic and immunologic findings in 18 patients. Pathology 1987;19:178–85.

ELSEVIER
SAUNDERS

Clin Chest Med 29 (2008) 149–164

CLINICS
IN CHEST
MEDICINE

Pulmonary Complications of Connective Tissue Diseases

Felix Woodhead, MBBChir, MRCP[a],
Athol U. Wells, MD, FRACP, FRCR[a],
Sujal R. Desai, MD, FRCP, FRCR[b],*

[a]Royal Brompton Hospital, Sydney Street, London SW3 6NP, UK
[b]Department of Radiology, King's College Hospital, Denmark Hill, London SE5 9RS, UK

Connective tissue diseases (CTDs) are characterized by immune-mediated involvement of a variety of organs. The joints are the principal sites of disease, but pulmonary manifestations also are common, particularly in systemic sclerosis (SSc), rheumatoid arthritis (RA) and polymyositis/dermatomyositis (PM/DM). A variety of intrathoracic disease processes can coexist in patients who have CTD, and this can confound the clinical, radiologic, and physiologic profile. Lung disease is a common cause of major morbidity and death in CTD, but the spectrum of severity ranges from trivial to life-threatening. Some processes are reversible, whereas others are irreversible but may be nonprogressive or may deteriorate inexorably with or without treatment; thus, the identification of reversible disease and, as a separate issue, progressive disease is a key clinical issue.

In this article, following a general overview of pathologic processes and their associated imaging features, we review the five CTDs (RA, SSc, PM/DM, systemic lupus erythematosus [SLE], and Sjögren's syndrome [SS]) commonly associated with interstitial lung disease. There is a particular focus on high resolution CT (HRCT) profiles but in selected CTDs, key clinical problems most applicable to that disease (but also relevant to other CTDs) are identified with discussion of the contribution made by imaging to accurate management.

*Corresponding author.
E-mail address: sujal.desai@kch.nhs.uk (S.R. Desai).

Histopathological aspects of lung disease in connective tissue disease

Interstitial lung disease

The spectrum of lung disease in CTDs includes all of the disease processes sub-classified in the idiopathic interstitial pneumonias (IIPs) [1], but the prevalence of individual processes differs greatly between the CTDs and the IIPs. The most prevalent form of interstitial lung disease in the IIPs is usual interstitial pneumonia (UIP), which is characterized by a patchy distribution often affecting the periphery of the acinus or lobule, the presence of fibroblastic foci, and often honeycombing and architectural destruction [2,3]. However, UIP is less frequent in CTDs (with the exception of RA, in which UIP is probably the most frequent histologic pattern) [4]. By contrast, nonspecific interstitial pneumonia (NSIP) is the most common pattern of lung fibrosis in CTDs other than RA. Although it had been increasingly apparent in recent decades that some patients had a pattern of interstitial involvement that was not typical of UIP, the entity of NSIP was not fully formulated until 1994 [5]. In contrast to UIP, NSIP is characterized by the absence or low profusion of fibroblastic foci, and lung involvement throughout a biopsy specimen is uniform with respect to the distribution and apparent age of the disease process. The subclassification of NSIP has evolved to a widely-used dichotomy: "cellular NSIP" (in which inflammation predominates and the outcome is almost universally good), and "fibrotic NSIP" (in which fibrosis and inflammation are equally severe or fibrosis predominates, and the outcome is often good) [3,5,6].

Organizing pneumonia (OP) is also a frequent complication of CTDs, corresponding to cryptogenic organizing pneumonia (COP) in the IIP spectrum. Histopathologically, the cardinal feature is foci of organizing granulation tissue within the alveoli and alveolar ducts. In some cases, the terminal bronchioles also are involved, which leads to occlusion by intraluminal polyps [7–9]. COP also was known previously as bronchiolitis obliterans organizing pneumonia, a term now discarded by expert groups. COP usually responds well to corticosteroid therapy, but evolution of OP to fibrosis occurs in some cases. This phenomenon appears to be more prevalent in CTDs, which probably accounts for a higher mortality than seen in COP.

Lymphocytic interstitial pneumonia (LIP) was included among the IIPs in the reclassification in 2002 [1] but almost always has an underlying cause, including the presence of a CTD. The defining feature of LIP is a dense interstitial infiltrate of lymphocytes, plasma cells, and histiocytes, which often are associated with enlarged lymphoid follicles [1]. Respiratory bronchiolitis associated with interstitial lung disease and desquamative interstitial pneumonia also are occasionally encountered in smokers who have CTD.

Sudden catastrophic decline is well recognized in IIP and, less frequently, in CTD-related interstitial lung disease, which occasionally occurs as the presenting feature. The histologic picture is diffuse alveolar damage (DAD) [10–12], which evolves from an exudative phase with edema, acute interstitial inflammation, and hyaline membranes, to an organizing phase with organizing fibrosis and type II pneumocyte hyperplasia. Apart from the presence of background chronic fibrotic disease, the features at biopsy are those of the acute respiratory distress syndrome (also known as acute interstitial pneumonitis when idiopathic).

Intrinsic airways disease

The manifestations of intrinsic airways disease in CTD include bronchiectasis [13] and bronchiolitis [14]. Bronchiectasis frequently is present on HRCT in RA but is often clinically silent [15]. The involvement of small airways in a variety of CTDs is increasingly recognized [16,17] and can be subdivided into constrictive bronchiolitis, inflammatory bronchiolitis, and follicular bronchiolitis. Constrictive bronchiolitis, which is rare and

largely confined to patients who have RA [18], has been linked to penicillamine therapy in some cases and is irreversible and often fatal. HRCT appearances compatible with inflammatory bronchiolitis (ie, filling of bronchioles by secretions and inflammatory cells) are documented best in a subset of patients who have RA [19,20], but therapeutic outcomes have yet to be explored. In follicular bronchiolitis (reported in RA and SS) there is lymphoid hyperplasia and the formation of germinal centers. Regression of disease is reported with corticosteroid therapy in some patients, but the outcome is highly variable.

Pulmonary vascular disease

Pulmonary vasculopathy may result from pulmonary vasculitis (medium or large vessel vasculitis or capillaritis with diffuse alveolar hemorrhage), acute or chronic thromboembolism [21] (as in the antiphospholipid syndrome), or a noninflammatory ablative process histologicly indistinguishable from idiopathic pulmonary arterial hypertension [22]. Pulmonary vascular processes tend to be silent on chest radiography until pulmonary arteries and the right ventricle become dilated in late disease. Furthermore, vasculopathies also are difficult to detect clinically, especially when there is coexistent pulmonary fibrosis.

Extrapulmonary disease

A number of extrapulmonary complications of CTDs also can cause breathlessness or confound the diagnosis of coexisting lung disease. Involvement of the joints of the thoracic cage (as in ankylosing spondylitis) may lead to extrapulmonary restriction with a restrictive pattern of lung function and often near normal DL_{CO} with a raised K_{CO} [23]. A similar physiologic pattern can arise from obesity (which is not uncommon among patients treated with corticosteroids), severe pleural involvement, or muscle involvement. Pleural effusions are often a manifestation of an underlying serositis and when moderate or large may be apparent on plain chest radiographs. Smaller effusions and sequelae of previous episodes of serositis only may be apparent on CT. Other causes of breathlessness in patients who have CTDs include cardiac disease, anemia, and the increased work of breathing associated with inefficient locomotion (caused by severe musculoskeletal impairment).

Radiologic detection of lung disease

Chest radiography

Historically, plain chest radiography has been used to detect and monitor interstitial lung disease. Chest radiography is relatively cheap, readily available, and associated with a low radiation burden. However, conventional radiography is insensitive [24], has a low diagnostic accuracy [25], and interpretation is often difficult, as judged by the high level of interobserver variability reported in several studies [26–28]. Furthermore, the severity of disease often is difficult to quantify with confidence on chest radiography because of the two-dimensional superimposition of anatomic abnormalities. Thus, chest radiography often is useful in identifying overt interstitial lung disease, but HRCT should be performed to identify the likely histospecific diagnosis, quantify severity, and exclude radiographically occult interstitial lung disease as a cause of respiratory symptoms or lung function impairment.

High resolution computed tomography

HRCT is regarded as a central investigation in the assessment of interstitial lung disease and has played an increasingly important role in discriminating between individual IIPs in patients unable to undergo surgical biopsy. With accumulated experience, the radiologic correlates of the histopathologic patterns of airways and parenchymal disease are increasingly useful in clinical practice.

Interstitial lung disease

The typical HRCT features of the UIP pattern, as defined in idiopathic pulmonary fibrosis (IPF), are a predominantly basal and subpleural reticular pattern with honeycombing (Fig. 1) [1,29] often associated with architectural distortion and tractional dilatation of segmental and subsegmental airways [30,31]. Ground-glass opacification is present but is never more extensive than reticulation in typical UIP. When based on the cardinal HRCT features, a confident diagnosis of UIP by an experienced observer is correct in over 95% of cases [30–32]. However, atypical HRCT appearances, present in around one third of UIP cases, will not allow a confident HRCT diagnosis to be established [33].

Over the last decade, NSIP has evolved from a pathologic "waste basket" diagnosis to an identifiable and relatively common pattern of IIP. With the reclassification of IIPs and an increasing familiarity with the possible range of morphologic appearance, some of the initial difficulties with the HRCT diagnosis of NSIP have been resolved [34,35]. In contrast to a UIP pattern, the most prevalent finding at HRCT in patients who have NSIP is ground-glass opacification, which is commonly bilateral, symmetric, and subpleural in distribution (Fig. 2) [34,36–38].

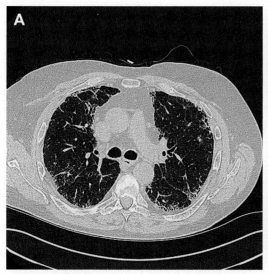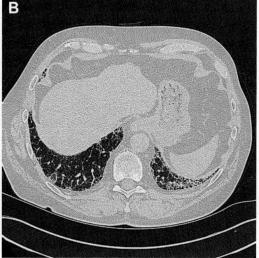

Fig. 1. (*A*, *B*) Typical appearance of the UIP pattern on CT in a patient who has RA at (*A*) the level of the carina and (*B*) through the lower lobes, demonstrating subpleural reticulation, microcystic honeycombing, and parenchymal distortion.

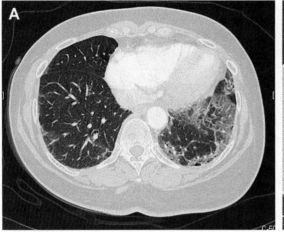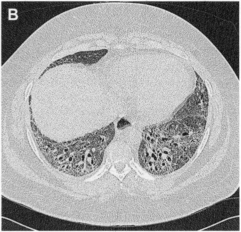

Fig. 2. (*A*, *B*) The NSIP pattern on CT in patients who have (*A*) RA and (*B*) SS. The common theme is the predominant ground-glass opacification and relative absence of honeycombing. There is also CT evidence of fine reticulation associated with traction bronchiectasis.

Irregular reticular opacities are seen in many cases, but it is the relative absence of honeycombing that distinguishes the NSIP pattern from UIP [39,40].

The HRCT findings in organizing pneumonia, which mirror the macroscopic histopathologic changes, consist of bilateral foci of consolidation (generally most pronounced in the lower zones, but all zones are potentially affected) (Fig. 3) [41–44]. The consolidation may be strikingly broncho- or

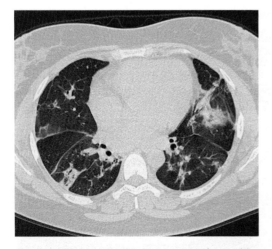

Fig. 3. CT at the level of the pulmonary venous confluence demonstrating bilateral foci of consolidation in a patient who has organizing pnemonia on a background of SLE. There is also evidence of parenchymal distortion, possibly attributable to pulmonary fibrosis.

bronchiolocentric, a pattern that is sometimes seen in patients who have organizing pneumonia occurring in the context of PM/DM (see below). Admixed reticular abnormalities are indicative of progression to fibrosis.

The HRCT features of LIP are nonspecific. However, the most common findings are ground-glass opacification (of variable extent) and multiple centrilobular nodules, which were seen in all 22 patients reported by Johkoh and colleagues [45]. Additional HRCT findings include multiple thin-walled cysts, thickening of bronchovascular bundles, prominent interlobular septa, and lymph node enlargement (Fig. 4). In occasional patients who have LIP on a background of SS, there is a combination of ground-glass opacification, thin-walled cysts, and large irregular nodules (with or without calcification), representing amyloid deposits [46]. Serial CT studies have shown that abnormalities in LIP either may resolve or progress, with cysts forming in areas with previous nodules and honeycombing in areas of ground-glass opacification [45].

DAD is the pathologic correlate of acute IIP; the clinico-radiologic findings of DAD are indistinguishable from those in patients who have acute respiratory distress syndrome. The key HRCT features of DAD are widespread but sometimes patchy ground-glass opacification with areas of dense parenchymal opacification (Fig. 5) [47,48]. Foci of consolidation are present in approximately two-thirds of patients [49] and there is occasional septal thickening. Increasingly

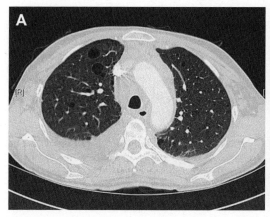
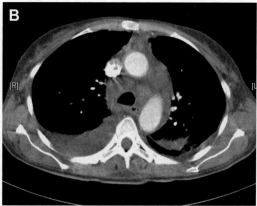

Fig. 4. (*A, B*) Two CT images at the level of the aortic arch in a patient who has RA and LIP. (*A*) On lung parenchymal window settings, there is a generalized increase in lung parenchymal attenuation. In addition, there are multiple thin-walled cysts of varying size in both lungs. (*B*) On soft-tissue window settings there are enlarged mediastinal lymph nodes and pleural effusions.

extensive ground-glass opacification or consolidation appears to denote a poor outcome when associated with traction bronchiectasis/bronchiolectasis and architectural distortion [50].

Airways disease

Airway pathology including bronchiectasis, obliterative bronchiolitis ,and exudative bronchiolitis is common in RA and SS. The HRCT features of these airways diseases have been documented. The cardinal HRCT sign of bronchiectasis, bronchial dilatation [51], is associated variably with bronchial wall thickening, patchy decreased parenchymal density (ie, mosaic

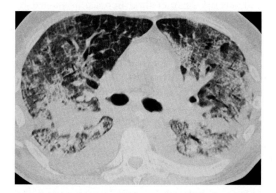

Fig. 5. CT at the level of the carina in a patient who has a presumed (but clinically-undeclared at the time of scanning) CTD and DAD. There is widespread ground-glass opacification and patchy foci of consolidation intermingled with regions of apparently normal aerated lung parenchyma.

attenuation), plugging of large and small airways, volume loss, and crowding of airways. Bronchiectasis is also a feature of constrictive (obliterative) bronchiolitis, but the most striking abnormality is mosaic attenuation, which is enhanced on scans taken at residual volume [52] and associated with a decrease in the number/calibre of vessels in regions of decreased density. Exudative bronchiolitis manifests on HRCT as a "tree-in-bud" appearance [53]; the peripheral airways, which are invisible in normal subjects, are delineated by an inflammatory exudate in their walls and lumina.

Vascular disease

Plain chest radiography makes little contribution to the evaluation of patients who have suspected vascular disease in CTDs. By contrast, HRCT often shows abnormalities [54], including a mosaic attenuation pattern (comprising intermingled zones of increased and decreased attenuation), ground-glass opacification, consolidation, nodule,s and interlobular septal thickening. HRCT features also supplement Doppler echocardiographic findings in the detection of pulmonary arterial hypertension. The normal range of main pulmonary artery diameters on CT has been defined [55,56]; a pulmonary artery diameter greater than 29mm [57] and a ratio of pulmonary artery to ascending aortic diameter greater than 1 mm [58] have been predictive of pulmonary hypertension. These promising data merit further study with multi-slice CT, which allows the pulmonary vessels and cardiac chambers to be examined concurrently.

Other imaging procedures

In specific scenarios, nuclear medicine tests have value in the evaluation of patients who have CTDs. For instance, the clearance of [99m]technetium-labeled diethylenetriamine penta-acetic acid (^{99m}Tc-DTPA) from the lung in different interstitial lung disease has been explored [59–63]. However, while ^{99m}Tc-DTPA clearance has been suggested to indicate the chance of decline, at least in idiopathic disease [64], the technique has never gained widespread clinical use. Gallium (^{67}Ga) scintigraphy also has also been used in the detection of lung disease in SS [65] ; however, as is often the case with such nuclear medicine investigations, the lack of spatial resolution is problematic.

Disease-specific findings

Rhematoid arthritis

In RA, the most common of CTDs, lung involvement can take the form of a variety of interstitial lung processes, including UIP, NSIP, organizing pneumonia, acute interstitial pneumonia, LIP, and intra-parenchymal rheumatoid nodule formation. Bronchiectasis and the various bronchiolitides outlined earlier also can complicate RA. Pleural disease is common and is usually self-limited. Pulmonary vasculopathy is rare.

In RA, alone among the CTDs, UIP appears to be at least as common as NSIP; even in patients who have biopsy-proven NSIP, the HRCT pattern often is suggestive of UIP with prominence of reticular abnormalities and, a paucity of ground-glass. It recently has been reported that severity-adjusted survival in RA is worse than in other CTDs for both NSIP and UIP (indicating that pulmonary fibrosis is, on average, more progressive in RA) [66]. Furthermore, fatal acute exacerbations caused by DAD appear to be more prevalent in RA than in other CTDs, but it probably occurs less frequently than in IPF [67,68].

Increasingly extensive interstitial disease on HRCT has been linked to higher titers of rheumatoid factor and older age, but no relationship has been found between HRCT disease extent and duration of disease [68]. Common HRCT findings in RA include interstitial thickening, honeycombing, and ground-glass opacification, which coincides with the observation of sizeable subgroups with histologic NSIP and UIP [19,20,68,69].

In RA, honeycombing and ground-glass opacification on HRCT are compatible with UIP on biopsy [19,20]. However, although there is some overlap between the radiologic features of UIP and NSIP, the radiological diagnosis is correct in most cases [4,20]. Consolidation usually is indicative of organizing pneumonia, but chronic eosinophilic pneumonia is an occasional finding [19]. Although consolidation regresses on serial imaging, there is HRCT progression to honeycombing in a significant proportion of cases; in general, disease progression on CT in RA manifests as increasing honeycombing [19,70].

Key clinical problems in connective tissue disease: the deconstruction of coexisting disease processes

Among CTDs, the variety of underlying lung pathologies is greatest in RA. Reversible interstitial lung processes, irreversible interstitial disease, variably reversible airway-centered disease, and pleural involvement seldom all coexist in the same patient. However, combinations of two or even three disorders are not infrequent. Furthermore, it is widely believed (although not yet proven) that smoking promotes the onset and progression of interstitial lung disease in RA—many patients who have "rheumatoid lung" also have smoking-related centrilobular emphysema. Chest radiographic evaluation often is misleading when it comes to quantifying disease severity in isolated pulmonary fibrosis and is not equal to the task of estimating the relative clinical importance of admixed disease processes. For example, the presence of pleural disease may mask the presence and severity of interstitial fibrosis, as judged by chest radiography, and both of these disorders may conceal radiographic evidence of bronchiectasis. Pulmonary function tests are equally confounded by the coexistence of two or more disease processes. In RA, an admixture of pulmonary fibrosis and emphysema commonly results in spurious preservation of lung volumes and a disproportionate reduction in measures of gas transfer, exactly as reported in IPF [71]. Pleural disease and interstitial disease give rise to restrictive ventilatory defects: although major reductions in DL_{CO} sometimes identify interstitial fibrosis as the more clinically important problem, admixed disease processes often are difficult to deconstruct using finely nuanced pulmonary function profiles.

The problem of coexisting disease processes must be confronted in other CTDs, although the number of possible disease processes and the frequency of their coexistence are both lower than in RA. The more common combinations include pulmonary fibrosis and pulmonary hypertension in SSc, pulmonary fibrosis and respiratory muscle weakness in PM/DM, and pulmonary hypertension and pleural disease in SLE.

The use of HRCT scoring in clinical studies of CTD has provided invaluable insights into the morphologic significance of routine pulmonary function variables. For example, the observation that DL_{CO} levels correlate more closely with disease extent on HRCT than other variables in SSc [72] has reinforced the view that DL_{CO} estimation should play a central role in the staging of the severity of pulmonary fibrosis. By contrast, arterial hypoxia at rest develops only when disease is extensive on HRCT [72] and arterial gases are largely unhelpful in quantifying less severe disease.

Formal HRCT scoring is not practicable in the outpatient setting in individual patients, but an informal evaluation of the extent of interstitial lung disease often is invaluable when disease processes coexist. With approximate knowledge of the extent of morphologic abnormalities on HRCT, the clinician can begin to understand if the severity and pattern of functional impairment is ascribable to pulmonary fibrosis or if additional disease processes must be invoked to rationalize the pulmonary function profile. For RA, in particular, knowledge of CT appearances allows the clinician to ascribe reductions in lung volumes to interstitial or pleural disease, as appropriate, and also to understand if disproportionate reduction in gas transfer is likely to represent pulmonary hypertension or the concurrence of pulmonary fibrosis and emphysema.

Systemic sclerosis

Although SSc is less prevalent than RA, pulmonary fibrosis is a much more frequent and widely studied complication in SSc [73] than in other CTDs. With SSc, there is microvascular damage and deposits of excess collagen and extracellular matrix in the skin and other organs and the presence of autoantibodies, most commonly against the centromere, topoisomerase 1, and RNA polymerase I and III [74]. The extent of skin involvement defines the two major clinical subtypes of disease; in limited cutaneous scleroderma (lcSSc), skin involvement is distal to the elbows, whereas in diffuse cutaneous disease (dcSSc), proximal skin disease is present. The reported prevalence of

lung involvement in SSc varies between 40% to 80% of patients, depending on the methods employed for disease detection [75,76], but lung involvement is more common in dcSSc than lcSSc [75,77–82] and anti-topoisomerase I (previously known as Scl-70) positive disease [74,75,77–81]. NSIP is the usual histologic pattern of lung disease in SSc, but UIP is present in a significant minority of SSc patients, and organizing pneumonia and DAD also have been reported [83–86].

The HRCT findings in SSc are indistinguishable from those in idiopathic NSIP, with a similar prominence of ground-glass opacification and little honeycombing [87,88]. Mediastinal lymph node enlargement is also fairly common [87] and seems to correlate with the extent of interstitial disease on CT, but it does not differentiate between lcSSc and dcSSc [89]. In an early HRCT study, predominant reticulation was strongly indicative of fibrotic histologic appearances at a surgical biopsy [90]. However, ground-glass opacification in this study was equally likely to represent fibrotic and inflammatory tissue [90]. There is a misconception that ground-glass opacification on HRCT almost always represents inflammation. In reality, ground-glass opacification often is more indicative of "fine fibrosis" [88], and the important clue on CT is the presence of traction bronchiectasis in regions of ground-glass infiltration (Fig. 6). With time, ground-glass

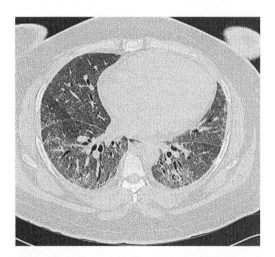

Fig. 6. CT through the lower zones showing widespread ground-glass opacification. Crucially, there are dilated segmental and subsegmental airways in both lower lobes, which indicates that the ground-glass opacification is likely to represent fibrosis and unlikely to represent "treatable" inflammation.

opacification and honeycombing increase as disease becomes more extensive [91]. In a very recent study, regression of ground-glass opacification on HRCT was seen in only 5% of SSc patients, despite aggressive treatment in some cases [92].

Key clinical problem in connective tissue disease: is lung disease clinically significant?

As discussed earlier, HRCT consistently is more sensitive than chest radiography in interstitial lung disease, and this applies equally to CTD. In SSc, HRCT is much more sensitive than chest radiography [93], and in SS [94,95] and SLE [96], HRCT discloses parenchymal abnormalities in a majority or large minority of patients. In RA, the prevalence of interstitial abnormalities on HRCT is approximately 25% [97]. It is now widely accepted that HRCT is the most accurate routine noninvasive means of detecting pulmonary fibrosis.

However, many patients have trivial interstitial lung disease, which must be distinguished from clinically important interstitial lung disease if accurate management decisions are to be made. The high sensitivity of HRCT sometimes creates difficulties for the clinician. Although interstitial abnormalities on HRCT commonly are present on HRCT in SS and SLE [95,96,98], clinically important interstitial disease is infrequent in both disorders. In a large study of SSc patients who had pulmonary fibrosis, only 13% of the lung was abnormal on HRCT on average and, in many cases, abnormalities were limited in extent and confined to the lower lung zones [76].

No published studies exist in which a cut-off for HRCT disease extent has been identified, above which disease can be regarded as clinically significant. Thus, in many cases, it is impossible to distinguish between subclinical and clinically significant disease based on HRCT appearances in isolation. Informal evaluation of the extent of disease on HRCT is useful, because in many other cases, abnormalities clearly either are limited or extensive. However, in a large subgroup of SSc patients who have disease on HRCT that cannot be categorized as obviously limited or extensive, HRCT findings must be integrated with pulmonary function tests to evaluate the clinical significance of disease.

Polymyositis/dermatomyositis

Idiopathic inflammatory myopathies are characterized by inflammation of striated muscle and a wide variety of systemic complications that are not specified in formal diagnostic criteria [99]. The typical skin rash of dermatomyositis is absent in polymyositis, but the range of pulmonary complications is identical in both disorders. Involvement of the respiratory muscles is seen in at least 5% of cases, and bulbar dysfunction predisposes to aspiration pneumonia. Interstitial lung disease is a common complication, occurring in 50% or more of patients [100,101], whereas clinically significant pulmonary vascular disease is rare (although self-limited subclinical pulmonary vascular limitation is not infrequent).

Interstitial lung disease more commonly follows the onset of musculoskeletal manifestations but precedes these in up to a third of PM/DM cases [102]. In an early biopsy series, it was evident that organizing pneumonia was more common than in other CTDs and was associated with the best outcome. A fibrotic disorder, viewed as UIP at that time, was equally frequent, and DAD also was observed [103]. In a more recent study, postdating the reclassification of the IIPs, fibrotic NSIP was much more prevalent than other patterns [102].

The natural history and treated course of interstitial lung disease in PM/DM is highly variable, reflecting the heterogeneity of HRCT appearances. Overall, there is a higher prevalence of consolidation and a lower prevalence of honeycombing in PM/DM than in other CTDs [104]. Subpleural consolidation on HRCT generally represents organizing pneumonia [104–106] and often responds to anti-inflammatory therapy [105]. However, in a minority of cases, consolidation evolves to honeycomb change [106,107], which is always fibrotic when biopsied. This patient group includes the small subgroup of PM/DM patients who have underlying UIP [104]. In other cases, extensive consolidation represents DAD; a precipitous decline caused by DAD may complicate any pre-existing radiologic pattern in PM/DM [106].

Based on a very broad overview of published series, it appears that the presenting HRCT profiles in PM/DM can be divided into three recognizable groups. The first group includes cases in which consolidation on HRCT is a prominent feature, but the overall picture is not one of DAD. In this group, appearances often resemble those in COP. However, consolidation in PM/DM is more often bronchocentric than in COP, and there is a higher likelihood of progression to fibrotic disease and, sometimes, a fatal outcome, despite aggressive treatment (Fig. 7). Consolidation and

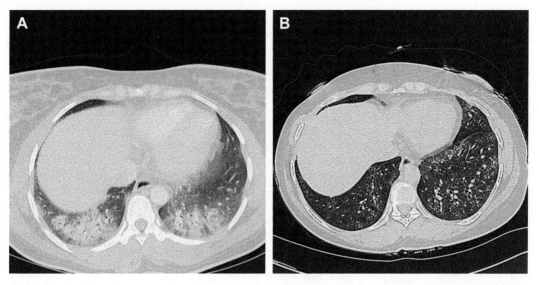

Fig. 7. (*A*, *B*) "Fibrotic" organizing pneumonia in polymyositis despite treatment. (*A*) CT image through the lower lobes at presentation shows bilateral peripheral and basal consolidation typical of the organizing pneumonia pattern. (*B*) At follow-up seven months later, there is a fine reticular pattern, traction bronchiolectasis, and limited ground-glass opacification.

overt fibrotic change sometimes are admixed on HRCT at presentation. The second group includes cases with acute onsets and HRCT appearances that show an extensive process with some features of DAD but also are admixed with more extensive consolidation than usually seen in DAD. In these cases, the treated outcome is sometimes excellent, especially when serum levels of muscle enzymes are strikingly increased; but in a roughly equal proportion of cases, disease is resistant to therapy and a fatal outcome often ensues. Normal or minimally elevated serum levels of muscle enzymes are an ominous sign in this context. The third group includes cases in which fibrotic disease (as shown by ground-glass abnormalities with prominent traction bronchiectasis/bronchiolectasis, reticular abnormalities, or, occasionally, honeycombing) predominates on HRCT. In the absence of honeycombing, fibrotic abnormalities on HRCT generally denote fibrotic NSIP. Predominantly fibrotic disease on HRCT is sometimes admixed with consolidation, but it also may be an isolated finding. It is sometimes argued that in PM/DM, isolated fibrotic disease is a post-inflammatory phenomenon. In a study of PM/DM patients who had biopsy-proven NSIP, ground-glass opacification and reticulation on HRCT regressed (to a greater or lesser degree) in 13 of 14 treated cases [108]. It appears that, unlike idiopathic NSIP and NSIP associated with SSc, the apparently fibrotic features of NSIP in PM/DM often are responsive to therapy.

Key clinical problem in connective tissue disease: prognostic evaluation

Among CTDs, outcomes from interstitial disease in PM/DM appear to be the most diverse. In principle, the prognostic use of HRCT has much to offer the clinician in PM/DM, but the prognostic value of HRCT in IIPs should not be extrapolated uncritically to PM/DM and needs to be nuanced carefully in RA and SSc. Other CTDs are insufficiently studied in this regard.

The subgroup of patients who have reversible disease are contained mostly within the subgroup that has consolidation or predominant ground-glass opacification on HRCT. However, unlike idiopathic disease, an HRCT pattern of organizing pneumonia (most often seen in PM/DM and RA) is not always associated with reversibility and a good outcome, especially when admixed with reticular abnormalities. Progression of consolidation to overt fibrosis on HRCT is not infrequent in PM/DM and RA. Thus, this HRCT profile justifies cautious optimism, a definitive trial of high dose therapy (usually corticosteroid therapy), and a longer term lower dose therapy to preserve therapeutic gains.

Prominent ground-glass attenuation on HRCT poses particular management difficulties in CTDs. In SSc, the view that this profiles equates to "alveolitis on HRCT" has been largely discredited. However, it is clear that a minority of patients who have this HRCT presentation do, in reality, have a predominantly inflammatory process (variably LIP, cellular NSIP, or desquamative interstitial pneumonia). As in idiopathic disease [90,109], the presence of admixed fine reticular abnormalities or traction bronchiectasis is useful ancillary signs that indicate a much higher likelihood of fibrotic disease. Although a trial of high dose corticosteroid therapy may, nonetheless, be warranted, this approach should not be instituted as a "knee-jerk reaction," solely because ground-glass opacification is prominent on HRCT.

Caveats notwithstanding, it appears that HRCT often plays a valuable role in CTDs by identifying important inflammation and an urgent need for high-dose therapy. By contrast, the accuracy of HRCT in identifying likely future progression in fibrotic disease has yet to be determined. There are tantalizing clues that this use of HRCT eventually will prove to be fruitful. In a large recent placebo-controlled study of oral cyclophosphamide in SSc, the treatment effect prevented progression in patients who had more extensive reticular abnormalities on HRCT [110]. In rheumatoid lung there is preliminary evidence that mortality is higher when HRCT appearances suggest underlying UIP [4]. However, despite outcome differences recently reported in RA, the prognostic distinction between UIP and NSIP appears to be less acute in CTDs than in idiopathic disease, and the true prognostic use of HRCT in fibrosis needs better definition.

Systemic lupus erythematosus

SLE is a multisystem CTD characterized by high titers of serum autoantibodies directed to the normal components of the nucleus (hence the label, anti-nuclear antibodies), most typically the so-called Smith antigen and native double-stranded DNA [111]. Immunopathologic studies indicate that immune complex formation is at the heart of tissue damage [112]: multiple-organ involvement including the skin, joints, kidneys and the central nervous system [113]. Serositis is more prevalent in SLE and RA than in other CTDs. Pleural disease is a particular problem and, in one study of 1000 patients, clinically-apparent pleuritis or pericarditis was documented

in over one third of patients, compared with a 7% prevalence of parenchymal disease [114].

Parenchymal lung disease in SLE is less well studied than in other CTDs but, when it does occur, may be life threatening because of diffuse pulmonary hemorrhage or DAD ("acute lupus pneumonitis"). Interstitial fibrosis is a less frequent complication and, on CT, a pattern of NSIP or UIP may be seen; the imaging of features of parenchymal disease associated with SLE were reviewed previously [115–118]. The other reported manifestations of SLE in the thorax include bronchiectasis [96], intra-alveolar hemorrhage [119,120], mediastinal lymph node enlargement [96], organizing pneumonia [121], so-called "shrinking lungs" [122], and in rare instances, amyloidosis [123].

Key clinical problem in connective tissue disease: differential diagnosis of lung disease

A frequent challenge in SLE (in particular), and in CTDs (in general), is to distinguish between expected pulmonary processes caused by CTDs and other disorders. Radiologists often are asked whether an abnormality is caused by the underlying rheumatologic disorder, is a complication of its treatment (ie, opportunistic infection caused by immunosuppression or drug induced lung disease), or is entirely unrelated. This problem often is difficult, as illustrated by the scenario of "new" air space opacities seen on chest radiography or CT.

Multifocal air space opacification is a nonspecific radiologic sign of pathology in the alveolar ducts and alveoli. In this context, CT often offers little diagnostic advantage over chest radiography. In SLE and to a lesser degree in other CTDs, new foci of air space opacification may denote pulmonary hemorrhage, organizing pneumonia, or the earliest signs of DAD. Opportunistic infection also may present with this radiologic profile. A multifocal area of consolidation may represent adenocarcinoma/broncho-alveolar cell carcinoma or lymphoma. Finally, the diagnosis of drug-induced lung disease is made more difficult by a lack of a consistent temporal relationship between the duration of therapy and the onset of pulmonary complications [124], because the range of histopathologic responses is narrow and non-specific drug-induced lung injury cannot always be distinguished from lung disease caused by CTD. Interstitial fibrosis, organizing pneumonia, hypersensitivity reactions, and DAD are all known histopathologic responses to drug-induced damage, and their radiologic correlates are equally nonspecific [124]. Thus, the diagnosis of drug-induced disease seldom is established on the basis of radiologic findings taken in isolation; it requires a multidisciplinary approach involving clinician, radiologist, and pathologist.

Sjögren's syndrome

SS is characterized clinically by dry eyes and dry mouth and often by salivary gland enlargement caused by lymphocytic infiltration of the exocrine glands. SS may occur in isolation (termed primary Sjögren's symdrome [pSS]) or in association with other CTDs, particularly RA, where it is known as secondary SS. Extraglandular involvement (which includes the lungs) may occur, and lymphoma occurs with a higher than expected frequency [125].

Infiltration, inflammation, and subsequent atrophy of the tracheo-bronchial mucosa leads to reduced respiratory secretions [126], and cough is a common complaint. However, the most significant thoracic abnormalities in SS are in the lung parenchyma; an almost full gamut of interstitial (with NSIP predominanting) and airways diseases have been reported [127–129]. Bronchiectasis and bronchiolitis are recognized findings in pSS. On HRCT, evidence of small airways disease and linear opacities is surprisingly prevalent; there was evidence of bronchiolectasis and bronchial/bronchiolar wall thickening in over two thirds of the patients reported by Franquet and colleagues [94]. Finally, it should be stressed that a spectrum of benign to frankly malignant lymphocytic infiltration is a worrying potential complication in SS [129–131].

Key clinical problem in Sjögren's syndrome: the detection of proliferative disease

The radiologic patterns seen in SS reflect the diverse range of pathology [94,95,132–134]. There is nonspecific ground-glass opacification and centrilobular nodules [45] in patients who have lymphocytic interstitial infiltration. In some patients who have SS, there is intrapulmonary cyst formation, occasionally which is associated with the deposition of amyloid nodules [132,134]. The pathophysiology of cyst formation is not entirely clear, but it seems likely that these are related to

lymphocytic infiltration per se and not, as has often previously been hypothesized, to a "check-valve" effect caused by partial bronchiolar obstruction. Honeycombing and radiologic evidence of fibrosis is uncommon.

Franquet and colleagues have confirmed the bronchiolocentric nature of the parenchymal disease in SS; airway changes and evidence of air trapping were present [135]. More recently, two studies comprising a total of 97 patients have reported CT changes in SS [132,134]. Ground-glass opacification (typically in the lower zones), interlobular septal thickening, and small nodules (centrilobular or subpleural) were typical HRCT finings in these two studies. Airway disease (bronchiectasis and bronchial wall thickening) was present in approximately one third of cases in one of these studies [132].

The index of suspicion, particularly when there are new findings on imaging, must remain high in patients who have SS because of the association with pulmonary lymphoma. In one small review of CT appearances in five patients who had lymphoma (and incidentally amyloidosis), there were variably-sized, irregular pulmonary nodules, and multiple cysts [136]. In another study of 10 patients who had extranodal marginal zone B-cell lymphoma, 7 patients also had SS [137]. The authors of this study noted the dramatic radiologic findings despite the indolent clinical course; multiple masses and areas of consolidation with or without air bronchograms.

Summary

Lung involvement is common in patients who have CTDs and causes considerable morbidity and mortality. Imaging tests and HRCT have a variety of roles in diagnosis and management. HRCT has a pivotal role in the detection of lung fibrosis. For patients who have coexistent pathologic processes, HRCT often allows the predominant process to be identified. The extent of interstitial disease also can be informally evaluated with HRCT, which provides insights into the likely pathophysiologic and prognostic significance of lung involvement. HRCT has an important role in detecting possible complications, such as opportunistic infection or the development of malignancy. However, the limitations of HRCT should not be overlooked. In many cases, HRCT appearances are nonspecific and may or may not be related to an underlying CTD. Thus, radiologic findings should never be interpreted without knowledge of the clinical picture.

References

[1] American Thoracic Society/European Respiratory Society. International Multidisciplinary Consensus Classification of the Idiopathic Interstitial Pneumonias. This Joint Statement of the American Thoracic Society (ATS), and the European Respiratory Society (ERS) was adopted by the ATS Board of Directors, June 2001 and by The ERS Executive Committee, June 2001. Am J Respir Crit Care Med 2002;165(2):277–304.

[2] Katzenstein AL, Myers JL. Idiopathic pulmonary fibrosis: clinical relevance of pathologic classification. Am J Respir Crit Care Med 1998;157(4 Pt 1): 1301–15.

[3] Travis WD, Matsui K, Moss J, et al. Idiopathic nonspecific interstitial pneumonia: prognostic significance of cellular and fibrosing patterns: survival comparison with usual interstitial pneumonia and desquamative interstitial pneumonia. Am J Surg Pathol 2000;24(1):19–33.

[4] Lee HK, Kim DS, Yoo B, et al. Histopathologic pattern and clinical features of rheumatoid arthritis-associated interstitial lung disease. Chest 2005; 127(6):2019–27.

[5] Katzenstein AL, Fiorelli RF. Nonspecific interstitial pneumonia/fibrosis. Histologic features and clinical significance. Am J Surg Pathol 1994;18(2): 136–47.

[6] Nagai S, Kitaichi M, Itoh H, et al. Idiopathic nonspecific interstitial pneumonia/fibrosis: comparison with idiopathic pulmonary fibrosis and BOOP. Eur Respir J 1998;12(5):1010–9.

[7] Colby TV. Pathologic aspects of bronchiolitis obliterans organizing pneumonia. Chest 1992; 102(Suppl 1):38S–43S.

[8] Epler GR, Colby TV, McLoud TC, et al. Bronchiolitis obliterans organizing pneumonia. N Engl J Med 1985;312(3):152–8.

[9] Izumi T, Kitaichi M, Nishimura K, et al. Bronchiolitis obliterans organizing pneumonia. Clinical features and differential diagnosis. Chest 1992;102(3): 715–9.

[10] Katzenstein AL, Myers JL, Mazur MT. Acute interstitial pneumonia. A clinicopathologic, ultrastructural, and cell kinetic study. Am J Surg Pathol 1986;10(4):256–67.

[11] Olson J, Colby TV, Elliott CG. Hamman-Rich syndrome revisited. Mayo Clin Proc 1990;65(12): 1538–48.

[12] Tomashefski JF Jr. Pulmonary pathology of acute respiratory distress syndrome. Clin Chest Med 2000;21(3):435–66.

[13] Barker AF. Bronchiectasis. N Engl J Med 2002; 346(18):1383–93.

[14] Visscher DW, Myers JL. Bronchiolitis: the pathologist's perspective. Proc Am Thorac Soc 2006;3(1): 41–7.

[15] Despaux J, Manzoni P, Toussirot E, et al. Prospective study of the prevalence of bronchiectasis in rheumatoid arthritis using high-resolution computed tomography. Rev Rhum Engl Ed 1998; 65(7–9):453–61.

[16] Cohen M, Sahn SA. Bronchiectasis in systemic diseases. Chest 1999;116(4):1063–74.

[17] White ES, Tazelaar HD, Lynch JP III. Bronchiolar complications of connective tissue diseases. Semin Respir Crit Care Med 2003;24(5):543–66.

[18] Geddes DM, Corrin B, Brewerton DA, et al. Progressive airway obliteration in adults and its association with rheumatoid disease. Q J Med 1977; 46(184):427–44.

[19] Akira M, Sakatani M, Hara H. Thin-section CT findings in rheumatoid arthritis-associated lung disease: CT patterns and their courses. J Comput Assist Tomogr 1999;23(6):941–8.

[20] Tanaka N, Kim JS, Newell JD, et al. Rheumatoid arthritis-related lung diseases: CT findings. Radiology 2004;232(1):81–91.

[21] Auger WR, Kim NH, Kerr KM, et al. Chronic thromboembolic pulmonary hypertension. Clin Chest Med 2007;28(1):255–69, x.

[22] Carreira PE. Pulmonary hypertension in autoimmune rheumatic diseases. Autoimmun Rev 2004; 3(4):313–20.

[23] Wright PH, Hanson A, Kreel L, et al. Respiratory function changes after asbestos pleurisy. Thorax 1980;35(1):31–6.

[24] Epler GR, McLoud TC, Gaensler EA, et al. Normal chest roentgenograms in chronic diffuse infiltrative lung disease. N Engl J Med 1978;298(17): 934–9.

[25] Mathieson JR, Mayo JR, Staples CA, et al. Chronic diffuse infiltrative lung disease: comparison of diagnostic accuracy of CT and chest radiography. Radiology 1989;171(1):111–6.

[26] Garland LH, Cochrane AL. Results of an international test in chest roentgenogram interpretation. JAMA 1952;149(7):631–4.

[27] Garland LH. Studies on the accuracy of diagnostic procedures. AJR Am J Roentgenol 1959;82(1): 25–38.

[28] Tuddenham WJ. Problems in perception in chest roentgenology: facts and fallacies. Radiol Clin North Am 1963;1:277–89.

[29] Lynch DA, Travis WD, Muller NL, et al. Idiopathic interstitial pneumonias: CT features. Radiology 2005;236(1):10–21.

[30] Hunninghake GW, Zimmerman MB, Schwartz DA, et al. Utility of a lung biopsy for the diagnosis of idiopathic pulmonary fibrosis. Am J Respir Crit Care Med 2001;164(2):193–6.

[31] Raghu G, Mageto YN, Lockhart D, et al. The accuracy of the clinical diagnosis of new-onset

idiopathic pulmonary fibrosis and other interstitial lung disease: A prospective study. Chest 1999; 116(5):1168–74.

[32] Swensen SJ, Aughenbaugh GL, Myers JL. Diffuse lung disease: diagnostic accuracy of CT in patients undergoing surgical biopsy of the lung. Radiology 1997;205(1):229–34.

[33] Flaherty KR, Thwaite EL, Kazerooni EA, et al. Radiological versus histological diagnosis in UIP and NSIP: survival implications. Thorax 2003; 58(2):143–8.

[34] Hartman TE, Swensen SJ, Hansell DM, et al. Nonspecific interstitial pneumonia: variable appearance at high-resolution chest CT. Radiology 2000; 217(3):701–5.

[35] Johkoh T, Muller NL, Cartier Y, et al. Idiopathic interstitial pneumonias: diagnostic accuracy of thin-section CT in 129 patients. Radiology 1999; 211(2):555–60.

[36] Cottin V, Donsbeck AV, Revel D, et al. Nonspecific interstitial pneumonia. Individualization of a clinicopathologic entity in a series of 12 patients. Am J Respir Crit Care Med 1998;158(4):1286–93.

[37] Johkoh T, Muller NL, Colby TV, et al. Nonspecific interstitial pneumonia: correlation between thin-section CT findings and pathologic subgroups in 55 patients. Radiology 2002;225(1):199–204.

[38] Kim EY, Lee KS, Chung MP, et al. Nonspecific interstitial pneumonia with fibrosis: serial high-resolution CT findings with functional correlation. AJR Am J Roentgenol 1999;173(4):949–53.

[39] Elliot TL, Lynch DA, Newell JD Jr, et al. High-resolution computed tomography features of nonspecific interstitial pneumonia and usual interstitial pneumonia. J Comput Assist Tomogr 2005;29(3): 339–45.

[40] Sumikawa H, Johkoh T, Ichikado K, et al. Usual interstitial pneumonia and chronic idiopathic interstitial pneumonia: analysis of CT appearance in 92 patients. Radiology 2006;241(1):258–66.

[41] Lee KS, Kullnig P, Hartman TE, et al. Cryptogenic organizing pneumonia: CT findings in 43 patients. AJR Am J Roentgenol 1994;162(3):543–6.

[42] Muller NL, Staples CA, Miller RR. Bronchiolitis obliterans organizing pneumonia: CT features in 14 patients. AJR Am J Roentgenol 1990;154(5): 983–7.

[43] Nishimura K, Itoh H. High-resolution computed tomographic features of bronchiolitis obliterans organizing pneumonia. Chest 1992;102(Suppl 1): 26S–31S.

[44] Arakawa H, Kurihara Y, Niimi H, et al. Bronchiolitis obliterans with organizing pneumonia versus chronic eosinophilic pneumonia: high-resolution CT findings in 81 patients. AJR Am J Roentgenol 2001;176(4):1053–8.

[45] Johkoh T, Ichikado K, Akira M, et al. Lymphocytic interstitial pneumonia: follow-up CT findings in 14 patients. J Thorac Imaging 2000;15(3):162–7.

[46] Desai SR, Nicholson AG, Stewart S, et al. Benign pulmonary lymphocytic infiltration and amyloidosis: computed tomographic and pathologic features in three cases. J Thorac Imaging 1997;12(3): 215–20.

[47] Johkoh T, Muller NL, Taniguchi H, et al. Acute interstitial pneumonia: thin-section CT findings in 36 patients. Radiology 1999;211(3):859–63.

[48] Primack SL, Hartman TE, Ikezoe J, et al. Acute interstitial pneumonia: radiographic and CT findings in nine patients. Radiology 1993;188(3):817–20.

[49] Tomiyama N, Muller NL, Johkoh T, et al. Acute respiratory distress syndrome and acute interstitial pneumonia: comparison of thin-section CT findings. J Comput Assist Tomogr 2001;25(1):28–33.

[50] Ichikado K, Suga M, Muller NL, et al. Acute interstitial pneumonia: comparison of high-resolution computed tomography findings between survivors and nonsurvivors. Am J Respir Crit Care Med 2002;165(11):1551–6.

[51] Naidich DP, McCauley DI, Khouri NF, et al. Computed tomography of bronchiectasis. J Comput Assist Tomogr 1982;6(3):437–44.

[52] Hansell DM, Rubens MB, Padley SP, et al. Obliterative bronchiolitis: individual CT signs of small airways disease and functional correlation. Radiology 1997;203(3):721–6.

[53] Pipavath SJ, Lynch DA, Cool C, et al. Radiologic and pathologic features of bronchiolitis. AJR Am J Roentgenol 2005;185(2):354–63.

[54] Hansell DM. Small-vessel diseases of the lung: CT-pathologic correlates. Radiology 2002;225(3): 639–53.

[55] Kuriyama K, Gamsu G, Stern RG, et al. CT-determined pulmonary artery diameters in predicting pulmonary hypertension. Invest Radiol 1984; 19(1):16–22.

[56] Edwards PD, Bull RK, Coulden R. CT measurement of main pulmonary artery diameter. Br J Radiol 1998;71(850):1018–20.

[57] Tan RT, Kuzo R, Goodman LR, et al. Utility of CT scan evaluation for predicting pulmonary hypertension in patients with parenchymal lung disease. Medical College of Wisconsin Lung Transplant Group. Chest 1998;113(5):1250–6.

[58] Ng CS, Wells AU, Padley SP. A CT sign of chronic pulmonary arterial hypertension: the ratio of main pulmonary artery to aortic diameter. J Thorac Imaging 1999;14(4):270–8.

[59] Gabbay E, Tarala R, Will R, et al. Interstitial lung disease in recent onset rheumatoid arthritis. Am J Respir Crit Care Med 1997;156(2 Pt 1):528–35.

[60] Harrison NK, Glanville AR, Strickland B, et al. Pulmonary Involvement in Systemic-Sclerosis - the Detection of Early Changes by Thin-Section Ct Scan, Bronchoalveolar Lavage and Tc-99M-Dtpa Clearance. Respir Med 1989;83(5):403–14.

[61] Kaushik VV, Lynch MP, Dawson JK. Tc-DTPA clearance and rheumatoid arthritis-associated

fibrosing alveolitis. Rheumatology (Oxford) 2002;
41(6):712–3.

[62] Kon OM, Daniil Z, Black CM, et al. Clearance of
inhaled technetium-99m-DTPA as a clinical index
of pulmonary vascular disease in systemic sclerosis.
Eur Respir J 1999;13(1):133–6.

[63] Okudan B, Sahin M, Ozbek FM, et al. Detection of
alveolar epithelial injury by Tc-99m DTPA radio-
aerosol inhalation lung scan in rheumatoid arthritis
patients. Ann Nucl Med 2005;19(6):455–60.

[64] Mogulkoc N, Brutsche MH, Bishop PW, et al. Pulmonary (99m)Tc-DTPA aerosol clearance and survival in usual interstitial pneumonia (UIP). Thorax
2001;56(12):916–23.

[65] Deheinzelin D, Capelozzi VL, Kairalla RA, et al.
Interstitial lung disease in primary Sjogren's syndrome. Clinical-pathological evaluation and response to treatment. Am J Respir Crit Care Med
1996;154(3 Pt 1):794–9.

[66] Park JH, Kim DS, Park IN, et al. Prognosis of fibrotic interstitial pneumonia: idiopathic versus collagen vascular disease-related. Am J Respir Crit
Care Med 2007;175:705–11.

[67] Park IN, Kim DS, Shim TS, et al. Acute exacerbation of interstitial pneumonia other than idiopathic
pulmonary fibrosis. Chest 2007;132(1):214–20.

[68] Zrour SH, Touzi M, Bejia I, et al. Correlations between high-resolution computed tomography of
the chest and clinical function in patients with rheumatoid arthritis. Prospective study in 75 patients.
Joint Bone Spine 2005;72(1):41–7.

[69] Biederer J, Schnabel A, Muhle C, et al. Correlation
between HRCT findings, pulmonary function tests
and bronchoalveolar lavage cytology in interstitial
lung disease associated with rheumatoid arthritis.
Eur Radiol 2004;14(2):272–80.

[70] Dawson JK, Fewins HE, Desmond J, et al. Predictors of progression of HRCT diagnosed fibrosing
alveolitis in patients with rheumatoid arthritis.
Ann Rheum Dis 2002;61(6):517–21.

[71] Cottin V. Combined pulmonary fibrosis and emphysema: a distinct underrecognised entity. Eur
Respir J 2005;26(4):586–93.

[72] Wells AU, Hansell DM, Rubens MB, et al. Fibrosing alveolitis in systemic sclerosis: indices of lung
function in relation to extent of disease on computed tomography. Arthritis Rheum 1997;40(7):
1229–36.

[73] Mayes M, Reveille JD. Epidemiology, Demo-
graphics, and Genetics. In: Clements PJ,
Furst DE, editors. Systemic sclerosis. 2nd edition.
Philadelphia: Lippincott Williams & Wilkins;
2004. p. 1–16.

[74] Ho KT, Reveille JD. The clinical relevance of autoantibodies in scleroderma. Arthritis Res Ther 2003;
5(2):80–93.

[75] Steen VD, Conte C, Owens GR, et al. Severe restrictive lung-disease in systemic-sclerosis. Arthritis
Rheum 1994;37(9):1283–9.

[76] Goh NS, Veeraraghavan S, Desai SR, et al. Bronchoalveolar lavage cellular profiles in patients
with systemic sclerosis-associated interstitial lung
disease are not predictive of disease progression.
Arthritis Rheum 2007;56(6):2005–12.

[77] Greidinger EL, Flaherty KT, White B, et al. Afri-
can-American race and antibodies to topoisomerase I are associated with increased severity of
scleroderma lung disease. Chest 1998;114(3):801–7.

[78] Jacobsen S, Halberg P, Ullman S, et al. Clinical features and serum antinuclear antibodies in 230 Danish patients with systemic sclerosis. Br J Rheumatol
1998;37(1):39–45.

[79] Manoussakis MN, Constantopoulos SH, Gharavi
AE, et al. Pulmonary involvement in systemic sclerosis. Association with anti-Scl 70 antibody and
digital pitting. Chest 1987;92(3):509–13.

[80] McNearney TA, Reveille JD, Fischbach M, et al.
Pulmonary involvement in systemic sclerosis: asso-
ciations with genetic, serologic, sociodemographic,
and behavioral factors. Arthritis Rheum 2007;
57(2):318–26.

[81] Meyer OC, Fertig N, Lucas M, et al. Disease subsets, antinuclear antibody profile, and clinical features in 127 French and 247 US adult patients with
systemic sclerosis. J Rheumatol 2007;34(1):104–9.

[82] Steen VD, Medsger TA. Severe organ involvement
in systemic sclerosis with diffuse scleroderma. Arthritis Rheum 2000;43(11):2437–44.

[83] Bouros D, Wells AU, Nicholson AG, et al. Histopathologic subsets of fibrosing alveolitis in patients
with systemic sclerosis and their relationship to outcome. Am J Respir Crit Care Med 2002;165(12):
1581–6.

[84] Kim DS, Yoo B, Lee JS, et al. The major histopathologic pattern of pulmonary fibrosis in scleroderma
is nonspecific interstitial pneumonia. Sarcoidosis
Vasc Diffuse Lung Dis 2002;19(2):121–7.

[85] Bridges AJ, Hsu KC, as-Arias AA, et al. Bronchiolitis obliterans organizing pneumonia and scleroderma. J Rheumatol 1992;19(7):1136–40.

[86] Muir TE, Tazelaar HD, Colby TV, et al. Organizing diffuse alveolar damage associated with progressive systemic sclerosis. Mayo Clin Proc 1997;
72(7):639–42.

[87] Warrick JH, Bhalla M, Schabel SI, et al. High resolution computed tomography in early scleroderma lung disease. J Rheumatol 1991;18(10):
1520–8.

[88] Remy-Jardin M, Remy J, Wallaert B, et al. Pulmonary involvement in progressive systemic sclerosis:
sequential evaluation with CT, pulmonary function
tests, and bronchoalveolar lavage. Radiology 1993;
188(2):499–506.

[89] Wechsler RJ, Steiner RM, Spirn PW, et al. The relationship of thoracic lymphadenopathy to pulmonary interstitial disease in diffuse and limited
systemic sclerosis: CT findings. AJR Am J Roentgenol 1996;167(1):101–4.

[90] Wells AU, Hansell DM, Corrin B, et al. High resolution computed tomography as a predictor of lung histology in systemic sclerosis. Thorax 1992;47(9): 738–42.

[91] Kim EA, Johkoh T, Lee KS, et al. Interstitial pneumonia in progressive systemic sclerosis: serial high-resolution CT findings with functional correlation. J Comput Assist Tomogr 2001;25(5):757–63.

[92] Shah RM, Jimenez S, Wechsler R. Significance of ground-glass opacity on HRCT in long-term follow-up of patients with systemic sclerosis. J Thorac Imaging 2007;22(2):120–4.

[93] Schurawitzki H, Stiglbauer R, Graninger W, et al. Interstitial lung disease in progressive systemic sclerosis: high-resolution CT versus radiography. Radiology 1990;176(3):755–9.

[94] Franquet T, Gimenez A, Monill JM, et al. Primary Sjogren's syndrome and associated lung disease: CT findings in 50 patients. AJR Am J Roentgenol 1997;169(3):655–8.

[95] Matsuyama N, Ashizawa K, Okimoto T, et al. Pulmonary lesions associated with Sjogren's syndrome: radiographic and CT findings. Br J Radiol 2003;76(912):880–4.

[96] Fenlon HM, Doran M, Sant SM, et al. High-resolution chest CT in systemic lupus erythematosus. AJR Am J Roentgenol 1996;166(2):301–7.

[97] Remy-Jardin M, Remy J, Cortet B, et al. Lung changes in rheumatoid arthritis: CT findings. Radiology 1994;193(2):375–82.

[98] Franquet T. High-resolution CT of lung disease related to collagen vascular disease. Radiol Clin North Am 2001;39(6):1171–87.

[99] Bohan A, Peter JB. Polymyositis and dermatomyositis (first of two parts). N Engl J Med 1975;292(7): 344–7.

[100] Fathi M, Dastmalchi M, Rasmussen E, et al. Interstitial lung disease, a common manifestation of newly diagnosed polymyositis and dermatomyositis. Ann Rheum Dis 2004;63(3):297–301.

[101] Selva-O'Callaghan A, Labrador-Horrillo M, Munoz-Gall X, et al. Polymyositis/dermatomyositis-associated lung disease: analysis of a series of 81 patients. Lupus 2005;14(7):534–42.

[102] Douglas WW, Tazelaar HD, Hartman TE, et al. Polymyositis-dermatomyositis-associated interstitial lung disease. Am J Respir Crit Care Med 2001;164(7):1182–5.

[103] Tazelaar HD, Viggiano RW, Pickersgill J, et al. Interstitial lung disease in polymyositis and dermatomyositis. Clinical features and prognosis as correlated with histologic findings. Am Rev Respir Dis 1990;141(3):727–33.

[104] Ikezoe J, Johkoh T, Kohno N, et al. High-resolution CT findings of lung disease in patients with polymyositis and dermatomyositis. J Thorac Imaging 1996;11(4):250–9.

[105] Mino M, Noma S, Taguchi Y, et al. Pulmonary involvement in polymyositis and dermatomyositis:

sequential evaluation with CT. AJR Am J Roentgenol 1997;169(1):83–7.

[106] Akira M, Hara H, Sakatani M. Interstitial lung disease in association with polymyositis-dermatomyositis: long-term follow-up CT evaluation in seven patients. Radiology 1999;210(2):333–8.

[107] Bonnefoy O, Ferretti G, Calaque O, et al. Serial chest CT findings in interstitial lung disease associated with polymyositis-dermatomyositis. Eur J Radiol 2004;49(3):235–44.

[108] Arakawa H, Yamada H, Kurihara Y, et al. Nonspecific interstitial pneumonia associated with polymyositis and dermatomyositis: serial high-resolution CT findings and functional correlation. Chest 2003;123(4):1096–103.

[109] Remy-Jardin M, Giraud F, Remy J, et al. Importance of ground-glass attenuation in chronic diffuse infiltrative lung disease: pathologic-CT correlation. Radiology 1993;189(3):693–8.

[110] Tashkin DP, Elashoff R, Clements PJ, et al. Cyclophosphamide versus placebo in scleroderma lung disease. N Engl J Med 2006;354(25):2655–66.

[111] D'Cruz DP, Khamashta MA, Hughes GR. Systemic lupus erythematosus. Lancet 2007; 369(9561):587–96.

[112] Davidson A, Aranow C. Pathogenesis and treatment of systemic lupus erythematosus nephritis. Curr Opin Rheumatol 2006;18(5):468–75.

[113] Quismorio FP Jr. Clinical and pathologic features of lung involvement in systemic lupus erythematosus. Semin Respir Med 1988;9(3):297–304.

[114] Cervera R, Khamashta MA, Font J, et al. Systemic lupus erythematosus: clinical and immunologic patterns of disease expression in a cohort of 1,000 patients. The European Working Party on Systemic Lupus Erythematosus. Medicine (Baltimore) 1993;72(2):113–24.

[115] Murin S, Wiedemann HP, Matthay RA. Pulmonary manifestations of systemic lupus erythematosus. Clin Chest Med 1998;19(4):641–65, viii.

[116] Lalani TA, Kanne JP, Hatfield GA, et al. Imaging findings in systemic lupus erythematosus. Radiographics 2004;24(4):1069–86.

[117] Kim JS, Lee KS, Koh EM, et al. Thoracic involvement of systemic lupus erythematosus: clinical, pathologic, and radiologic findings. J Comput Assist Tomogr 2000;24(1):9–18.

[118] Keane MP, Lynch JP III. Pleuropulmonary manifestations of systemic lupus erythematosus. Thorax 2000;55(2):159–66.

[119] Santos-Ocampo AS, Mandell BF, Fessler BJ. Alveolar hemorrhage in systemic lupus erythematosus: presentation and management. Chest 2000;118(4): 1083–90.

[120] Badsha H, Teh CL, Kong KO, et al. Pulmonary hemorrhage in systemic lupus erythematosus. Semin Arthritis Rheum 2004;33(6):414–21.

[121] Min JK, Hong YS, Park SH, et al. Bronchiolitis obliterans organizing pneumonia as an initial

manifestation in patients with systemic lupus erythematosus. J Rheumatol 1997;24(11):2254–7.

[122] Alberto CJ, Diana D, Guillermo NG. Shrinking lungs syndrome, a rare manifestation of systemic lupus erythematosus. Int J Clin Pract 2006;60(12): 1683–6.

[123] Marenco JL, Sanchez-Burson J, Ruiz CJ, et al. Pulmonary amyloidosis and unusual lung involvement in SLE. Clin Rheumatol 1994;13(3):525–7.

[124] Akira M, Ishikawa H, Yamamoto S. Drug-induced pneumonitis: thin-section CT findings in 60 patients. Radiology 2002;224(3):852–60.

[125] Tonami H, Matoba M, Kuginuki Y, et al. Clinical and imaging findings of lymphoma in patients with Sjogren syndrome. J Comput Assist Tomogr 2003; 27(4):517–24.

[126] Mathieu A, Cauli A, Pala R, et al. Tracheo-bronchial mucociliary clearance in patients with primary and secondary Sjogren's syndrome. Scand J Rheumatol 1995;24(5):300–4.

[127] Yamadori I, Fujita J, Bandoh S, et al. Nonspecific interstitial pneumonia as pulmonary involvement of primary Sjogren's syndrome. Rheumatol Int 2002;22(3):89–92.

[128] Parambil JG, Myers JL, Lindell RM, et al. Interstitial lung disease in primary Sjogren syndrome. Chest 2006;130(5):1489–95.

[129] Ito I, Nagai S, Kitaichi M, et al. Pulmonary manifestations of primary Sjogren's syndrome: a clinical, radiologic, and pathologic study. Am J Respir Crit Care Med 2005;171(6):632–8.

[130] Papiris SA, Kalomenidis I, Malagari K, et al. Extranodal marginal zone B-cell lymphoma of the lung in Sjogren's syndrome patients: reappraisal of clinical, radiological, and pathology findings. Respir Med 2007;101(1):84–92.

[131] Jeong YJ, Lee KS, Chung MP, et al. Amyloidosis and lymphoproliferative disease in Sjogren syndrome: thin-section computed tomography findings and histopathologic comparisons. J Comput Assist Tomogr 2004;28(6):776–81.

[132] Koyama M, Johkoh T, Honda O, et al. Pulmonary involvement in primary Sjogren's syndrome: spectrum of pulmonary abnormalities and computed tomography findings in 60 patients. J Thorac Imaging 2001;16(4):290–6.

[133] Lohrmann C, Uhl M, Warnatz K, et al. High-resolution CT imaging of the lung for patients with primary Sjogren's syndrome. Eur J Radiol 2004;52(2):137–43.

[134] Uffmann M, Kiener HP, Bankier AA, et al. Lung manifestation in asymptomatic patients with primary Sjogren syndrome: assessment with high resolution CT and pulmonary function tests. J Thorac Imaging 2001;16(4):282–9.

[135] Franquet T, Diaz C, Domingo P, et al. Air trapping in primary Sjogren syndrome: correlation of expiratory CT with pulmonary function tests. J Comput Assist Tomogr 1999;23(2):169–73.

[136] Jeong YJ, Lee KS, Chung MP, et al. Amyloidosis and lymphoproliferative disease in Sjogren syndrome: thin-section computed tomography findings and histopathologic comparisons. J Comput Assist Tomogr 2004;28:776–81.

[137] Papiris SA, Kalomenidis I, Malagari K, et al. Extranodal marginal zone B-cell lymphoma of the lung in Sjogren's syndrome patients: reappraisal of clinical, radiological, and pathology findings. Respir Med 2007;101:84–92.

CLINICS
IN CHEST
MEDICINE

Clin Chest Med 29 (2008) 165–179

Imaging of Small Airways Disease and Chronic Obstructive Pulmonary Disease

David A. Lynch, MD

Division of Radiology, National Jewish Medical and Research Center, 1400 Jackson Street, Denver, CO 80206, USA

CT has an increasingly important role in the diagnosis and differential diagnosis of obstructive lung diseases. The purposes of this chapter are to describe imaging techniques for small airways disease, to illustrate the distinction between inflammatory and fibrotic forms of small airways disease, and to discuss the role of CT in characterization of chronic obstructive pulmonary disease (COPD).

Imaging techniques

When imaging the patient who has suspected small airways disease, inspiratory and expiratory high resolution CT images should be obtained, using thin collimation (1.25 mm or less). The inspiratory high resolution images either may be obtained as noncontiguous images acquired at intervals of 1 or 2 cm or may be reconstructed from a volumetric spiral acquisition. Although noncontiguous thin collimation images are associated with a substantially lower radiation dose, volumetric acquisition offers several advantages, including the ability to evaluate the larger airways for associated bronchiectasis, and the possibility of reconstructing multiplanar or postprocessed images to facilitate detection and characterization of airway-related abnormalities [1].

It is important to include expiratory imaging as part of the routine high resolution CT acquisition. However, the number of expiratory CT images acquired in studies of small airway disease is variable [2,3]. There is no clear consensus on the optimal expiratory maneuver for expiratory CT. The majority of studies acquire images at the

end of a deep expiration, presumably close to residual volume [4–6]. However, others have used an acquisition at the end of a tidal volume expiration or after a forceful expiration [7]. Continuous acquisition of images during a forced or slow expiratory maneuver [8–12] (dynamic expiratory CT) is not only more sensitive for detection of air trapping but also leads to identification of air trapping in normal individuals [9]. Spirometric confirmation of the level of expiration [13,14] usually is not obtained, because spirometric control is quite cumbersome and technically complex. However, in the absence of a spirometric tracing, it can be difficult sometimes to determine whether an adequate expiratory effort has been made.

Normal anatomy and CT findings

The description of the small airways requires anatomic precision. The anatomic terminology used in this article is summarized in Box 1.

In healthy individuals, the small airways are too thin-walled to be recognizable on CT. The identification of abnormal small airways is facilitated by knowledge of lobular anatomy, best seen at the lung periphery. In normal subjects, only a small dot or fine branching structure, representing the centrilobular pulmonary arteriole, may be seen at the center of the lobule, separated from the pleura by 2–5 mm (Fig. 1). In patients who have inflammatory small airways diseases, the centrilobular structures are markedly accentuated.

Several studies have found that air trapping, particularly lobular air trapping, may be found on end-expiratory CT in a substantial proportion of normal subjects (Fig. 2), particularly in cigarette smokers [10,15–17]. Clinical interpretation of the CT finding of air trapping, therefore, must consider

E-mail address: lynchd@njc.org

0272-5231/08/$ - see front matter © 2008 Elsevier Inc. All rights reserved.
doi:10.1016/j.ccm.2007.11.008

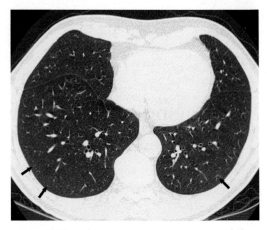

Fig. 1. Normal appearances on HRCT. A few small dots or branching structures are identified in the periphery of the lung (*arrows*). They are recognized as centrilobular because they are separated by 2–5 mm from the pleural surface.

the extent of abnormality, associated CT findings of bronchial abnormalities or mosaic attenuation, and physiologic evidence of obstruction.

Classification of small airways diseases

The spectrum of diseases that involve the small airways can be understood most easily by understanding the related pathology. Evolving understanding of small airways disease has led to repeated revisions of the classification of this group of disorders [18–20]. Initial pathologic descriptions of the small airways diseases tended to lump these conditions together under the descriptor bronchiolitis obliterans. However, it soon became clear that this category included a spectrum of diseases with markedly different clinical, radiologic, and physiologic features (Table 1). Older

classification systems for small airways disease were complicated by the inclusion of bronchiolitis obliterans organizing pneumonia, which presents radiologically with an appearance of lung consolidation. This entity has been reclassified as organizing pneumonia [21], and it is no longer included as a small airways disease. The related entity of bronchiolitis with organizing polyps still is included in some pathology-based classifications of small airways disease [22], but the imaging correlate of this entity is not clear.

Because the small airways are a critical part of the conducting system of the lungs, focal disease centered on the small airways may result in severe

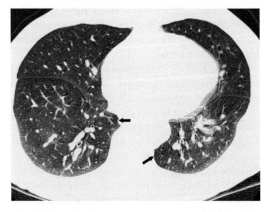

Fig. 2. Normal end-expiratory CT. Most of the lung has become homogenously gray as it is partially emptied of air. However, there are some small poorly defined areas of air trapping.

Table 1
Imaging-based classification of bronchiolitis

Classification	Radiologic pattern	Pathologic features	Characteristic radiologic features	Prototype disease	Other causes	Differential diagnosis
Inflammatory	Cellular bronchiolitis	Acute or chronic inflammatory infiltration of bronchiolar wall	Centrilobular nodularity Tree-in-bud pattern Bronchiectasis (with more chronic disease)	Acute infection (viral, mycoplasma)	Chronic infection (mycobacterial) Chronic aspiration	Hypersensitivity pneumonitis
	Panbronchiolitis	Severe transmural inflammation of bronchiolar wall.	Tree-in-bud pattern Bronchiolectasis Bronchiectasis	Diffuse panbronchiolitis	Inflammatory bowel disease Thymoma	Cystic fibrosis Immune deficiency Mycobacterial infection
	Respiratory bronchiolitis	Macrophage accumulation in bronchiolar lumen and adjacent alveoli	Poorly defined centrilobular nodules Patchy ground-glass attenuation	Smokers' lung	Other inhalation exposures	
	Follicular bronchiolitis	Lymphoid follicles adjacent to bronchioles	Centrilobular nodules. Peribronchial nodules Ground glass opacity	Rheumatoid disease	Sjogren syndrome Other collagen vascular diseases Immunodeficiency	
Fibrotic	Constrictive bronchiolitis	Circumferential thickening of bronchiolar wall, with narrowing or obliteration of lumen	Diffuse or geographic air trapping/mosaic pattern Cylindric bronchial dilation	Cryptogenic bronchiolitis obliterans	Rheumatoid disease Chronic rejection Prior viral/mycoplasma infection Toxic inhalation (fumes, diacetyl)	
	Neuroendocrine hyperplasia		Diffuse or geographic air trapping/mosaic pattern, with nodules	Neuroendocrine hyperplasia		

symptoms and physiologic impairment with little, if any, chest radiographic abnormality. CT scanning provides excellent insight into the morphology of these entities [23].

For the imager, the most helpful working classification of small airways disease divides these entities into inflammatory and fibrotic forms. This classification system is presented in Table 1.

CT signs of bronchiolitis

Bronchiolitis is manifested on CT by direct and indirect signs [24]. Direct signs include centrilobular thickening, tree-in-bud pattern, and later bronchiolar dilation [23]. The earliest sign of bronchiolar inflammation is centrilobular thickening, usually best identified at the periphery of the lung (Fig. 3). Tree-in-bud pattern is a reflection of more marked bronchiolar inflammation and mucoid impaction, where inflamed or impacted bronchioles are visible as centrilobular branching structures terminating in a tiny nodule (Fig. 4). Bronchiolar dilation (bronchiolectasis) may be identified when a cystic or tubular structure is identified within the secondary pulmonary lobule (Fig. 5). Differential diagnosis of bronchiolitis is facilitated by evaluation of the pattern of centrilobular thickening and the presence of associated features such as ground glass attenuation, as shown in Table 1.

When the bronchiole is not inflamed but narrowed by fibrosis, indirect signs of bronchiolitis predominate. The primary indirect sign of bronchiolitis is air trapping on expiratory CT (Fig. 6).

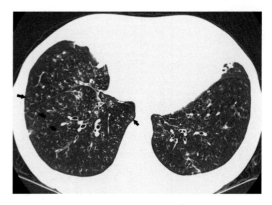

Fig. 4. Tree-in-bud pattern in a patient who has diffuse panbronchiolitis. Diffuse tree-in-bud pattern is present (*arrows*).

On inspiratory imaging, mosaic attenuation is commonly seen, characterized by alternating geographic areas of decreased and increased lung attenuation. The areas of decreased attenuation (blacker lung) are usually associated with decreased vascularity, reflecting hypoxic vasoconstriction in areas of poor ventilation. Diffuse decrease in lung attenuation (Fig. 7) is more difficult to detect, unless one is accustomed to viewing lung CT scans at constant window settings. Cylindric bronchial dilation is commonly associated with several forms of constrictive bronchiolitis, including those related to transplantation (see Fig. 7), collagen vascular disease, previous infection, and toxic fume inhalation. The mechanism of this form of cylindric bronchiectasis is not clear, but it is often helpful as a further indirect sign suggesting this diagnosis.

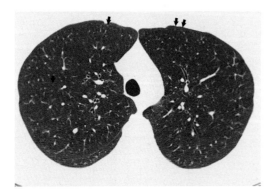

Fig. 3. Centrilobular nodules in respiratory bronchiolitis. Multiple poorly defined nodules are scattered through the lung parenchyma. The nodules at the periphery of the lung (*arrows*) are recognized as centrilobular because they are separated by 2–5 mm from the pleural surface.

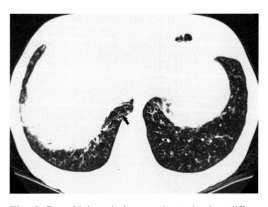

Fig. 5. Bronchiolectasis in a patient who has diffuse panbronchiolitis. In addition to widespread tree-in-bud pattern, a cylindric dilated bronchus is seen within a secondary pulmonary lobule (*arrow*).

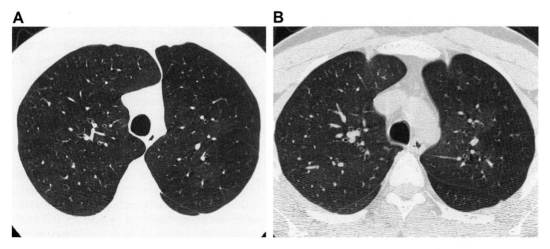

Fig. 6. Mosaic attenuation and air trapping in a patient who has postinfectious bronchiolitis obliterans. (*A*) Inspiratory image shows patchy decreased attenuation (ie, blacker lung), mainly in the left lung. (*B*) End-expiratory image shows air trapping in the same area.

Inflammatory small airways diseases

Acute cellular bronchiolitis is characterized histologically by a pattern of acute bronchiolar injury, with epithelial necrosis and inflammation of the bronchiolar walls and intraluminal exudates [23]. This inflammatory material in the walls and lumina of the bronchioles leads to abnormal visibility of the centrilobular structures on CT. The tree-in-bud pattern is the primary sign of cellular bronchiolitis, whether acute or chronic.

Cellular bronchiolitis is most commonly caused by infection or aspiration. Acute viral or mycoplasma infection (ie, atypical pneumonia) may present with a CT pattern of cellular bronchiolitis (Fig. 8), often associated with ground glass abnormality or consolidation [25]. Immunocompromised patients may develop bronchiolitis caused by viral infection or aspergillus, or less commonly, mycobacteria. If a pattern of patchy cellular bronchiolitis is seen in a patient who has more chronic illness, tuberculous, or nontuberculous, mycobacterial infection should be considered (Fig. 9). If the abnormality is marked most at the lung bases in an older patient, aspiration is very likely. Any of these forms of chronic cellular bronchiolitis may be associated with bronchiectasis.

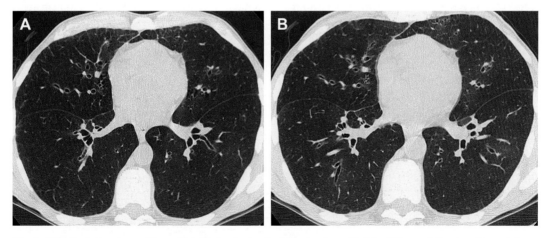

Fig. 7. Diffuse air trapping and bronchial dilation in a patient who has bronchiolitis obliterans following allogeneic bone marrow transplant. (*A*) Inspiratory image shows diffuse decrease in lung attenuation and widespread bronchial dilation. Mild interlobular septal thickening is seen anteriorly. (*B*) End-expiratory image shows diffuse air trapping.

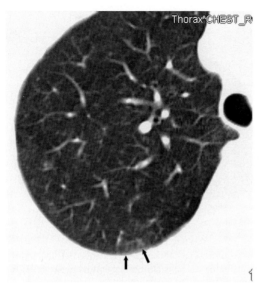

Fig. 8. Mycoplasma pneumonia in liver transplant patient. CT through right upper lobe shows centrilobular nodularity with tree-in-bud pattern (*arrows*).

Although cellular bronchiolitis is a common manifestation of hypersensitivity pneumonitis (HP), the centrilobular nodules of HP differ from those of infectious cellular bronchiolitis in that they are usually diffuse, poorly defined, and of ground-glass attenuation rather than soft tissue attenuation (Fig. 10). The tree-in-bud pattern is uncommon, but areas of mosaic attenuation caused by air trapping are frequent [26,27].

Diffuse panbronchiolitis most commonly occurs in Asian patients, particularly in Japanese adults. Though most widely recognized in Japan, it has been described in most parts of the world [28–33]. Indeed, it may be under-recognized in non-Asian people [28]. High resolution CT findings are pivotal in the diagnosis of diffuse panbronchiolitis, and chest CT may provide the initial suspicion of this diagnosis. The CT features include centrilobular nodules, tree-in-bud pattern, cystic bronchiolar dilation, and bronchiectasis (Fig. 11). Mosaic attenuation may be seen, and air trapping may be seen on expiratory images. The abnormalities almost always predominate in the lower lobes. When correlated with pathology, the centrilobular nodules correlate with inflamed bronchioles, the tree-in-bud pattern correlates with secretion-filled bronchioles, and the cystic structures represent dilated bronchioles and bronchi [34]. Other imaging findings may include patchy consolidation (perhaps indicating pseudomonas pneumonia), mucoid impaction in bronchi, and segmental atelectasis [35].

Akira and colleagues [36]. developed an imaging-based classification of panbronchiolitis:

Type I: centrilobular nodules
Type II: centrilobular nodules connected by branching lines
Type III: bronchiolectasis
Type IV: bronchiectasis.

Classification of panbronchiolitis in this way correlates with the clinical stage and pathologic severity of disease. CT may help monitor the course of patients who have diffuse panbronchiolitis. On serial evaluation in untreated patients [37], centrilobular nodules progress, with development of bronchiolectasis and bronchiectasis; conversely, in patients treated with erythromycin, the nodules decrease in size and number, though areas

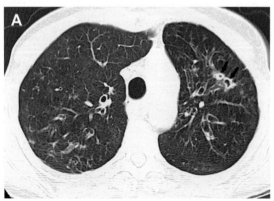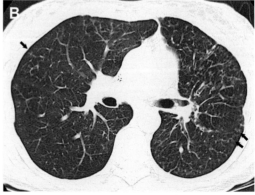

Fig. 9. Nontuberculous mycobacterial infection in a middle-aged woman. (*A*) CT through the upper lobes shows two small cavities (*arrows*) and widespread bronchiectasis. (*B*) CT through the lower lobes shows diffuse tree-in-bud pattern (*arrows*).

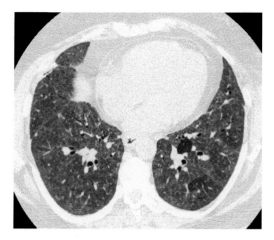

Fig. 10. Hypersensitivity pneumonitis. CT through the lower lobes shows profuse poorly defined centrilobular nodules associated with ground glass abnormality. The scattered lobular areas of decreased attenuation are an important clue to the diagnosis of HP.

of decreased attenuation may persist (see Fig. 11) [37,38]. Bronchiolectasis also improves on treatment, but bronchiectasis does not change significantly [39]. Improvement in the extent of centrilobular nodules on treatment correlates with physiologic evidence of decreased air trapping [39].

A similar clinical and imaging pattern to diffuse panbronchiolitis may be seen in patients who have inflammatory bowel disease and some patients who have thymoma. Other differential diagnostic considerations include chronic infection (particularly mycobacterial infection), cystic fibrosis, ciliary dysmotility, immune deficiency, and chronic aspiration.

Follicular bronchiolitis is a benign polyclonal lymphoid proliferative condition, defined by the presence of abundant hyperplastic lymphoid follicles, distributed along the bronchioles [40,41]. Although follicular bronchiolitis may be idiopathic, it is frequently associated with underlying collagen vascular disease (especially Sjögren syndrome and rheumatoid arthritis) and immunodeficiency states including acquired immunodeficiency syndrome [42]. It also has been described as the salient lesion in workers exposed to nylon or polyethylene flock [43,44].

On CT scanning of patients who have follicular bronchiolitis, centrilobular nodules are present universally, and are usually the predominant feature [40,41]. They may be associated with tree-in-bud pattern. The nodules are typically small (less than 3 mm), but nodules measuring up to 10 mm also may be seen. Peribronchial nodules are common, being found in three of six cases in one study [40], and in 5 of 12 patients in another study [41]. Ground-glass abnormality is more variable, being seen in 1 of 6 and 9 of 12 patients in these two studies. The presence of ground-glass abnormality probably is indicative of histologic interstitial inflammation in addition to the peribronchiolar abnormalities.

Acute or chronic injury to the bronchioles may be caused by a wide variety of inhaled substances. The clinical course of acute inhalational injury has been well-characterized in individuals who have silo-fillers' lung, caused by inhalation of oxides of nitrogen accumulating in a partially filled silo, just above the surface of the grain. Significant exposure typically results in the development of cough, dyspnea, and fever after a latent period of 3 to 24

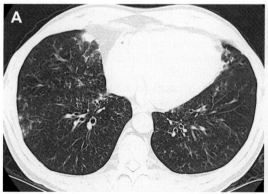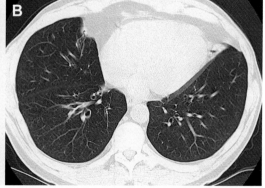

Fig. 11. Diffuse panbronchiolitis. (A) Baseline CT through the lower lungs shows diffuse tree-in-bud pattern and moderate cylindric bronchiectasis. There is a small patch of consolidation in the right middle lobe. (B) Follow-up CT one year later, following treatment with macrolide antibiotic and steroids, shows near-normal CT with some residual bronchiectasis.

hours. Bronchospasm is common, with wheezing on examination. Initial chest radiograph is often normal, but noncardiac pulmonary edema may develop. CT may show ground-glass abnormality caused by edema or evidence of bronchiolitis. Following recovery from the acute phase of lung injury, some patients develop a relapse of symptoms within 3 to 6 weeks, characterized by severe, progressive airway obstruction, and histologic and imaging findings of bronchiolitis obliterans.

Respiratory bronchiolitis related to cigarette smoking is the most common form of chronic bronchiolitis. This lesion is an almost invariable histologic feature of cigarette smokers found at autopsy. The histologic features include inflammation and mild fibrosis of the wall of the respiratory bronchiole and accumulation of dusky pigmented macrophages in the adjacent alveoli. In respiratory bronchiolitis, centrilobular prominence (without tree-in-bud pattern) usually is associated with patchy ground-glass opacity caused by accumulation of pigmented macrophages in the alveoli (Fig. 12) [45]. Respiratory bronchiolitis may be difficult to differentiate from hypersensitivity pneumonitis, but most patients who have hypersensitivity pneumonitis are non-smokers. The extent and severity of respiratory bronchiolitis ranges from asymptomatic minor abnormalities discovered in chronic smokers to symptomatic diffuse abnormality found in patients who have respiratory bronchiolitis interstitial lung disease (RB-ILD). The CT features of

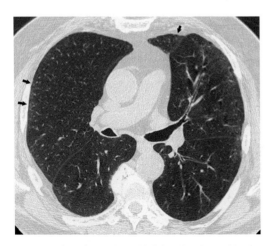

Fig. 12. Respiratory bronchiolitis related to cigarette smoking. CT through the mid-lungs shows patchy poorly defined centrilobular nodules (*arrows*). The bronchi are markedly thick walled, and subpleural ground-glass abnormality is present in the lateral left lung.

asymptomatic smokers' lung, symptomatic RB-ILD, and desquamative interstitial pneumonitis overlap significantly [46]. Respiratory bronchiolitis is discussed further below in the section on smoking-related lung disease.

One of the most common forms of inhalational lung injury worldwide is related to inhalation of burning biomass fuels. The term "hut lung" has been applied to the domestically acquired particulate lung disease related to inhalation of burning biomass fuels [47,48] The imaging features of hut lung and related anthracotic conditions have been evaluated in several case reports and two series [47–50]. In the initial description of 25 patients by Grobbelaar and colleagues [47], the findings on chest radiographs were similar to those of silicosis, with features ranging from a fine nodular pattern to a pattern of progressive massive fibrosis. Indeed, some of these patients had previously been assumed to have silicosis from grinding grain ("Transkei silicosis"). On CT scanning, the nodules may be centrilobular [48] or distributed along the bronchovascular bundle [49]. Septal thickening and lymphadenopathy also may be seen [49]. Ground-glass abnormality, fibrotic bands, and irregular pleural interfaces also may be seen [50].

Fibrotic/constrictive small airways diseases

Constrictive bronchiolitis occurs in patients who have collagen vascular disease, toxic fume inhalation, previous infection, lung transplant rejection, and graft-versus-host disease in allogeneic bone marrow transplant recipients.

In patients who have constrictive bronchiolitis, the bronchiolar wall is often only mildly thickened, but the lumen is markedly narrowed or obliterated by concentric inflammation and fibrosis. The resultant air trapping is manifested on CT as geographic or diffuse decrease in lung attenuation, associated with decreased vascularity caused by hypoxic vasoconstriction (see Figs. 6 and 7) [19,51]. Because the bronchiolar wall is not markedly thickened, the centrilobular structures usually are not visible. If the air trapping is geographic, it results in a mosaic pattern. Diffuse air trapping may be more difficult to detect on CT. Many forms of constrictive bronchiolitis are associated with bronchial dilation and bronchiectasis. Constrictive bronchiolitis can be very subtle, with a normal or near-normal inspiratory CT, even in patients who have severe physiologic impairment.

In children and young adults, constrictive bronchiolitis most commonly occurs as a sequel of a severe adenoviral or mycoplasma bronchiolitis [52]. Postinfectious constrictive bronchiolitis is characterized by patchy mosaic attenuation almost always associated with cylindric bronchiectasis. Lobar atelectasis also may be present [52]. When postinfectious bronchiolitis is predominantly unilateral, it is called Swyer-James syndrome and is characterized on the chest radiograph by unilateral hyperlucency with decreased vascularity (Fig. 13). CT in patients who have Swyer-James syndrome confirms predominantly unilateral decrease in attenuation with bronchiectasis, but it invariably shows smaller patches of similar abnormality in the contralateral lung [53].

In lung transplant recipients, constrictive bronchiolitis occurs as a manifestation of chronic rejection. The CT features of post-transplant bronchiolitis obliterans include bronchial dilation, decreased lung attenuation, and expiratory air trapping [7,54–62]. Of these, the most sensitive manifestations are bronchial dilation and expiratory air trapping. However, in general, these abnormalities are less sensitive and specific than physiologic evaluation for diagnosis of bronchiolitis obliterans syndrome [63]. The reasons for this relatively low sensitivity remain unclear. However, a recent article suggested that the use of a composite CT visual score, incorporating scores for bronchiectasis, mucus plugging, airway

wall thickening, consolidation, mosaic pattern, and air trapping, correlated with FEV1 in patients who had post-transplant bronchiolitis obliterans syndrome [64]. It also is possible that dynamic expiratory CT [65] or quantitative measurement of air trapping [66] may be more sensitive than visual scoring. MRI with hyperpolarized 3-Helium or other gases is probably more sensitive than CT for detecting air trapping, and this technique might be useful if it becomes more widely available [67].

Constrictive bronchiolitis also occurs as a manifestation of graft-versus-host disease in recipients of allogeneic bone marrow transplants. The CT features of constrictive bronchiolitis related to bone marrow transplants resemble those in lung transplants (see Fig. 7) [68,69].

Collagen vascular diseases, particularly rheumatoid arthritis, may cause bronchiolitis obliterans [70,71], and indeed bronchiolitis obliterans may precede other manifestations of rheumatoid arthritis [72]. The CT features of this entity are similar to those of other forms of constrictive bronchiolitis, and bronchial dilation is often a salient feature (Fig. 14). In making this diagnosis, one must be aware that diffuse panbronchiolitis [73] and follicular bronchiolitis [74] also may be seen in patients who have rheumatoid arthritis.

It may be difficult to distinguish clinically between refractory asthma and constrictive bronchiolitis. Jensen and colleagues [75] compared the CT findings of patients who had refractory severe

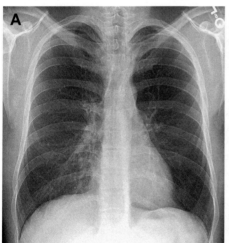
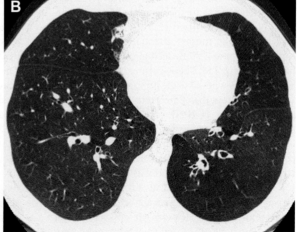

Fig. 13. Swyer-James syndrome (unilateral postinfectious bronchiolitis obliterans). (*A*) Chest radiograph shows a diffusely hyperlucent left lung with decreased vascularity. (*B*) CT confirms diffuse decrease in attenuation of the left lung with some focal areas of sparing. There is moderate cylindric bronchial dilation.

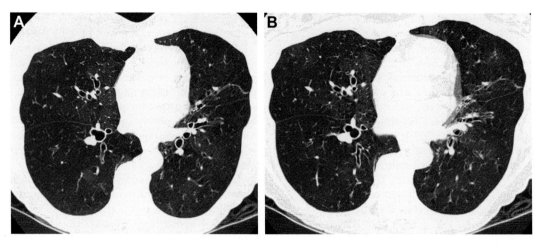

Fig. 14. Constrictive bronchiolitis related to rheumatoid arthritis. (*A*) Inspiratory CT shows mosaic attenuation with more normal attenuation in the medial right lung. There is widespread cylindric bronchiectasis. (*B*) Expiratory CT shows marked patchy air trapping.

asthma with those in constrictive bronchiolitis. Both groups of patients showed air trapping on expiratory images, but patients who had constrictive bronchiolitis were more likely to have ground-glass attenuation and a mosaic pattern of CT attenuation on inspiratory images. About 50% of patients who had constrictive bronchiolitis were indistinguishable from patients who had severe asthma. The presence of marked air trapping may favor the diagnosis of severe asthma.

Inhalational exposures may result in bronchiolitis. This may occur as a sequel of acute toxic exposure. More recently, bronchiolitis obliterans has been described as a consequence of chronic occupational exposure to diacetyl, a flavoring compound [76]. This entity is characterized by airway wall thickening, mosaic attenuation, and expiratory air trapping [77]. Bronchial dilation also may be present (Fig. 15). These features can be diagnostic in workers who have the appropriate exposure.

Diffuse idiopathic pulmonary neuroendocrine cell hyperplasia (DIPNECH) is an uncommon syndrome occurring in women 40 years or older, who typically present with a history of chronic cough and physiologic evidence of airway obstruction. DIPNECH usually is associated with CT features of constrictive bronchiolitis with airway wall thickening, mosaic attenuation, and air trapping [78,79]. However, at least half the patients who have this condition have pulmonary nodules consisting of carcinoid tumors. The nodules are typically less than 5 mm in diameter, but they may be larger. DIPNECH should be

strongly considered in women who have a pattern of constrictive bronchiolitis associated with pulmonary nodules (Fig. 16).

Chronic obstructive pulmonary disease and smoking-related airways disease

Several distinct components of COPD may be evaluated on CT; these include emphysema, large airway inflammation, and small airways abnormality. Less wel characterized components of COPD are bronchiectasis and tracheobronchomalacia.

CT is substantially more sensitive than spirometry for detecting emphysema [4,80]. In a study by Omori and colleagues [81] of 615 subjects who underwent lung cancer screening CT, 116 of 380 current cigarette smokers showed emphysema on CT; 91 (78%) of these subjects had normal spirometry. The prevalence of spirometric impairment appeared to increase with age. Emphysema may be classified on CT as centrilobular, panlobular, distal acinar, and cicatricial [82].

Both qualitative (radiologist scoring) and quantitative (computerized image analysis) approaches have been used to analyze the severity of emphysema and its distribution through the lungs. Many studies of emphysema have used a visual approach to quantification, asking observers to score the extent of lung abnormality along a semiquantitative four-point or five-point scale (eg, 0%–25%, 26%–50%, 51%–75%, 76%–100%). Multiple independent studies have shown good correlation between the grading of

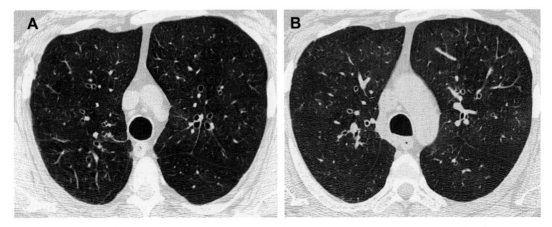

Fig. 15. Constrictive bronchiolitis related to occupational exposure to diacetyl. (*A*) Inspiratory CT shows mosaic attenuation, bronchial wall thickening, and bronchial dilation. (*B*) Expiratory CT shows patchy air trapping.

emphysema on CT and the pathology "gold standard" [83–88]. High resolution, thin section CT demonstrates improved sensitivity when compared with 10mm CT in the diagnosis of mild emphysema [88,89].

Evaluation of the extent of small airways abnormality is a critical component of assessing a patient who has COPD. Respiratory bronchiolitis related to cigarette smoking is probably the most common form of smoking related lung disease. Abnormalities are seen on HRCT in at least 50% of cigarette smokers [90]. The typical smoking-related abnormalities are prominence of the centrilobular structures and patchy ground-glass opacity. Airway wall thickening from chronic bronchitis also is very common. In a study

of patients who had respiratory bronchiolitis interstitial lung disease [91], our group demonstrated that the extent of centrilobular nodularity was correlated with the extent of macrophages in respiratory bronchioles and with chronic inflammation of respiratory bronchioles. The extent of ground-glass opacity correlated with the amount of macrophage accumulation in the alveoli and alveolar ducts. Similar findings were reported by Remy-Jardin and colleagues [92]. The changes of smokers' lung are commonly reversible in those who stop smoking, but centrilobular nodules usually either increase in profusion or progress to emphysema in those who continue to smoke [93]. The presence of emphysema and ground-glass abnormality on a baseline

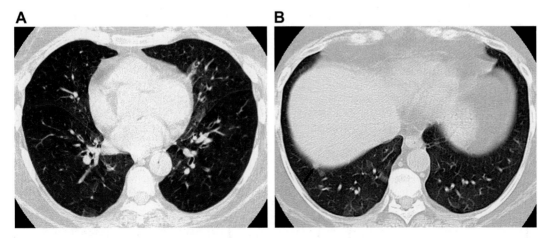

Fig. 16. Diffuse pulmonary neuroendocrine hyperplasia (DIPNECH) in a middle aged woman. (*A*) Inspiratory CT shows mosaic attenuation. Expiratory CT (not shown) showed widespread air trapping, suggesting constrictive bronchiolitis. (*B*) CT at a lower level shows a nodule adjacent to the diaphragm.

scan is associated with a significantly more rapid decline in physiologic indices of airway obstruction [93]. Thus, CT is a useful noninvasive marker of the extent of inflammation in the small airways and adjacent interstitium, which may be a precursor of emphysema and physiologic deterioration.

Evaluation of air trapping on expiratory CT has been helpful in assessing air trapping caused by small airway disease [94–98]. Availability of scans performed at total lung capacity and functional residual capacity with multi-channel CT spiral datasets also can enable evaluation of airway compliance by comparing airway geometry at the two different lung volumes. The contribution of tracheobronchomalacia to the physiologic impairment of COPD has not been documented systematically.

A further component of COPD that may be evaluated by volumetric CT is the thickness of the airway walls. Increased thickness of airway walls (see Fig. 12) is associated with the presence of COPD [99], the reversibility of airway obstruction [100], and symptoms of chronic bronchitis [101]. In patients who have COPD, bronchial wall thickening is an important independent predictor of FEV_1 [102,103]. Visual assessment of airway wall thickening is quite subjective, but it can be assessed quantitatively by measuring the percentage wall area as a proportion of total bronchial area.

References

[1] Beigelman-Aubry C, Hill C, Guibal A, et al. Multidetector row CT and postprocessing techniques in the assessment of diffuse lung disease. Radiographics 2005;25(6):1639–52.

[2] Chooi WK, Morcos SK. High resolution volume imaging of airways and lung parenchyma with multislice CT. Br J Radiol 2004;77(Spec No 1): S98–105.

[3] Hashimoto M, Tate E, Watarai J, et al. Air trapping on computed tomography images of healthy individuals: effects of respiration and body mass index. Clin Radiol 2006;61(10):883–7.

[4] Spaggiari E, Zompatori M, Verduri A, et al. Early smoking-induced lung lesions in asymptomatic subjects. Correlations between high resolution dynamic CT and pulmonary function testing. Radiol Med (Torino) 2005;109(1-2):27–39.

[5] Kauczor HU, Hast J, Heussel CP, et al. Focal air-trapping at expiratory high-resolution CT: comparison with pulmonary function tests. Eur Radiol 2000;10(10):1539–46.

[6] Leung AN, Fisher K, Valentine V, et al. Bronchiolitis obliterans after lung transplantation: detection using expiratory HRCT. Chest 1998;113(2): 365–70.

[7] Lee ES, Gotway MB, Reddy GP, et al. Early bronchiolitis obliterans following lung transplantation: accuracy of expiratory thin-section CT for diagnosis. Radiology 2000;216(2):472–7.

[8] Stern EJ, Webb WR. Dynamic imaging of lung morphology with ultrafast high-resolution computed tomography. J Thorac Imaging 1993;8(4): 273–82.

[9] Webb WR, Stern EJ, Kanth N, et al. Dynamic pulmonary CT: findings in healthy adult men. Radiology 1993;186(1):117–24.

[10] Stern EJ, Webb WR, Gamsu G. Dynamic quantitative computed tomography. A predictor of pulmonary function in obstructive lung diseases. Invest Radiol 1994;29(5):564–9.

[11] Gotway MB, Lee ES, Reddy GP, et al. Low-dose, dynamic, expiratory thin-section CT of the lungs using a spiral CT scanner. J Thorac Imaging 2000;15(3):168–72.

[12] Zhang J, Hasegawa I, Hatabu H, et al. Frequency and severity of air trapping at dynamic expiratory CT in patients with tracheobronchomalacia. AJR Am J Roentgenol 2004;182(1):81–5.

[13] Zeidler MR, Goldin JG, Kleerup EC, et al. Small airways response to naturalistic cat allergen exposure in subjects with asthma. J Allergy Clin Immunol 2006;118(5):1075–81.

[14] Goldin JG, Tashkin DP, Kleerup EC, et al. Comparative effects of hydrofluoroalkane and chlorofluorocarbon beclomethasone dipropionate inhalation on small airways: assessment with functional helical thin-section computed tomography. J Allergy Clin Immunol 1999;104(6):S258–67.

[15] Mastora I, Remy-Jardin M, Sobaszek A, et al. Thin-section CT finding in 250 volunteers: assessment of the relationship of CT findings with smoking history and pulmonary function test results. Radiology 2001;218(3):695–702.

[16] Tanaka N, Matsumoto T, Miura G, et al. Air trapping at CT: high prevalence in asymptomatic subjects with normal pulmonary function. Radiology 2003;227(3):776–85.

[17] Lee KW, Chung SY, Yang I, et al. Correlation of aging and smoking with air trapping at thin-section CT of the lung in asymptomatic subjects. Radiology 2000;214(3):831–6.

[18] Colby T, Myers J. Clinical and histologic spectrum of bronchiolitis obliterans, including bronchiolitis obliterans organizing pneumonia. Semin Resp Med 1992;13:119–33.

[19] Garg K, Lynch DA, Newell JD, et al. Proliferative and constrictive bronchiolitis: classification and radiologic features. AJR Am J Roentgenol 1994; 162(4):803–8.

[20] Colby TV. Bronchiolitis. Pathologic considerations. Am J Clin Pathol 1998;109(1):101–9.

[21] American Thoracic Society/European Respiratory Society. International multidisciplinary consensus classification of the idiopathic interstitial

pneumonias. Am J Respir Crit Care Med 2002; 165(2):277–304.

[22] Couture C, Colby TV. Histopathology of bronchiolar disorders. Semin Respir Crit Care Med 2003; 24(5):489–98.

[23] Muller NL, Miller RR. Diseases of the bronchioles: CT and histopathologic findings. Radiology 1995; 196(1):3–12.

[24] Pipavath S, Lynch D, Cool C, et al. Radiologic and pathologic features of bronchiolitis. AJR Am J Roentgenol 2005;185:354–63.

[25] Reittner P, Muller NL, Heyneman L, et al. Mycoplasma pneumoniae pneumonia: radiographic and high-resolution CT features in 28 patients. AJR Am J Roentgenol 2000;174(1):37–41.

[26] Adler BD, Padley SP, Muller NL, et al. Chronic hypersensitivity pneumonitis: high-resolution CT and radiographic features in 16 patients. Radiology 1992;185(1):91–5.

[27] Ando M, Arima K, Yoneda R, et al. Japanese summer-type hypersensitivity pneumonitis. Geographic distribution, home environment, and clinical characteristics of 621 cases. Am Rev Respir Dis 1991;144(4):765–9.

[28] Krishnan P, Thachil R, Gillego V. Diffuse panbronchiolitis: a treatable sinobronchial disease in need of recognition in the United States. Chest 2002;121(2):659–61.

[29] Fisher MS Jr, Rush WL, Rosado-de-Christenson ML, et al. Diffuse panbronchiolitis: histologic diagnosis in unsuspected cases involving North American residents of Asian descent. Arch Pathol Lab Med 1998;122(2):156–60.

[30] Fitzgerald JE, King TE Jr, Lynch DA, et al. Diffuse panbronchiolitis in the United States. Am J Respir Crit Care Med 1996;154(2 Pt 1): 497–503.

[31] Souza R, Kairalla RA, Santos Ud Ude P, et al. Diffuse panbronchiolitis: an underdiagnosed disease? Study of 4 cases in Brazil. Rev Hosp Clin Fac Med Sao Paulo 2002;57(4):167–74.

[32] Gulhan M, Erturk A, Kurt B, et al. Diffuse panbronchiolitis observed in a white man in Turkey. Sarcoidosis Vasc Diffuse Lung Dis 2000;17(3): 292–6.

[33] Naalsund A, Foerster A, Aasebo U, et al. [An answer to an inquiry on diffuse panbronchiolitis. Now it has found its way here!]. Lakartidningen 1995;92(35):3119–21 [in Swedish].

[34] Nishimura K, Kitaichi M, Izumi T, et al. Diffuse panbronchiolitis: correlation of high-resolution CT and pathologic findings. Radiology 1992; 184(3):779–85.

[35] Sueyasu Y. Diffuse panbronchiolitis–a thin-section CT scoring system. Kurume Med J 1996;43(1): 63–71.

[36] Akira M, Kitatani J, Yong-Sik L, et al. Diffuse panbronchiolitis: evaluation with high-resolution CT. Radiology 1988;168:433–8.

[37] Akira M, Higashihara T, Sakatani M, et al. Diffuse panbronchiolitis: follow-up CT examination. Radiology 1993;189(2):559–62.

[38] Ichikawa Y, Hotta M, Sumita S, et al. Reversible airway lesions in diffuse panbronchiolitis. Detection by high-resolution computed tomography. Chest 1995;107(1):120–5.

[39] Yamada G, Igarashi T, Itoh E, et al. Centrilobular nodules correlate with air trapping in diffuse panbronchiolitis during erythromycin therapy. Chest 2001;120(1):198–202.

[40] Romero S, Barroso E, Gil J, et al. Follicular bronchiolitis: clinical and pathologic findings in six patients. Lung 2003;181(6):309–19.

[41] Howling SJ, Hansell DM, Wells AU, et al. Follicular bronchiolitis: thin-section CT and histologic findings. Radiology 1999;212(3):637–42.

[42] Exley CM, Suvarna SK, Matthews S. Follicular bronchiolitis as a presentation of HIV. Clin Radiol 2006;61(8):710–3.

[43] Boag AH, Colby TV, Fraire AE, et al. The pathology of interstitial lung disease in nylon flock workers. Am J Surg Pathol 1999;23(12):1539–45.

[44] Eschenbacher WL, Kreiss K, Lougheed MD, et al. Nylon flock-associated interstitial lung disease. Am J Respir Crit Care Med 1999;159(6):2003–8.

[45] Holt R, Schmidt R, Godwin J, et al. High resolution CT in respiratory bronchiolitis-associated interstitial lung disease. J Comput Assist Tomogr 1993;1993:46–50.

[46] Heyneman LE, Ward S, Lynch DA, et al. Respiratory bronchiolitis, respiratory bronchiolitis-associated interstitial lung disease, and desquamative interstitial pneumonia: different entities or part of the spectrum of the same disease process? AJR Am J Roentgenol 1999;173(6):1617–22.

[47] Grobbelaar JP, Bateman ED. Hut lung: a domestically acquired pneumoconiosis of mixed aetiology in rural women. Thorax 1991;46(5):334–40.

[48] Gold JA, Jagirdar J, Hay JG, et al. Hut lung. A domestically acquired particulate lung disease. Medicine (Baltimore) 2000;79(5):310–7.

[49] Diaz JV, Koff J, Gotway MB, et al. Case report: a case of wood-smoke-related pulmonary disease. Environ Health Perspect 2006;114(5):759–62.

[50] Kara M, Bulut S, Tas F, et al. Evaluation of pulmonary changes due to biomass fuels using high-resolution computed tomography. Eur Radiol 2003; 13(10):2372–7.

[51] Sweatman MC, Millar AB, Strickland B, et al. Computed tomography in adult obliterative bronchiolitis. Clin Radiol 1990;41:116–9.

[52] Chang AB, Masel JP, Masters B. Post-infectious bronchiolitis obliterans: clinical, radiological and pulmonary function sequelae. Pediatr Radiol 1998;28(1):23–9.

[53] Marti-Bonmati L, Ruiz Perales F, Catala F, et al. CT findings in Swyer-James syndrome. Radiology 1989;172:477–80.

[54] Morrish WF, Herman SJ, Weisbrod GL, et al. Bronchiolitis obliterans after lung transplantation: findings at chest radiography and high-resolution CT. Radiology 1991;179:487–90.

[55] Loubeyre P, Revel D, Delignette A, et al. Bronchiectasis detected with thin-section CT as a predictor of chronic lung allograft rejection [see comments]. Radiology 1995;194(1):213–6.

[56] Worthy SA, Park CS, Kim JS, et al. Bronchiolitis obliterans after lung transplantation: high-resolution CT findings in 15 patients. AJR Am J Roentgenol 1997;169(3):673–7.

[57] Lau DM, Siegel MJ, Hildebolt CF, et al. Bronchiolitis obliterans syndrome: thin-section CT diagnosis of obstructive changes in infants and young children after lung transplantation. Radiology 1998; 208(3):783–8.

[58] Medina LS, Siegel MJ. CT of complications in pediatric lung transplantation. Radiographics 1994; 14(6):1341–9.

[59] Ikonen T, Kivisaari L, Taskinen E, et al. High-resolution CT in long-term follow-up after lung transplantation. Chest 1997;111(2):370–6.

[60] Miller WT Jr, Kotloff RM, Blumenthal NP, et al. Utility of high resolution computed tomography in predicting bronchiolitis obliterans syndrome following lung transplantation: preliminary findings. J Thorac Imaging 2001;16(2):76–80.

[61] Bankier AA, Van Muylem A, Scillia P, et al. Air trapping in heart-lung transplant recipients: variability of anatomic distribution and extent at sequential expiratory thin-section CT. Radiology 2003;229(3):737–42.

[62] Berstad AE, Aalokken TM, Kolbenstvedt A, et al. Performance of long-term CT monitoring in diagnosing bronchiolitis obliterans after lung transplantation. Eur J Radiol 2006;58(1):124–31.

[63] Konen E, Gutierrez C, Chaparro C, et al. Bronchiolitis obliterans syndrome in lung transplant recipients: can thin-section CT findings predict disease before its clinical appearance? Radiology 2004;231(2):467–73.

[64] de Jong PA, Dodd JD, Coxson HO, et al. Bronchiolitis obliterans following lung transplantation: early detection using computed tomographic scanning. Thorax 2006;61(9):799–804.

[65] Knollmann FD, Kapell S, Lehmkuhl H, et al. Dynamic high-resolution electron-beam CT scanning for the diagnosis of bronchiolitis obliterans syndrome after lung transplantation. Chest 2004; 126(2):447–56.

[66] Bankier AA, Schaefer-Prokop C, De Maertelaer V, et al. Air trapping: comparison of standard-dose and simulated low-dose thin-section CT techniques. Radiology 2007;242(3):898–906.

[67] Gast KK, Viallon M, Eberle B, et al. MRI in lung transplant recipients using hyperpolarized 3He: comparison with CT. J Magn Reson Imaging 2002;15(3):268–74.

[68] Worthy SA, Flint JD, Muller NL. Pulmonary complications after bone marrow transplantation: high- resolution CT and pathologic findings. Radiographics 1997;17(6):1359–71.

[69] Ooi GC, Peh WC, Ip M. High-resolution computed tomography of bronchiolitis obliterans syndrome after bone marrow transplantation. Respiration 1998;65(3):187–91.

[70] Kim EA, Lee KS, Johkoh T, et al. Interstitial lung diseases associated with collagen vascular diseases: radiologic and histopathologic findings. RadioGraphics 2002;22(Spec No):S151–65.

[71] Tanaka N, Kim JS, Newell JD, et al. Rheumatoid arthritis-related lung diseases: CT findings. Radiology 2004;232(1):81–91.

[72] Schwarz MI, Lynch DA, Tuder R. Bronchiolitis obliterans: the lone manifestation of rheumatoid arthritis? Eur Respir J 1994;7(4):817–20.

[73] Sugiyama Y, Ohno S, Kano S, et al. Diffuse panbronchiolitis and rheumatoid arthritis: a possible correlation with HLA-B54. Intern Med 1994; 33(10):612–4.

[74] Kinoshita M, Higashi T, Tanaka C, et al. Follicular bronchiolitis associated with rheumatoid arthritis. Intern Med 1992;31(5):674–7.

[75] Jensen SP, Lynch DA, Brown KK, et al. High-resolution CT features of severe asthma and bronchiolitis obliterans. Clin Radiol 2002;57(12): 1078–85.

[76] Kreiss K, Gomaa A, Kullman G, et al. Clinical bronchiolitis obliterans in workers at a microwave-popcorn plant. N Engl J Med 2002;347(5): 330–8.

[77] Akpinar-Elci M, Travis WD, Lynch DA, et al. Bronchiolitis obliterans syndrome in popcorn production plant workers. Eur Respir J 2004;24(2): 298–302.

[78] Lee JS, Brown KK, Cool C, et al. Diffuse pulmonary neuroendocrine cell hyperplasia: radiologic and clinical features. J Comput Assist Tomogr 2002;26(2):180–4.

[79] Brown MJ, English J, Muller NL. Bronchiolitis obliterans due to neuroendocrine hyperplasia: high-resolution CT–pathologic correlation. AJR Am J Roentgenol 1997;168(6):1561–2.

[80] Klein JS, Gamsu G, Webb WR, et al. High-resolution CT diagnosis of emphysema in symptomatic patients with normal chest radiographs and isolated low diffusing capacity. Radiology 1992; 182(3):817–21.

[81] Omori H, Nakashima R, Otsuka N, et al. Emphysema detected by lung cancer screening with low-dose spiral CT: prevalence, and correlation with smoking habits and pulmonary function in Japanese male subjects. Respirology 2006;11(2): 205–10.

[82] Foster WL Jr, Gimenez EI, Roubidoux MA, et al. The emphysemas: radiologic-pathologic correlations. Radiographics 1993;13(2):311–28.

[83] Goddard PR, Nicholson EM, Laszlo G, et al. Computed tomography in pulmonary emphysema. Clin Radiol 1982;33:379–87.

[84] Foster WL Jr, Pratt PC, Roggli VL, et al. Centrilobular emphysema: CT-pathologic correlation. Radiology 1986;159(1):27–32.

[85] Bergin C, Muller N, Nichols DM, et al. The diagnosis of emphysema. A computed tomographic-pathologic correlation. Am Rev Respir Dis 1986; 133(4):541–6.

[86] Coddington R, Mera SL, Goddard PR, et al. Pathological evaluation of computed tomography images of lungs. J Clin Pathol 1982;35(5):536–40.

[87] Hruban RH, Meziane MA, Zerhouni EA, et al. High resolution computed tomography of inflation-fixed lungs. Pathologic-radiologic correlation of centrilobular emphysema. Am Rev Respir Dis 1987;136(4):935–40.

[88] Kuwano K, Matsuba K, Ikeda T, et al. The diagnosis of mild emphysema. Correlation of computed tomography and pathology scores. Am Rev Respir Dis 1990;141(1):169–78.

[89] Sanders C, Nath PH, Bailey WC. Detection of emphysema with computed tomography. Correlation with pulmonary function tests and chest radiography. Invest Radiol 1988;23(4):262–6.

[90] Remy-Jardin M, Remy J, Boulenguez C, et al. Morphologic effects of cigarette smoking on airways and pulmonary parenchyma in healthy adult volunteers: CT evaluation and correlation with pulmonary function tests. Radiology 1993;186: 107–15.

[91] Park JS, Brown KK, Tuder RM, et al. Respiratory bronchiolitis-associated interstitial lung disease: radiologic features with clinical and pathologic correlation. J Comput Assist Tomogr 2002;26(1):13–20.

[92] Remy-Jardin M, Remy J, Gosselin B, et al. Lung parenchymal changes secondary to cigarette smoking: pathologic-CT correlations. Radiology 1993; 186(3):643–51.

[93] Remy-Jardin M, Edme JL, Boulenguez C, et al. Longitudinal follow-up study of smoker's lung with thin-section CT in correlation with pulmonary function tests. Radiology 2002;222(1):261–70.

[94] Zeidler MR, Kleerup EC, Goldin JG, et al. Montelukast improves regional air-trapping due to small airways obstruction in asthma. Eur Respir J 2006; 27(2):307–15.

[95] Jain N, Covar RA, Gleason MC, et al. Quantitative computed tomography detects peripheral airway disease in asthmatic children. Pediatr Pulmonol 2005;40(3):211–8.

[96] Grenier PA, Beigelman-Aubry C, Fetita C, et al. New frontiers in CT imaging of airway disease. Eur Radiol 2002;12(5):1022–44.

[97] Goldin J. Quantitative CT of the lung. Radiol Clin North Am 2002;40:145–62.

[98] Newman KB, Lynch DA, Newman LS, et al. Quantitative computed tomography detects air trapping due to asthma. Chest 1994;106(1):105–9.

[99] Berger P, Perot V, Desbarats P, et al. Airway wall thickness in cigarette smokers: quantitative thin-section CT assessment. Radiology 2005;235(3): 1055–64.

[100] Kitaguchi Y, Fujimoto K, Kubo K, et al. Characteristics of COPD phenotypes classified according to the findings of HRCT. Respir Med 2006; 100(10):1742–52.

[101] Orlandi I, Moroni C, Camiciottoli G, et al. Chronic obstructive pulmonary disease: thin-section CT measurement of airway wall thickness and lung attenuation. Radiology 2005;234(2):604–10.

[102] Aziz ZA, Wells AU, Desai SR, et al. Functional impairment in emphysema: contribution of airway abnormalities and distribution of parenchymal disease. AJR Am J Roentgenol 2005;185(6):1509–15.

[103] Hasegawa M, Nasuhara Y, Onodera Y, et al. Airflow limitation and airway dimensions in chronic obstructive pulmonary disease. Am J Respir Crit Care Med 2006;173(12):1309–15.

ELSEVIER
SAUNDERS

Clin Chest Med 29 (2008) 181–193

CLINICS
IN CHEST
MEDICINE

Imaging of the Large Airways

Phillip M. Boiselle, MD

Department of Radiology, Beth Israel Deaconess Medical Center, Harvard Medical School,
330 Brookline Avenue, Boston, MA 02115, USA

Recent advances in multidetector-row CT technology and advances in post-processing techniques have revolutionized the ability to noninvasively image the large airways. This article provides a comprehensive review of imaging of the large airways. Introductory sections covering airway anatomy and CT imaging methods are followed by a review of tracheobronchial stenoses, neoplasms, tracheobronchomalacia, and congenital large airway abnormalities. Throughout, an emphasis is placed upon the complementary role of axial CT images and multiplanar reformation and three-dimensional reconstruction images for noninvasively assessing the large airways.

Anatomy

The trachea is a cartilaginous and fibromuscular tubular structure that extends from the inferior aspect of the cricoid cartilage to the level of the carina, a ridge that marks the origin of the main bronchi (Fig. 1) [1–3]. The trachea is comprised of 16 to 22 C-shaped cartilages, which are linked longitudinally by annular ligaments of fibrous and connective tissue [1–3]. The cartilages compose the anterior and lateral walls of the trachea and are connected posteriorly by the membranous wall of the trachea, which lacks cartilage and is supported by the trachealis muscle [1–3]. This muscle is composed of transverse smooth muscle fibers that narrow the tracheal lumen upon contraction [1–3]. The cartilaginous rings play a supportive function and help to maintain an adequate tracheal lumen during expiration. The posterior wall of the trachea either flattens or bows slightly forward during expiration

in normal subjects (Fig. 2) [4,5]. During forced expiration, normal subjects have been shown to demonstrate a mean decrease in anteroposterior dimension of the tracheal lumen of about 35% [4]; however, in the setting of weakening or deficiency of the cartilaginous or membranous components of the airway, excessive expiratory collapsibility (>50% reduction), also referred to as tracheobronchomalacia, may be observed.

The trachea does not derive its blood supply from a single main vessel. Rather, it is supplied by a variety of vessels, including superiorly from the inferior thyroid arteries and right intercostal artery, and inferiorly from branches of the bronchial and intercostals arteries [2].

Normal tracheal measurements are reviewed in Box 1. The trachea is generally midline in position, but it is often displaced slightly to the right at the level of the aortic arch, with greater degree of displacement in the setting of a markedly tortuous, atherosclerotic aorta. The proximal trachea lies close to the skin surface, but the trachea angles posteriorly as it courses inferiorly in the thorax, eventually achieving a midcoronal location at the level of the carina (Fig. 3). Because of the angled course of the trachea, axial CT images do not provide a true perpendicular cross section of its lumen.

On axial CT images, the normal tracheal lumen usually demonstrates an oval, round (see Fig. 2a), or horseshoe shape [6]. The tracheal index can be calculated by dividing the coronal diameter (mm) by the sagittal diameter (mm). The normal value is approximately 1 [1,3–5]. A "saber-sheath" trachea (Fig. 4) refers to a configuration in which there is marked coronal narrowing and accentuation of the sagittal diameter (sagittal:coronal ratio >2) [10,11]. This finding is frequently associated with chronic obstructive

E-mail address: pboisell@bidmc.harvard.edu

0272-5231/08/$ - see front matter © 2008 Elsevier Inc. All rights reserved.
doi:10.1016/j.ccm.2007.11.002

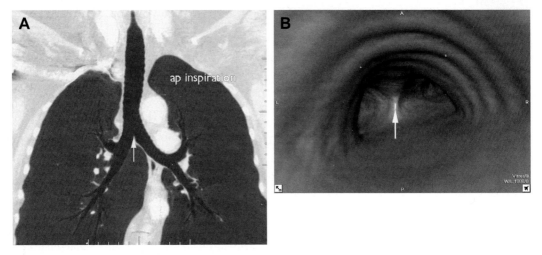

Fig. 1. Normal trachea. (*A*) Minimum intensity projection coronal oblique reformation CT image of the normal trachea and bronchi. Main bronchi originate from inferior trachea at level of carina (*arrow*). (*B*) Virtual bronchoscopic image shows internal perspective of lower trachea, carina (*arrow*), and proximal main bronchi.

lung disease. In contrast, a "lunate" trachea (Fig. 5a) refers to accentuation of the coronal diameter with a relative narrowing of the sagittal diameter (coronal:sagittal ratio >1) [12]. This finding is frequently associated with airway malacia (excessive expiratory collapsibility of the airway lumen) (see Fig. 5b).

The tracheal wall is composed of several layers, including an inner mucosa layer, followed by submucosa, cartilage or muscle, and an outer adventitia layer [13]. On axial CT images, the tracheal wall is usually visible as a 1- to 3-mm soft-tissue density stripe, demarcated internally

by the air-filled tracheal lumen and externally by the adjacent fat-density of the mediastinum (Fig. 6) [13]. The posterior wall is typically thinner than the anterior and lateral walls. Cartilage within the tracheal wall may normally appear slightly denser than surrounding soft tissue and fat [13]. Calcification of cartilage may be observed in older patients, especially women [13].

Thickening of the airway wall (with or without calcification) is an important sign of tracheal pathology (Figs. 7 and 8). Importantly, axial images are the reference standard for assessing tracheal wall thickening, a finding that may be

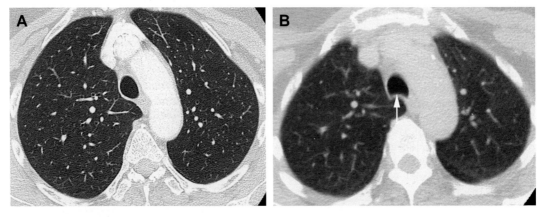

Fig. 2. Normal tracheal dynamics. (*A*) End-inspiratory image shows a round configuration of the tracheal lumen. (*B*) At end-expiration, the tracheal lumen has narrowed slightly, with anterior bowing of the posterior membranous wall (*arrow*).

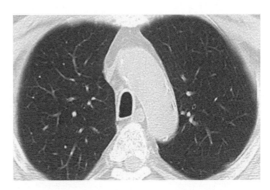

Fig. 4. Saber sheath trachea. Axial CT image demonstrates elongated sagittal dimension of trachea with relative narrowing in the coronal plane, consistent with saber sheath configuration.

overlooked at conventional bronchoscopy and three dimensional (3D) reconstruction images. The distribution of wall thickening can be helpful in limiting the differential diagnosis of the various causes of tracheal stenosis. For example, disorders of cartilage, such as relapsing polychondritis (see Fig. 7) and tracheobronchopathia osteochondroplastica (TBO), will spare the posterior membranous wall of the trachea, whereas other

disorders generally result in circumferential thickening (see Fig. 8).

The main bronchi arise from the trachea at the level of the carina (see Fig. 1) and course obliquely to the axial plane. Because of the limitations of axial images for assessing structures that course obliquely, multiplanar and 3D reconstruction images are particularly helpful for evaluating caliber changes in the mainstem bronchi.

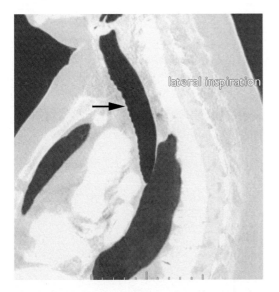

Fig. 3. Normal trachea. Minimum intensity projection sagittal oblique reformation CT image of the normal trachea (*arrow*) shows typical angled course of trachea from proximal anterior location to midcoronal position at level of carina.

CT imaging methods

The recent advent of multidetector-row CT (MDCT) imaging has revolutionized noninvasive imaging of the central airways. With the latest generation of MDCT scanners, thin-section images of the entire central airways can be obtained in only a few seconds, creating an isotropic dataset in which the resolution is the same in the axial, coronal, and sagittal planes. Compared with standard helical CT scanners, MDCT provides higher spatial resolution, faster speed, greater anatomic coverage, and higher quality multiplanar reformation and 3D reconstruction images.

Axial CT images provide important anatomical information about the airway lumen, airway wall, and adjacent mediastinal and lung structures. Although axial CT images are still the reference standard for airway imaging, they have several important limitations, including limited ability to detect subtle airway stenoses, underestimation of the craniocaudad extent of disease, difficulty displaying complex 3D relationships of the airway, and inadequate representation of airways oriented obliquely to the axial plane

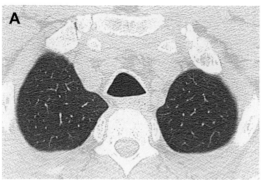
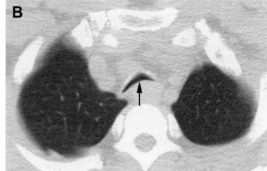

Fig. 5. Lunate trachea. (*A*) Axial end-inspiratory CT image shows elongated coronal dimension of trachea. (*B*) Axial dynamic expiratory CT image shows severe malacia, with excessive expiratory collapse of the tracheal lumen (*arrow*).

[14–22]. These limitations have important implications for assessing airway stenoses and complex, congenital airway abnormalities. Fortunately, multiplanar and 3D reconstruction images can overcome these limitations by providing a more anatomically meaningful display of the airways and adjacent structures [14–21]. These images have been shown to enhance the detection of airway stenoses, to aid the assessment of the craniocaudad extent of stenoses (Fig. 9), and to clarify complex, congenital airway abnormalities [19]. They have also been shown to improve diagnostic confidence of interpretation, enhance preprocedural planning for bronchoscopy and surgery, and improve communication among radiologists, clinicians, and patients [14–16].

Anatomical imaging of the airways is performed at end-inspiration; however, an additional expiratory imaging sequence should be performed for suspected airway malacia, which escapes detection on routine end-inspiratory sequences. As reviewed later in this article, dynamic expiratory imaging (imaging during a forced expiration) is superior to end-expiratory imaging (imaging after exhalation) for eliciting airway malacia [23–27].

Tracheobronchial stenosis

Tracheobronchial stenosis is defined as focal or diffuse narrowing of the tracheal lumen. It may occur secondary to a wide variety of benign and malignant causes (Box 2).

Axial CT images provide a precise anatomical display of the tracheal wall and lumen; however, as noted earlier in this article, they have a limited

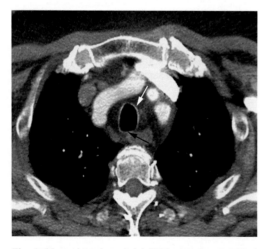

Fig. 6. Normal trachea. Axial CT image shows normal thickness of tracheal wall. Note the "paper thin" quality of the posterior membranous wall (*black arrow*) and the slightly thicker anterior (*white arrow*) and lateral walls.

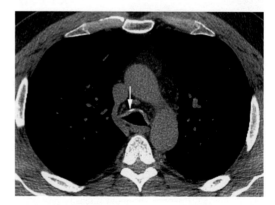

Fig. 7. Relapsing polychondritis. Axial CT image shows thickening of anterolateral tracheal walls with focal calcification (*arrow*). Note characteristic sparing of posterior membranous wall.

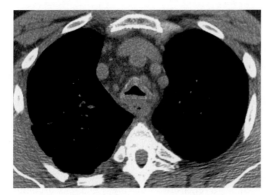

Fig. 8. Sarcoidosis. Axial CT image shows circumferential wall thickening of tracheal airway lumen.

ability to detect subtle airway stenoses, and frequently underestimate the craniocaudad extent of stenoses [14–20]. By providing a continuous anatomical display of the airways, multiplanar and 3D reconstruction images help to overcome these limitations [14]. In settings where such reconstructions are not possible, careful review of contiguous thin-section axial images can help to prevent the radiologist from overlooking stenoses.

CT evaluation of suspected tracheal stenosis is routinely performed at end-inspiration during a single breath hold. An additional sequence during dynamic expiration may be helpful to assess for tracheomalacia, which may coexist with tracheobronchial stenoses, especially among patients who have relapsing polychondritis, post-intubation stenosis, and airway narrowing secondary to long-standing extrinsic compression

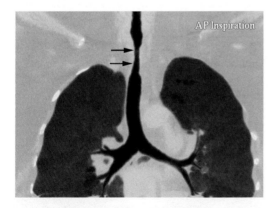

Fig. 9. Subglottic stenosis caused by prior tracheostomy tube. Minimum intensity projection, coronal reformation image of trachea shows moderate tracheal stenosis (*arrows*). Severity and craniocaudad length of stenosis were underestimated on axial CT images (not shown).

Box 2. Causes of tracheobronchial stenosis:

Iatrogenic
- Post-intubation[a]
- Lung transplantation

Idiopathic

Infection
- Laryngotracheal papillomatosis[b]
- Rhinoscleroma
- Tuberculosis

Neoplasm
- Primary tracheal neoplasm (squamous carcinoma, adenoid cystic carcinoma)
- Direct invasion (lung, esophagus, thyroid)
- Secondary neoplasm (breast, renal, melanoma, thyroid)

Saber sheath deformity

Systemic diseases
- Amyloidosis
- Inflammatory bowel disease
- Relapsing polychondritis
- Sarcoidosis
- Wegener granulomatosis

Tracheobronchopathia osteochondroplastica

Trauma

_____
[a] Most common etiology.
[b] Although papillomas represent growth of new tissue, laryngotracheal papillomatosis is most frequently categorized as a non-neoplastic disease.

(eg, thyroid enlargement or mediastinal aortic vascular anomalies) [28,29].

It is important to accurately assess the location, length, and distribution of the stenosis, as well as the presence, distribution, and type of wall thickening. A consideration of these factors, in combination with ancillary thoracic findings and pertinent clinical and laboratory data, will allow the radiologist to effectively narrow the broad differential diagnosis of tracheobronchial stenosis to a few likely entities. In certain cases, such as relapsing polychondritis or TBO, a confident diagnosis can be made on the basis of imaging findings alone.

Although there is significant overlap in the imaging features of many causes of tracheobronchial stenosis, several key imaging features can help to effectively narrow this broad differential diagnosis. These features include: sparing of the posterior membranous wall (typical of relapsing polychondritis and TBO) (see Fig. 7), "hourglass" configuration (post-intubation stenosis), and calcification (relapsing polychondritis, TBO, amyloid, and tuberculosis). Additionally, systemic disorders (eg, amyloid, inflammatory bowel disease, polychondritis, sarcoid [see Fig. 8], tuberculosis, Wegener granulomatosis) are often associated with characteristic ancillary imaging and laboratory findings that may suggest their diagnosis.

Post-intubation stenosis is by far the most common cause of acquired tracheal stenosis, and may occur following endotracheal intubation or tracheostomy tube placement (see Fig. 9) [30]. It typically occurs secondary to injury of the trachea from the high pressure of an endotracheal tube balloon against the wall of the trachea [30,31]. This initially results in mucosal necrosis, followed by scarring and stenosis [30,31].

A recent study comparing MDCT with the gold standard of bronchoscopy showed a high sensitivity (92%) and specificity (100%) for detection of post-intubation stenosis [32]. The most common CT finding in post-intubation stenosis is a focal area of proximal tracheal luminal narrowing measuring approximately 2 cm in craniocaudad length [13,30,31]. The focal nature and circumferential narrowing typically produces a characteristic hourglass configuration. Less common findings include a thin membrane projecting into the tracheal lumen or a long segment of eccentric soft-tissue thickening [30,31].

Tracheobronchial neoplasms

Tracheobronchial neoplasms are rare. For example, it has been estimated that a primary tracheal tumor is roughly 180 times less common than a primary lung cancer [33]. A neoplasm within the central airways is more likely caused by direct airway invasion by an adjacent secondary neoplasm originating from the thyroid, lung, or esophagus [34].

A majority of primary tracheal neoplasms in adults are malignant, whereas the opposite is true in children [30,35]. Although a wide variety of neoplasms may arise in the central airways, five histologies compose the majority of primary tracheobronchial neoplasms: squamous cell carcinoma, adenoid cystic carcinoma, carcinoid, mucoepidermoid carcinoma, and squamous cell papilloma [36]. The most common cell type is squamous cell carcinoma, which is associated with cigarette smoking [30,35]. The second most common cell type is adenoid cystic carcinoma (Fig. 10), which is not associated with smoking [30,35]. It has a better prognosis than squamous cell carcinoma, but late recurrence is relatively common. The most common benign tracheal neoplasm is squamous cell papilloma, which is associated with cigarette smoking [30,35]. Carcinoid tumors are neuroendocrine neoplasms that most commonly arise within the main and lobar bronchi (Fig. 11), but about 15% develop within the segmental bronchi or lung periphery [37,38]. They are not associated with cigarette smoking.

MDCT is the imaging modality of choice for detection and staging of central airway neoplasms. Multiplanar reformation and 3D reconstruction images complement conventional axial images by providing a more anatomically meaningful display of the neoplasm and its relationship to adjacent structures, and by accurately determining the craniocaudad extent of disease [14]. Virtual bronchoscopy images provide a unique intraluminal perspective of the tumor. These images also play a potentially complementary role to conventional bronchoscopy by providing assessment of distal airways beyond a high-grade luminal narrowing or obstruction. Moreover, this method can provide a more global perspective of an endoluminal lesion than conventional bronchoscopy.

Surgery is the optimal therapy for both benign and malignant airway neoplasms [35,39,40].

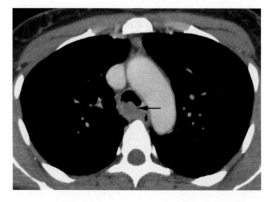

Fig. 10. Adenoid cystic carcinoma. Axial CT at level of aortic arch shows a lobulated, intraluminal mass (*black arrow*).

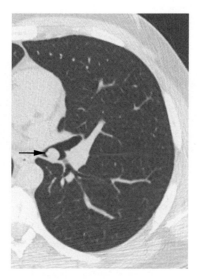

Fig. 11. Carcinoid tumor. Axial CT demonstrates a round, smoothly marginated, intraluminal lesion (*arrow*) in distal left main bronchus.

Radiation therapy may be administered to patients who have unresectable disease or as an adjunct to surgery, particularly in patients who have adenoid cystic carcinoma [39].

MDCT can determine whether a tumor is amenable to complete surgical resection, as well as the approach, type, and extent of surgical resection. MDCT provides critical information for the surgeon, including precise delineation of the 3D size of the neoplasm, including the craniocaudal length, and its relationship with other vital structures, including vascular structures. MDCT accurately defines the intraluminal and extraluminal extension of tumor, as well as post-obstructive complications such as atelectasis, pneumonia, and mucous plugging. Although MDCT can reliably detect the presence of lymphadenopathy, it cannot distinguish between hyperplastic and malignant nodes. Hyperplastic nodes are frequently seen in the setting of postobstructive pneumonitis from an endoluminal neoplasm. Additionally, MDCT does not reliably detect microscopic mediastinal invasion or neural invasion [41]. MDCT may detect pulmonary and extrapulmonary metastases, thereby enhancing tumor staging.

When a discrete tracheal mass is identified on imaging studies, the diagnosis of a primary tracheal neoplasm can usually be made with a high degree of confidence. CT can frequently suggest whether a tracheal lesion is malignant or benign [39]. Although some overlap exists, benign lesions are typically less than 2 cm in diameter, with well-defined, smooth borders, and without evidence of contiguous tracheal thickening or mediastinal invasion. In contrast, malignant lesions usually vary in size between 2 and 4 cm in diameter, with a flat or polypoid shape and irregular or lobulated borders (see Fig. 10). Contiguous tracheal wall thickening and mediastinal invasion are frequently observed. Although CT usually cannot distinguish between neoplastic cell types, detection of fat within a lesion on CT is nearly pathognomonic for a hamartoma or lipoma, and identification of calcification within a lesion is highly suggestive of a chondroid tumor (chondroma, chondrosarcoma). Vigorous enhancement of a bronchial neoplasm is typical of a carcinoid tumor.

In a minority of cases, tracheal neoplasms present as eccentric or circumferential tracheal wall thickening rather than a discrete mass. In such cases, the differential diagnosis includes tracheal stenosis from a variety of nonmalignant entities. In general, the presence of marked irregularity of tracheal wall thickening and the presence of extratracheal extension favor a primary tracheal neoplasm, but biopsy is usually necessary to establish the diagnosis.

Tracheobronchomalacia

Trachebronchomalacia refers to weakness of the airway walls or supporting cartilage, and is characterized by excessive expiratory collapse (see Figs. 5; Figs. 12 and 13) [28,29,42,43]. It may be either congenital or acquired. The acquired form is associated with a variety of risk factors and comorbidities, most notably chronic obstructive pulmonary disease (Box 3) [28,29,42]. Because it cannot be detected with routine end-inspiratory imaging studies, tracheobronchomalacia is widely considered an underdiagnosed condition [42,44–47].

Although bronchoscopy with functional maneuvers can reliably detect tracheobronchomalacia, it is not clinically feasible or desirable to perform this invasive test in all patients who present with chronic cough and other nonspecific respiratory symptoms. Recently, MDCT has been shown to noninvasively diagnose tracheobronchomalacia with similar sensitivity to conventional bronchoscopy [48–50].

Changes in size of malacic trachea and bronchi depend on the difference between the intraluminal

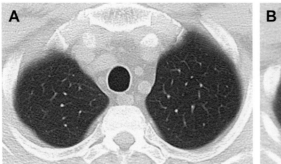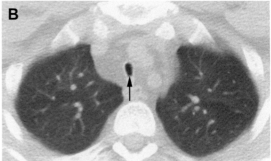

Fig. 12. Tracheomalacia. (*A*) End-inspiratory image of proximal trachea is normal. (*B*) Dynamic expiratory image shows excessive expiratory collapse with circumferential narrowing of trachea lumen (*arrow*).

pressure inside the airways and the pleural (intrathoracic) pressure outside [23,28]. Pleural pressure depends mostly on respiratory muscles, and is high during expiratory efforts. In contrast, intraluminal pressures are highly variable, and depend on airflow. When airflow is zero, intraluminal pressure equals alveolar pressure, and differs from pleural pressure only by the elastic recoil pressure of the lung, which depends on lung volume. At maximal lung volume with no flow (end-inspiration), the intraluminal pressure is 20 to 30 cm H_2O greater than pleural pressure, and the pressure difference expands the trachea. At low lung volumes with no flow (end-expiration), the intraluminal pressure is nearly equal to pleural pressure, and the trachea is unstressed. The trachea is most compressed during cough and dynamic

expiration at low lung volume, when pleural pressure is high (~ 100 cm H_2O), and expiratory flow limitation in the small airways prevents transmission of the high alveolar pressures to the central airways. Under these conditions, intraluminal pressure is nearly atmospheric, and the large transmural pressure causes tracheal collapse [51].

Baroni and colleagues [23] directly compared the ability of end-expiratory and dynamic expiratory CT imaging methods to elicit tracheobronchomalacia. Consistent with the principles of respiratory physiology, their study showed that dynamic expiratory CT elicited a significantly greater degree of tracheal collapse than end-expiratory CT.

The vast majority of studies reported in the literature support the use of a threshold of greater

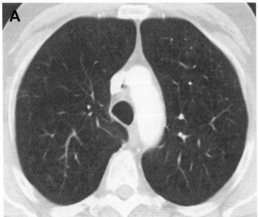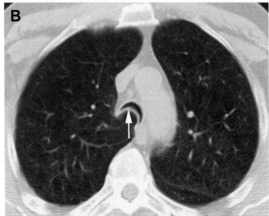

Fig. 13. Frown sign. (*A*) End-inspiratory image of the trachea is normal. Note the presence of emphysema. (*B*) Dynamic expiratory CT image demonstrates frownlike configuration of proximal trachea caused by excessive anterior displacement of posterior membranous wall that parallels the convex contour of the anterior wall, resulting in a characteristic crescentic lucency (*arrow*) that mimics a frown.

masses, in whom long-standing compression has been complicated by tracheomalacia.

The most accurate means for diagnosing malacia on CT is to use an electronic tracing tool to calculate the cross-sectional area of the airway lumen on images at the same anatomic level obtained at inspiration and dynamic expiration [29]. Such tools can be found on commercially available picture archival computer system (PACS) stations and dedicated post-processing workstations. Care should be taken to ensure that the same anatomical level is compared between the two sequences by comparing vascular structures and other anatomical landmarks.

In the setting of severe malacia, in which there is near complete collapse of the airway lumen during expiration, the diagnosis can be confidently made based on visual analysis of the images. It has recently been shown that about half of patients who have acquired tracheomalacia will demonstrate a characteristic expiratory "frownlike" configuration, in which the posterior membranous wall is excessively bowed forward and parallels the convex contour of the anterior wall with less than 6 mm distance between the anterior and posterior walls (see Fig. 13) [54]. This appearance, which has been termed the "frown sign," is highly suggestive of tracheomalacia, and can suggest the diagnosis of tracheomalacia on routine CT scans if patients inadvertently exhale [54]. Ideally, however, the diagnosis of tracheomalacia should be confirmed and quantified by a dedicated CT tracheal study.

When interpreting CT scans of patients who have tracheomalacia, it is important to report the severity, distribution, and morphology. These factors have an important impact upon treatment decisions, which are based upon a combination of symptoms, severity and distribution of disease, and underlying cause of tracheomalacia [55]. Patients who have severely symptomatic diffuse tracheomalacia characterized by excessive mobility and weakening of the posterior membranous wall may benefit from tracheoplasty, a surgical procedure that reinforces the posterior wall of the trachea with Marlex graft [56].

than or equal to 50% collapse as diagnostic of tracheobronchomalacia when using either bronchoscopy or CT; however, several studies have advocated the adoption of different threshold values, and there are only limited data in the literature regarding the normal range of dynamic expiratory collapse [2,52,53]. Based on available data in the literature, it is reasonable to employ a diagnostic threshold of greater than 50% expiratory luminal collapse, keeping in mind that some normal individuals may exceed this threshold.

Interpretation of CT images for the diagnosis of tracheobronchomalacia requires careful review and comparison of both end-inspiratory and dynamic expiratory images. The tracheal lumen is almost always normal in appearance on end-inspiration CT in patients who have tracheobronchomalacia (see Figs. 12a and 13a) [54]. Notable exceptions include: patients who have relapsing polychondritis who may demonstrate characteristic wall thickening and calcification that spares the posterior membranous wall of the trachea; patients who have lunate tracheal shape (coronal>sagittal dimension), which is frequently associated with tracheomalacia (see Fig. 5); and patients who have extrinsic tracheal compression from adjacent vascular anomalies or thyroid

Congenital anomalies

A variety of congenital anomalies may affect the central airways, including branching anomalies, congenital stenosis, congenital malacia, congenital tracheobronchomegaly, and congenital diverticula.

190   BOISELLE

Tracheal bronchus

Tracheal bronchus refers to an anomalous bronchial origin from the trachea, carina, or main bronchi. The anomalous origin is usually located within 2 cm of the carina [11,57–59]. Most commonly, this occurs as a displaced bronchus arising from the lower trachea and supplying the right upper lobe apical segment. Less commonly, the entire right upper lobe bronchus may be displaced, a configuration that is also referred to as a "pig bronchus" (Fig. 14). Although usually an asymptomatic and incidentally detected finding, impaired drainage may result in recurrent infections in some cases. Additionally, following endotracheal intubation, atelectasis may occur in the portion of lung supplied by the aberrant bronchus because of inadvertent obstruction by the balloon cuff.

Congenital tracheal stenosis

Congenital tracheal stenosis is a rare disorder that is characterized by complete tracheal rings associated with absent or deficient tracheal membranes [60–62]. It ranges in length from short to long segment stenosis. It typically presents during the first year of life and is associated with a high mortality rate. Symptoms include stridor, wheezing, cyanosis, and recurrent pneumonia. Adult presentation is rare, but is more common with short segment stenosis (Fig. 15) [62].

CT is highly sensitive for evaluating the length and extent of narrowing, as well as for identifying associated cardiopulmonary anomalies, including pulmonary artery sling. On axial CT images, there is narrowing of the tracheal lumen with an O-shaped configuration and absence of airway

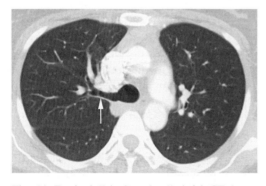

Fig. 14. Tracheal "pig bronchus." Axial CT image shows anomalous origin of entire right upper lobe bronchus (*arrow*) from the lower trachea.

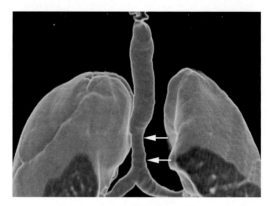

Fig. 15. Congenital tracheal stenosis. 3D external rendering of the trachea demonstrates a short-segment stenosis of the lower trachea (*arrows*).

wall thickening. Virtual bronchoscopy is diagnostic by showing concentric rings extending along the posterior wall of the trachea. Surgical treatment usually involves resection of the involved segment or a slide tracheoplasty [62]. Asymptomatic pediatric patients may be followed by CT to noninvasively monitor tracheal growth [63].

Congenital tracheomalacia

Congenital tracheomalacia refers to softening of the trachea secondary to weakening or deficiency of cartilage, resulting in increased tracheal compliance with excessive expiratory collapse [28]. This condition is most commonly identified in premature infants, likely related to inadequate maturation of the tracheobronchial cartilage. It may also be associated with diseases involving cartilage (eg, polychondritis, chondromalacia, Hunter and Hurler syndromes) [28]. Symptoms include expiratory stridor and a barking cough.

Intervention is unnecessary in most cases because tracheal cartilage strengthens and stiffens as the child grows. Patients who do not spontaneously improve may respond to continuous positive airway pressure (CPAP) or surgical intervention (eg, aortopexy or tracheoplasty).

Congenital tracheomegaly

Congenital tracheomegaly (also referred to as Mounier-Kuhn syndrome) is characterized by dilation of the trachea and main bronchi caused by severe atrophy of longitudinal elastic fibers and thinning of the muscularis mucosa [9,64]. Affected patients typically present during the third and fourth decades with recurrent respiratory

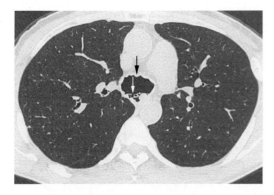

Fig. 16. Congenital tracheobronchomegaly. Axial CT image at carina level shows enlargement of tracheal lumen with corrugated configuration of anterior wall (*black arrow*) and small diverticuli posteriorly (*white arrow*).

infections. Tracheomegaly is defined in women as tracheal diameter greater than 21 mm in the coronal dimension and 23 mm in the sagittal dimension, and in men as tracheal diameter greater than 25 mm in the coronal dimension and 27 mm in the sagittal dimension [9].

On imaging studies, there is dilation of the tracheobronchial lumen, often associated with a corrugated appearance of the tracheal wall and frequent diverticula (Fig. 16). Bronchiectasis and tracheobronchomalacia are also frequently present.

Congenital tracheal diverticula

Congenital tracheal diverticula are less common than the acquired form [65]. They are characterized by single or multiple invaginations of the tracheal wall. They commonly arise 4 to 5 cm below the vocal cords or 2 to 3 cm above the carina on the right lateral aspect of the trachea. In the absence of symptoms, no treatment is necessary.

References

[1] Holbert JM, Strollo DC. Imaging of the normal trachea. J Thorac Imaging 1995;10:171–9.
[2] Naidich DP, Webb WR, Grenier PA, et al. Introduction to imaging methodology and airway anatomy. In: Naidich DP, Webb WR, Grenier PA, editors. Imaging of the airways: functional and radiologic correlations. Philadelphia: Lippincott, Williams and Wilkins; 2005. p. 1–28.
[3] Fraser RS, Colman N, Muller NL, et al. The airways and pulmonary ventilation. In: Fraser RS, Colman N, Muller NL, editors. Fraser and Pare's diagnosis of diseases of the chest. 4th edition. Philadelphia: W.B. Saunders; 1999. p. 3–70.
[4] Stern EJ, Graham CM, Webb WR, et al. Normal trachea during forced expiration: dynamic CT measurements. Radiology 1993;187(1):27–31.
[5] Naidich DP, Webb WR, Grenier PA, et al. Functional imaging of the airway. In: Naidich DP, Webb WR, Grenier PA, editors. Imaging of the airways: functional and radiologic correlations. Philadelphia: Lippincott, Williams and Wilkins; 2005. p. 181–2.
[6] Gamsu G, Webb WR. Computed tomography of the trachea: normal and abnormal. AJR Am J Roentgenol 1982;139:321–6.
[7] Vock P, Spiegel T, Fram EK, et al. CT assessment of the adult intrathoracic cross section of the trachea. J Comput Assist Tomogr 1984;8:1076–82.
[8] Breatnach E, Abbott GC, Fraser RG. Dimensions of the normal human trachea. AJR Am J Roentgenol 1983;141:903–6.
[9] Woodring JH, Smith Howard R, Rehn SR. Congenital tracheobronchomegaly (Mounier-Kuhn) syndrome: a report of 10 cases and review of the literature. J Thorac Imaging 1991;6:1–10.
[10] Greene R, Lechner GL. "Saber-sheath" trachea: a clinical and functional study of marked coronal narrowing of the intrathoracic trachea. Radiology 1975;115:265–8.
[11] Trigaux JP, Hermes G, Dubois P, et al. CT of saber-sheath trachea: correlation with clinical, chest radiographic and functional findings. Acta radiol 1994;35: 247–50.
[12] Lomasney L, Bergin CJ, Lomasney J, et al. CT appearance of lunate trachea. J Comput Assist Tomogr 1989;13:520–2.
[13] Webb EM, Elicker BM, Webb WR. Using CT to diagnose nonneoplastic tracheal abnormalities. Appearance of the tracheal wall. AJR Am J Roentgenol 2000;174:1315–21.
[14] Boiselle PM, Reynolds KF, Ernst A. Multiplanar and three-dimensional imaging of the central airways with multidetector CT. AJR Am J Roentgenol 2002;179:301–8.
[15] Boiselle PM, Lee KS, Ernst A. Multidetector CT of the central airways. J Thorac Imaging 2005;20: 186–95.
[16] Salvolini L, Secchi EB, Costarelli L, et al. Clinical applications of 2D and 3D CT imaging of the airways—a review. Eur J Radiol 2000;34:9–25.
[17] Naidich DP, Gruden JF, McGuiness GM, et al. Volumetric (helical/spiral) CT (VCT) of the airways. J Thorac Imaging 1997;12:11–28.
[18] Remy-Jardin M, Remy J, Artaud D, et al. Tracheobronchial tree: assessment with volume rendering—technical aspects. Radiology 1998;208:393–8.
[19] Remy-Jardin M, Remy J, Artaud D, et al. Volume rendering of the tracheobronchial tree: clinical evaluation of bronchographic images. Radiology 1998; 208:761–70.

[20] Remy-Jardin M, Remy J, Deschildre F, et al. Obstructive lesions of the central airways: evaluation by using spiral CT with multiplanar and three-dimensional reformations. Eur Radiol 1996;6:807–16.

[21] Rubin GD. Data explosion: the challenge of multidetector-row CT. Eur J Radiol 2000;36:74–80.

[22] Lucidarme O, Grenier PA, Coche E, et al. Bronchiectasis: comparative assessment with thin-section CT and helical CT. Radiology 1996;200:673–9.

[23] Baroni R, Feller-Kopman D, Nishino M, et al. Tracheobronchomalacia: comparison between end-expiratory and dynamic-expiratory CT methods for evaluation of central airway collapse. Radiology 2005;2:635–41.

[24] Nishino M, Hatabu H. Volumetric expiratory HRCT imaging with MSCT. J Thorac Imaging 2005;20:176–85.

[25] Choi SJ, Choi BK, Kim HJ, et al. Lateral decubitus HRCT: a simple technique to replace expiratory CT in children with air trapping. Pediatr Radiol 2002;32:179–82.

[26] Long FR, Williams RS, Adler BH, et al. Comparison of quiet breathing and controlled ventilation in the high-resolution CT assessment of airway disease in infants with cystic fibrosis. Pediatr Radiol 2005;35:1075–80.

[27] Goo HW, Kim HJ. Detection of air trapping on inspiratory and expiratory phase images obtained by 0.3-second cine CT in the lungs of free-breathing young children. AJR Am J Roentgenol 2006;187:1019–23.

[28] Carden K, Boiselle PM, Waltz D, et al. Tracheomalacia and tracheobronchomalacia in children and adults: an in-depth review of a common disorder. Chest 2005;127:984–1005.

[29] Boiselle PM, Feller-Kopman D, Ashiku S, et al. Tracheobronchomalacia: evolving role of mutlislice helical CT. Radiol Clin North Am 2003;41:627–36.

[30] Fraser RS, Colman N, Müller NL, et al. Upper airway obstruction. In: Fraser RS, Colman N, Müller NL, editors. Fraser and Pare's diagnosis of diseases of the chest. 4th edition. Philadelphia: W. B. Saunders Co; 1999. p. 2033–6.

[31] Prince JS, Duhamel DR, Levin DL, et al. Nonneoplastic lesions of the tracheobronchial wall: radiographic findings with bronchoscopic correlation. Radiographics 2002;22:S215–30.

[32] Sun M, Ernst A, Boiselle PM. MDCT of the central airways: comparison with bronchoscopy in the evaluation of complications of endotracheal and tracheostomy tubes. J Thorac Imaging 2007;22:136–42.

[33] Houston HE, Payne WS, Harrison EG Jr, et al. Primary cancers of the trachea. Arch Surg 1969;99:132–40.

[34] Dennie CJ, Coblentz CL. The trachea: pathologic conditions and trauma. Can Assoc Radiol J 1993;44:157–67.

[35] McCarthy MJ, Rosado-de-Christenson ML. Tumors of the trachea. J Thorac Imaging 1995;10:180–98.

[36] Grillo HC, Mathisen DJ. Primary tracheal tumors: treatment and results. Ann Thorac Surg 1990;49:69–77.

[37] Okike N, Bernatz PE, Woolner LB. Carcinoid tumors of the lung. Ann Thorac Surg 1976;22:270–7.

[38] Parsons RB, Milestone BN, Adler LP. Radiographic assessment of airway tumors. Chest Surg Clin N Am 2003;13:63–77.

[39] Kaminski JM, Langer CJ, Movsas B. The role of radiation therapy and chemotherapy in the management of airway tumors other than small-cell carcinoma and non-small-cell carcinoma. Chest Surg Clin N Am 2003;13:149–67.

[40] Kwong JS, Adler BD, Padley SPG, et al. Diagnosis of diseases of the trachea and main bronchi: chest radiography vs CT. AJR Am J Roentgenol 1993;161:519–22.

[41] Kwak SH, Lee KS, Chung MJ, et al. Adenoid cystic carcinoma of the airways: helical CT and histopathologic correlation. AJR Am J Roentgenol 2004;183:277–81.

[42] Johnson TH, Mikita JJ, Wilson RJ, et al. Acquired tracheomalacia. Radiology 1973;109:576–80.

[43] Jokinen K, Palva T, Sutinen S, et al. Acquired tracheobronchomalacia. Ann Clin Res 1977;9:52–7.

[44] Palombini BC, Villanova CA, Araujo E, et al. A pathogenic triad in chronic cough: asthma, postnasal drip syndrome and gastroesophageal reflux disease. Chest 1999;116:279–84.

[45] Ikeda S, Hanawa T, Konishi T, et al. Diagnosis, incidence, clinicopathology and surgical treatment of acquired tracheobronchomalacia. Nihon Kyobu Shikkan Gakkai Zasshi 1992;30:1028–103 [in Japanese].

[46] Hasegawa I, Boiselle PM, Hatabu H. Bronchial artery visualization on multislice CT in patients with acute PE: comparison with chronic or recurrent PE. AJR Am J Roentgenol 2004;182:67–72.

[47] Lee KS, Ernst A, Trentham D, et al. Prevalence of functional airway abnormalities in relapsing polychondritis. Radiology 2006;240:565–73.

[48] Gilkeson RC, Ciancibello LM, Hejal RB, et al. Tracheobronchomalacia: dynamic airway evaluation with multidetector CT. AJR Am J Roentgenol 2001;176:205–10.

[49] Zhang J, Hasegawa I, Feller-Kopman D, et al. Dynamic expiratory volumetric CT imaging of the central airways: comparison of standard-dose and low-dose techniques. Acad Radiol 2003;10:719–24.

[50] Lee KS, Sun ME, Ernst A, et al. Comparison of dynamic expiratory CT with bronchoscopy in diagnosing airway malacia. Chest 2007;131:758–64.

[51] Wilson TA, Rodarte JR, Butler JP. Wave speed and viscous flow limitation. In: Macklem PT, Mead J, editors. Handbook of physiology, the respiratory system. Mechanics of breathing, part 1, vol. 3. Bethesda (MD): The American Physiological Society; 1986. p. 55–61.

[52] Heussel CP, Hafner B, Lill J, et al. Paired inspiratory/expiratory spiral CT and continuous respiration cine CT in the diagnosis of tracheal instability. Eur Radiol 2001;11:982–9.

[53] Aquino SL, Shepard JA, Ginns LC, et al. Acquired tracheomalacia: detection by expiratory CT scan. J Comput Assist Tomogr 2001;25(3):394–9.

[54] Boiselle PM, Ernst A. Tracheal morphology in patients with tracheomalacia: prevalence of inspiratory "lunate" and expiratory "frown" shapes. J Thorac Imaging 2006;21:190–6.

[55] Murgu SD, Colt HG. Recognizing tracheobronchomalacia. J Respir Dis 2006;27:327–35.

[56] Baroni RH, Ashiku S, Boiselle PM. Dynamic-CT evaluation of the central airways in patients undergoing tracheoplasty for tracheobronchomalacia. AJR Am J Roentgenol 2005;184:1444–9.

[57] Ghaye B, Szapiro D, Fanchamps JM, et al. Congenital bronchial abnormalities revisited. Radiographics 2001;21:105–19.

[58] Zylak CJ, Eyler WR, Spizarny DL, et al. Developmental lung anomalies in the adult: radiologic-pathologic correlation. Radiographics 2002;22:S25–43.

[59] McGuinness G, Naidich DP, Garay SM, et al. Accessory cardiac bronchus: computed tomographic features and clinical significance. Radiology 1993;189:563–6.

[60] Ali MI, Brunson CD, Mayhew JF. Failed intubation secondary to complete tracheal rings: a case report and literature review. Paediatr Anaesth 2005;15:890–2.

[61] Faust RA, Stroh B, Rimell F. The near complete tracheal ring deformity. Int J Pediatr Otorhinolaryngol 1998;45:171–6.

[62] Boiselle PM, Ernst A, DeCamp M. CT diagnosis of complete tracheal rings in an adult patient. J Thorac Imaging 2007;22:169–71.

[63] Rutter MJ, Willging JP, Cotton RT. Nonoperative management of complete tracheal rings. Arch Otolaryngol Head Neck Surg 2004;130:450–2.

[64] Shin MS, Jackson RM, Ho K. Tracheobronchomegaly (Mounier-Kuhn syndrome): CT diagnosis. AJR Am J Roentgenol 1988;150:777–8.

[65] Soto-Hurtado EJ, Penuela-Ruiz L, Rivera-Sanchez I, et al. Tracheal diverticulum: a review of the literature. Lung 2006;184:303–7.

ELSEVIER
SAUNDERS

Clin Chest Med 29 (2008) 195–216

CLINICS
IN CHEST
MEDICINE

Functional Imaging: CT and MRI

Edwin J.R. van Beek, MD, PhD, FRCR*, Eric A. Hoffman, PhD

Department of Radiology, Carver College of Medicine, University of Iowa,
C-751 GH, 200 Hawkins Drive, Iowa City, IA 52242-1077, USA

The traditional approach to lung imaging, using so-called high resolution CT (HRCT) consisting of 1 mm slices, is replaced increasingly by novel methods. The introduction of multi-detector row CT (MDCT) has enabled coronal, sagital, and oblique reformatting at greater spatial resolution than before, while contrast-enhanced CT methods now allow assessment of vasculature and lung perfusion. Developments do not stop there; techniques using spirometric controlled MDCT allow for quantification of presence and distribution of parenchymal and airway pathology; xenon gas can be employed to assess regional ventilation of the lungs, and, although many such applications are currently still driven by research, it is expected that HRCT will become antiquated in the not too distant future as CT evolves from mere static assessment of morphology into a dynamic and quantifiable tool for regional assessment of the lung.

Complementary to CT of the lung, MRI of the lung, which previously was handicapped by field inhomogeneity and the lack of protons in lung tissue, is developing its own arsenal for lung assessment in terms of morphology, pulmonary circulation, ventilation, and right heart assessment. It is clear that the inherent advantage of MRI over CT—its lack of ionizing radiation—makes it of primary interest in the field of lung diseases that tend to be chronic with acute exacerbations and require multiple investigations during the life span of the patient. Unfortunately, availability of some of the tools required (such as gas polarizers) or MRI techniques (such as broadband upgrades) is

still somewhat limited. However, there is a significant drive toward making access easier, and in many centers, MRI already has become a main diagnostic tool.

This article describes some of the new features involving lung imaging from a CT and MRI perspective. It is the authors' intention that the reader should be familiar with the current available techniques and techniques that are expected to reach clinical applications in the near future.

CT

The scanners

Volumetric physiologic imaging by way of x-ray CT had its beginning in the mid 1970s with the dynamic spatial reconstructor (DSR), the prototype of dynamic volumetric x-ray CT designed and installed at the Mayo Clinic [1]. Much of the work establishing the accuracy and precision of volumetric lung imaging was performed on the DSR [1,2]. The primary lesson learned from the DSR was that lungs, in particular, must be studied dynamically and volumetrically. Commercial imaging technology significantly lagged behind this early work. The electron beam CT [3] used parallel x-ray targets to get improved scan speeds up to 50 ms per slice pair, acquiring eight stacked slices in approximately 224 milliseconds. There have been rapid advances in speed and resolution with the advent of MDCT [4]. Its cone-beam spiral CT uses a 2-dimensional detector array, allowing larger scanning range in shorter time with higher image resolution [5,6]. Acquiring multiple image slices per rotation and rotation speeds as short as 0.3 seconds allow for a significant reduction in acquisition time. Faster scan times will significantly impact functional imaging protocols where the rate of

* Correspondence.
E-mail address: edwin-vanbeek@uiowa.edu
(E.J.R. van Beek).

0272-5231/08/$ - see front matter © 2008 Elsevier Inc. All rights reserved.
doi:10.1016/j.ccm.2007.12.003

chestmed.theclinics.com

perfusion of a contrast agent is measured over time or gated imaging is needed. It is believed that the future of lung assessment resides with true dynamic low dose volumetric CT scanners that image at least 1/3 of the thorax with at least a 0.5 mm isotropic voxel, achieve a full rotation scan aperture of 150 milliseconds, and have superior contrast resolution for radiopaque gas and injected contrast detection. The system likely will be coupled with a low Tesla MR scanner that will be used to complement the information available from the CT image. Patients will be scanned frequently by low tesla MR and less frequently over time by the CT component.

With the introduction of dual source MDCT [7,8] into the clinical arena, scan apertures now fall below 150 milliseconds, but z-axis coverage with single rotation on these scanners remains at 2.4 cm. Other single source spiral scanners have advanced to as many as 256 rows of detectors [9,10] with a z-axis coverage of up to 12 cm. By the end of 2007, 128 rows and 4 cm z-axis coverage will be the minimum configuration of the high-end MDCT scanners. With the broader coverage, retrospective gating methods have emerged for cardiac and pulmonary imaging whereby, by way of a very low pitch, images are gathered during the respiratory or cardiac cycles while recording the physiologic signal together with the projection images. Prospectively [11], or retrospectively [10,12–17], the portions of the physiologic cycle of interest can be selected from within the slow pitch spiral data so that a volumetric image data set is reconstructed for just that location of the respiratory or cardiac cycle. Thus, multiple portions of the physiologic cycle can be reconstructed to yield a dynamic image sequence of the organ of interest [10,12–17]. In pulmonary applications, the earliest use of this method has been in oncology, tracking the maximum trajectory throughout a respiratory cycle for the purposes of treatment planning [15,18].

As the scanners become faster with more slices, some people have questioned how many slices is enough. The answer to this question is determined largely by the more advanced functional applications, such as retrospective gating technologies, ventilation, and perfusion imaging. Perfusion and ventilation imaging requires an axial mode of scanning to dynamically track the first pass of a sharp bolus of contrast agent (approximately 0.5 mL/kg over 2–3 seconds injected into the vena cava or right atrial junction). With axial dynamic scanning, the functional parameter under

investigation (ventilation or perfusion in the case of the lung) is evaluated only as broadly along the z-axis as the coverage of the multiple rows of detectors will permit (typically 4–12 cm). If it is important to evaluate dynamically the whole lung, then one must have long z-axis coverage; otherwise, the dynamic acquisition will have to be repeated at multiple levels to gain the z-axis coverage. There must be enough rows of detectors to maintain structural detail and apex-to-base coverage.

With the introduction of dual source CT, there is a growing interest in the use of dual energy [19–22] as a means of characterizing tissues regionally and quantitating local amounts of a contrast agent. Dual energy imaging permits mathematical separation of the contrast signal from the background tissue signal on a single scan acquisition. This simultaneous acquisition avoids the need for separate unenhanced and enhanced scans with associated or added radiation dose and alignment challenges caused by variations in breath hold, cardiogenic motion, alterations in chest wall configuration during a breath hold, normal stress relaxation occurring when the lung is held at a fixed inflation pressure, and so forth. In the case of a perfused blood volume scan used to assess pulmonary emboli, it is possible (through the use of dual energy whereby one x-ray source is set to 80kV and the other to 140kV) to generate a virtual contrast-only image and a virtual unenhanced image [20]. The accuracy of the Hounsfield units in the virtual unenhanced image remains untested, and it is not clear if this virtual image data set can be used, for instance, in a density mask analysis seeking to quantify presence and distribution of emphysema in a smoker being imaged with a contrast enhanced scan for the detection and characterization of lung nodules.

With the growing use of prolonged infusions of iodinated x-ray contrast agent to detect pulmonary emboli, the enhancement has been used as an index of regional pulmonary blood flow. This has been and should be dubbed a "perfused blood volume" scan [23–25], so as not to confuse this measure with the quantitative assessment of parenchymal perfusion. With dual energy imaging, it may be possible to obtain a volumetric image of regional ventilation and regional lung structure by imaging with dual energy spiral scanning during a single breath of xenon gas [21,22]. This is an experimental method yet to be validated against the dynamic xenon CT assessment of regional ventilation. The single breath dual energy xenon method has been employed successfully in rabbits using a synchrotron source [26–28].

Quantitative image analysis

The ability to evaluate objectively the information content of the images is critical to taking full advantage of MDCT (and MRI). In the case of the lung, the starting point is reliable detection of the lungs [29], lobes [30], airways [31–41], and blood vessels, which is followed by an analysis of parenchymal attenuation and texture, and is followed finally by a regional quantification of ventilation and perfusion parameters. The authors and colleagues have reviewed these capabilities elsewhere [42,43]. With the advent of MDCT and isotropic voxels, it is possible now to reliably segment the airway tree to approximately the 5th generation (trachea being generation 0), and many of the 6th and 7th generation branches are captured in the segmentation. Airway wall thickness is expressed commonly as wall area percent (percent of the area defined by the outer wall of the airway segment occupied by the airway wall) [44]. These measures are being used to assess airway remodeling in asthma and chronic obstructive pulmonary diseases (COPD). Fig. 1 shows a depiction of the airway tree and lobe segmentation from a normal non-smoker and a patient who has COPD. These images can be used not only to quantify the airway and parenchyma characteristics but also to provide a roadmap linking airway paths to sub-lobar segment.

Evaluation of the lung at its functional interface

Computer-based methods for objective quantitation of MDCT data sets to compare normal and diseased lung are being used increasingly in conjunction with 2-dimensional data sets. Methods have ranged from counting the number of voxels below a cut-off (-850HU, -910HU, -950HU) [45–56] to methods that make use of measures derived from the histogram, including skewness, kurtosis, and so forth [57]. HRCT enhances the resolving power of the image [58–62], allowing detection of less severe emphysema. Various computer-assisted texture based methods have been used successfully for tissue characterization. Traditional methods of texture analysis can be grouped into statistical, structural, and hybrid methods [63]. Methods for tissue classification typically rely on region gray scale statistical measures (ie, mean, variance, and frequency histogram) or textural measures (autocorrelation, co-occurrence matrices, run-length matrices, and so forth) [46,47,55,57,64–74]. Lung

tissue can be evaluated objectively by using the attenuation of lung tissue either as mean lung attenuation or by measuring the attenuation of lung falling below a set value (the density mask) [46,47,55,57,73]. It has been demonstrated that lung tissue mean attenuation can be an index of emphysema [46,47,55]. However, a later study showed significant lung attenuation variation in normal individuals that could be misleading [73]. To use attenuation distribution as a quantitative measure, much greater care must be taken to assure accurate scanner calibration in the air-water Hounsfield range and to standardize lung volumes at which scanning occurs [75–79]. Furthermore, one must consider that, in a longitudinal pharmaceutical study, lung attenuation is affected oppositely by changes in emphysema status and inflammation burden. A useful index of peripheral inflammation and airway disease has been a measure of air trapping. Quantitative tools used to access air trapping have been shown to be quite sensitive [80,81]. A density masking approach alone is not sufficient to distinguish normal lung from diseased lung, and Uppaluri and colleagues [82–84] have introduced what has been dubbed the "adaptive multiple feature method" (AMFM). This technique has used up to 26 different mathematical formulations to describe the gray scale heterogeneity of parenchymal regions within CT slices, and then it employed a Bayesian classifier to identify the best small number of mathematical formulations ("features") that distinguish one texture (pathologic state) from another.. More recently, Xu and colleagues [85,86] have shown that using volumetric images with isotropic voxels for 3-dimensional texture assessment provides significant improvements in the assessment of regional parenchymal pathology. In one test, Xu and colleagues used the AMFM method with appropriate training sets to accurately differentiate the CT scans of normal smokers from those of normal non-smokers. The use of the texture analysis method is only as good as the training sets developed, and if it is desirable to use the method for detection of parenchymal pathology undetectable by the human observer, training paradigms such as the one used by Xu and colleagues must be established. Even when the training sets come from CT findings identified by human observers, the computer-based AMFM is more consistent than human observers in its assessment of lung regions. Quantitation of lung images has become critical, because pharmaceutical and device manufacturers seek to reduce the development time and seek to

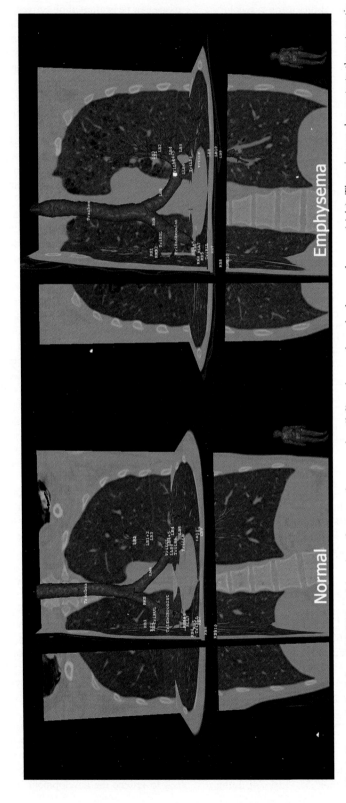

Fig. 1. Images derived from MDCT-based imaging of a normal non-smoker (*left*) and a smoker who has emphysema (*right*). These images demonstrate the automatic segmentation of the lungs, lobes and bronchial tree with automatic bronchial tree labeling. Segmentation and display was done by way of a Pulmonary Workstation Plus (VIDA Diagnostics, Coralville, Iowa).

use imaging as a tool for the detection of regional lung changes (either a desired effect or an unwanted side effect) not reflected in the traditional pulmonary function tests, which provide a global measure of the pulmonary physiology, but are relatively insensitive to regional changes. Fig. 2 demonstrates a whole lung classification in which the AMFM simultaneously identified areas of emphysema (red), honeycomb (pink), normal (blue), and ground glass (yellow).

Functional imaging

Numerous imaging-based methods have been developed to assess ventilation, perfusion, or their functional outcome (gas exchange). Examples of how MDCT imaging technology is used to probe normal and abnormal cardiopulmonary structure and function are discussed later. The authors argue that MDCT technology offers a unique and comprehensive approach to evaluating the structural and functional complexity of the respiratory sytems and cardiopulmonary systems.

Ventilation assessed by CT. The measurement of lung ventilation, lung volume, and tidal volume traditionally has been made for the entire lung, despite the fact that lung function in health and disease is inhomogeneous. Attempts have been made to quantify regional ventilation directly and indirectly with a variety of invasive techniques or radioisotope imaging [87–96], but these methods have been limited by invasiveness, poor spatial and temporal resolution, qualitative nature, or complexity. Xenon-enhanced MDCT (XE-MDCT) is a method for the noninvasive

measurement of regional pulmonary ventilation, which is determined from the wash-in or wash-out rates of the radiodense, nonradioactive gas xenon as measured in serially acquired axial MDCT scans. Little work had been done since the original description of this technique nearly 25 years ago [97–100], although the FDA approval of XE-MDCT for measurement of cerebral blood flow has met with moderate clinical acceptance [101]. Recently, however, the application of XE-MDCT for measurement of regional pulmonary ventilation has been updated, validated, and refined, including extension of the technique to estimate regional perfusion and ventilation/perfusion ratio [28,102–111]. In Fig. 3, the authors demonstrate a typical xenon wash-in wash-out attenuation curve in a sheep, along with a color coded image of regional ventilation. Scanning was accomplished through gated imaging (end-expiration), while a fixed concentration of xenon gas was inspired during the wash-in phase, and then room air was inspired during the wash-out phase. A mono-exponential curve is fitted to the wash-in or wash-out phase, providing a time constant as a measure of ventilation. Because the dynamic XE-MDCT method requires the gated acquisition of axial CT images, timed so that the images are gathered at the same point in a series of standardized tidal breaths, the method has been applied most effectively to research animals breathing by way of respirators. The transfer of this methodology to humans has required the development of sophisticated feedback devices that monitor respiration by way of flow meters and displays that provide the subject with information

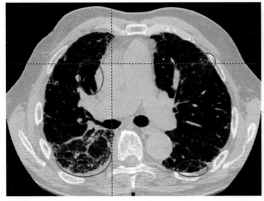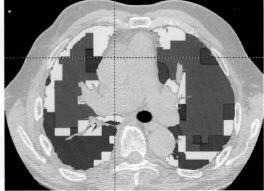

Fig. 2. Whole lung classification using the 3-dimensional AMFM. Ellipses in the original image slice (*left*) represent emphysema (red) and honeycomb (purple) patterns. The tissue types are color coded: red, emphysema; pink, honeycomb; blue; normal; yellow, ground glass. (*Data from* Ye Xu. Computer aided 3-D texture analysis for lung characterization using MDCT images. PhD dissertation, University of Iowa, 2007.)

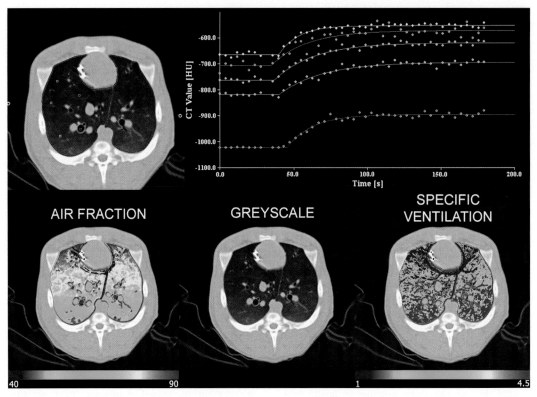

Fig. 3. Demonstration of the density changes occurring regionally across time as a result of the re-breathing of a constant concentration of xenon gas. Imaging is in the axial mode and scans are gated to end expiration. Data are from a supine anesthetized pig. In the upper panel, regions of interest are sampled, including parenchymal regions spaced from the dependent to the non-dependent lung regions, with one region of interest in a right sided bronchus. The exponential rise from the baseline is sharper in the dependent (yellow) region versus a much shallower exponential rise in the non-dependent region (blue). The sharp and shallow rise from the baseline represents a fast or slow gas turnover rate respectively. Note the gradient in specific ventilation (*lower right*), where specific ventilation is the gas turn over rate (time constant) normalized by the local amount of air in that region of lung.

related to targeted rate and depth of breathing information. Because of the complexity of such a system, there is considerable interest in the application of a single breath method using dual energy CT. With the introduction of dual source CT, it is possible to image a subject during a breath hold following the inhalation of a single breath of a mixture of xenon and oxygen. With the kV of the two x-ray sources set to 80kV and 140kV, it is possible to use material decomposition methods [19] to separate the xenon signal from the inherent x-ray attenuation of the lung [21,22]. Saba and colleagues [21] have demonstrated the feasibility of such an approach, using 80kV and 140 kV, during a single breath hold in a sheep. The images are presented in Fig. 4 and show the color coded xenon distribution superimposed upon the CT sections. In this sheep, a region of ventilation deficit in an area presenting with very subtle ground glass is demonstrated.

With the ability to retrospectively reconstruct 4-dimensional image data sets to represent a complete breathing cycle, it becomes possible to assess regional ventilation through the use of image matching algorithms [12–18,112]. Such image matching provides not only regional volume changes but also regional images of tissue strain, providing potential insights into local tissue properties such as early fibrosis and so forth. The use of such measures is being investigated only now.

Perfusion assessed by CT

Dynamic imaging methods have been used to estimate arterial, venous, and capillary transit times and capillary flow distributions [113–120]. These methods involve two types of image data collection regimes. Inlet-outlet detection is used typically for evaluating conducting vessels and whole organ analysis. The other data collection

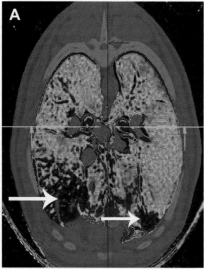

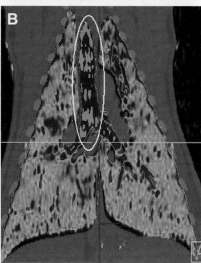

Fig. 4. Dual energy color coded images in axial (*A*) and coronal (*B*) planes demonstrate the presence of xenon gas following the inhalation of a single breath of 80% xenon. Imaging was accomplished in the prone position at 80kV and 140kV, allowing subtraction of the xenon signal while minimally changing the signal from the natural occurring tissue of the body. Note the region of low or no xenon ventilation (*white arrows*, upper panel). This region had a ground glass pattern indicative of regional small airway inflammation. (*Data from* Saba OI, Fuld MK, Krauss B, et al. Dual energy MDC for volumetric assessment of V/Q: initial experiences. American Thoracic Society Annual Meeting 2007;A938; and Fuld M, Saba O, Krauss B, et al. Dual energy Xe-MDCT for automated assessment of the central airway tree: initial Experiences. American Thoracic Society Annual Meeting 2007;A250.)

regime, referred to as residue detection, typically is used alone or in conjunction with inlet detection, because analysis of microvascular regions wherein the individual vessels are below the resolution of the imaging system. Various approaches for determining blood flow and mean transit time have been described [114,117–127]. A growing number of studies demonstrate the use of MDCT with infusion of iodinated contrast agent to assess the presence of pulmonary emboli by way of visualization of flow voids in peripheral lung segments; the improved ability to detect pulmonary emboli, aortic dissection, and coronary atherosclerosis have resulted in the "triple ruleout" method for use in patients who have chest pain [128]. One must take care not to confuse this method to assess "flowing blood volume" with an assessment of true perfusion parameters. To assess regional parenchymal perfusion by way of dynamic axial MDCT [129,130], the authors place a catheter in the right ventricular outflow tract in animals and place a catheter in the superior vena cava in humans. A sharp (0.5 mL/ kg over 2 seconds) bolus of iodinated contrast agent is delivered during ECG gated axial scanning. Scanning commences one to two heart beats before contrast injection, with lungs held at functional residual capacity. By sampling the reconstructed time-attenuation curves within the region of a pulmonary artery and the lung parenchyma as shown in Fig. 5, the authors were able to calculate regional mean transit times, blood flow normalized to air or tissue content [131]; the authors also were able to deconvolve the the signals to estimate the timing of flow within the microvascular bed [129]. In Fig. 5 a color coded image of a non-smoker and a smoker who has normal pulmonary function tests but early CT findings of emphysema can be seen. In Fig. 5, color coding provides a regional depiction of mean transit time. Using this approach, Alford and colleagues [132] have demonstrated that heterogeneity of mean transit times is increased significantly in lung regions of smokers who have normal pulmonary function tests but who have very early CT evidence of emphysema. Through a series of recent publications [133–135], Hoffman and colleagues have used functional CT imaging to demonstrate that hypoxic pulmonary vasoconstriction normally is blocked when hypoxic conditions are accompanied by inflammation. These observations have lead to the hypothesis that the failure of inherent mechanisms to block the normal hypoxic pulmonary vasoconstrictor response of the pulmonary vasculature in the presence of inflammatory

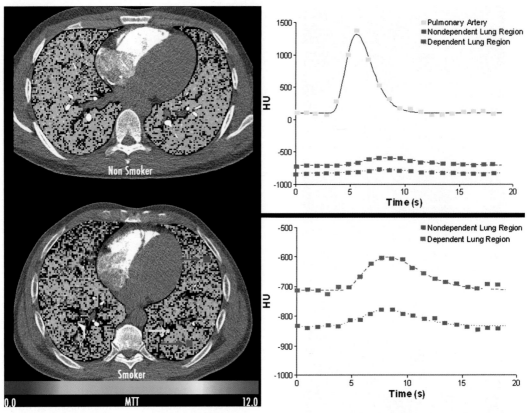

Fig. 5. Regional assessment of pulmonary blood flow mean transit times by use of temporally sequenced axial imaging, gated to the electrocardiogram during a sharp bolus contrast injection (0.5 mL/kg iodinated contrast agent) into the superior vena cava/right atrial junction in a normal non-smoker (*upper left*) and a smoker (*lower left*) with CT showing only findings of early emphysema. Regions of interest are highlighted in the lower left image showing an ROI placed in the pulmonary artery (yellow) and non-dependent (red) and dependent (purple) parenchymal regions. Associated time intensity curves are shown, from which mean transit times and pulmonary blood flow may be calculated, with the parenchymal curves expanded in the lower right graph. Studies have shown that the regional heterogeneity of pulmonary blood flow mean transit times is significantly increased in smokers who have CT findings of emphysema. (*Data from* Alford SK, Van Beek EJ, McLennan G, et al. Characterization of smoking related regional alterations in pulmonary perfusion via functional CT. Proceedings of the Annual Meeting of the American Thoracic Society, San Francisco, CA, 2007:A818.)

processes may lead to a failure of the normal response mechanisms serving to limit the inflammatory response, which will lead to the emphysema process. Fig. 6 provides a demonstration of an intact hypoxic pulmonary vasoconstrictor (HPV) response and an inflammation-based blocking of the HPV response in the same sheep. An endobronchial valve was placed in the animal, which allowed air out but did not allow air into a regional segment of the lung. At the same time, the animal arrived in the lab with regional pneumonia. Fig. 6 demonstrates that in the region of the valve, there is a shunting of blood flow away from the hypoxic lung region, whereas in the dependent regions of pneumonia, blood flow shunted away from the

valve region is distributed preferentially to the region of inflammation, because it presumably represents the path of least resistance. These images demonstrate the power of advanced MDCT imaging to provide a link between structure and function.

MRI

MRI has several advantages over CT, including the speed of imaging, the lack of ionizing radiation, the ability to identify tissue characteristics, and the potential to obtain information on different nuclei, which allows for novel approaches to lung function and micro-structure assessment.

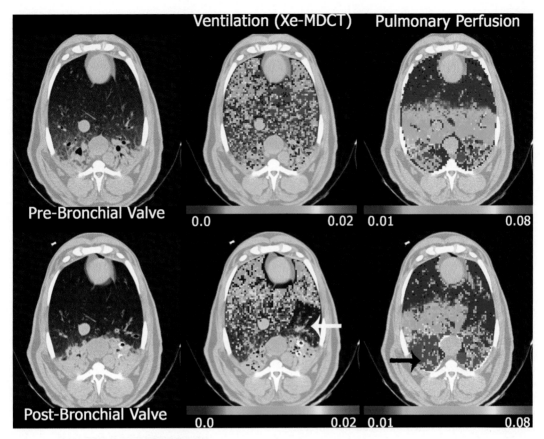

Fig. 6. Axial images from a sheep with native pneumonia (dependent lung regions) that was imaged supine and anesthetized in the MDCT scanner. Ventilation (*middle column*) and perfusion (*left column*) data sets were obtained before (*upper rows*) and after (*lower rows*) the placement of an endobronchial valve. The white arrow in the lower middle column marks the location of ventilation defect caused by the endobronchial valve. In this same region on the perfusion images (see *lower right*) there is a regional reduction in perfusion indicating regional, intact hypoxic pulmonary vasoconstriction. The black arrow in the lower right image marks a region that preferentially receives an increase in blood flow following the shunting of perfusion from the regional of the endobronchial valve, presumably because regional HPV is blocked in the presence of inflammation. (*Adapted from* Easley RB, Fuld MK, Fernandez-Bustamante A, et al. Mechanism of hypoxemia in acute lung injury evaluated by multidetector-row CT. Acad Radiol 2006;13:918; with permission.)

Technical requirements

Most modern MR systems will be capable of obtaining excellent quality proton images of the chest. This will lead to relatively black lungs and excellent delineation of the chest wall, mediastinum, and diaphragm. Parallel imaging sequences assist in obtaining images faster, within a single breath-hold, which allows for rapid image acquisition without the issue of motion artifact [136–138] A host of sequences are available, ranging from those focused on the diaphragm and mediastinum to those aimed at obtaining signal from the actual lungs themselves. Using intravenous gadolinium-based contrast agents, it is possible to delineate the pulmonary vascular tree and the right heart. Within the chest, MRIs almost always are obtained during a single breath-hold, although dynamic imaging during a respiratory cycle is feasible (for instance to demonstrate diaphragm excursions). Ultrafast imaging also is capable of obtaining dynamic contrast images, leading to interpretation of pulmonary perfusion.

Proton imaging

As with any MRI technique, proton imaging uses the large magnetic field and the free moving protons to derive signal from changes in proton orientation caused by radiofrequency pulses. The lungs are different from the rest of the body, because there are a relative low number of protons and most of the lung parenchyma consists of air. Although this is a problem, it can be used to advantage, because pathologic processes tend to increase the number of protons (hemorrhage, edema, inflammation, or tumor) or alternatively lead to relative voids of proton density (as with calcification or fibrosis).

The application of differently weighted sequences will lead to an increase or decrease in proton signal. For instance, water will lead to increased signal on T2-weighted sequences and decreased signal on T1-weighted sequences, whereas fat will have increased signal on both sequences. Moreover, it is possible to produce fat saturation pulses, resulting in complete depression of signal from fat.

To achieve faster imaging times, several techniques may be used. The oldest of these uses half-Fourier techniques that only reconstruct slightly more than half the data space and extrapolate the missing data. This led to the single breath-hold sequences, which tend to be slightly T2-weighted and are employed also in a variety of other body imaging applications, such as MR cholangiopancreatography. The newer MRI systems all have the ability to perform parallel imaging techniques, which is somewhat similar to MDCT in that multiple slices are excited and read out simultaneously, thus increasing temporal resolution by a factor of 2–8 [136–138].

Although MRI has never really played a major role in routine chest imaging, several pathologic processes can be evaluated using proton imaging, including pleural effusions, pneumonia, lung tumors (particularly useful in Pancoast tumors and for determination of tumor invasion in mesothelioma) and the assessment of the mediastinum (Fig. 7) [139–141]. The technique is complementary to CT, although tissue plane definition and characterization is better using MRI.

Assessment of respiratory dynamics has become feasible with the advent of ultrafast proton imaging capabilities. This has resulted in novel approaches for assessment of the diaphragm, chest wall motion assessment, and breathing mechanics [142,143].

Gadolinium-enhanced imaging

The use of gadolinium contrast has enabled a rapid expansion of chest MRI, because it became feasible to assess enhancement of pathologic processes and visualization of the pulmonary vascular tree (as a static component and as

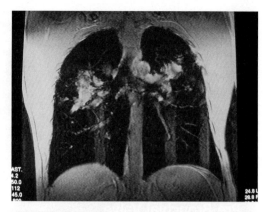

Fig. 7. Patient who has sarcoidosis. Coronal proton single shot fast spin echo sequence demonstrating black lungs with some interstitial markings and extensive mediastinal and bilateral hilar lymphadenopathy.

dynamics of perfusion) and the other large arteries [144]. This allowed MRI to become competitive with more traditional CT techniques in several aspects of chest imaging, particularly imaging of the large vessels, including congenital anomalies, such as patent ductus arteriosus (Fig. 8) and the assessment of pulmonary hypertension (Fig. 9) [145,146]. Although CT has maintained a primary

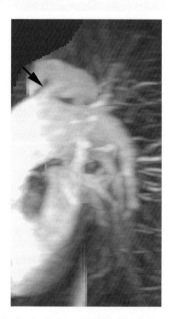

Fig. 8. Sagittal 3-dimensional gadolinium-enhanced MR angiogram demonstrates direct connection between aorta and pulmonary artery (*arrow*), consistent with patent ductus arteriosus in a patient who has pulmonary hypertension.

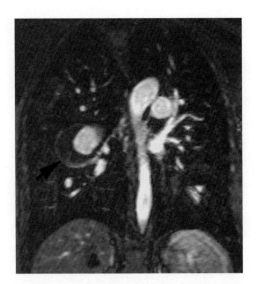

Fig. 9. Coronal 3-dimensional gadolinium-enhanced MR angiogram demonstrates enhancement of an aneurysm of the right pulmonary artery with a black rim of mural organized thrombus (*arrow*) in a patient who has pulmonary hypertension.

role in the diagnosis of pulmonary embolism, the application of MRI for subsets of patients (like pregnant women or patients who will require follow-up imaging to assess response to therapy) is now feasible with very high-resolution MR angiographic imaging [147–149].

In addition to the above described imaging techniques, MRI also offers the possibility to assess perfusion of the lung vascular bed by ultrafast imaging during the injection of gadolinium contrast [150,151]. This enables direct visualization of regional perfusion, with the possibility of some form of quantification (though this is notoriously difficult in MRI because of signal-noise properties). Several studies have demonstrated the feasibility of this technique for assessment of normal and pathologic processes [152–155]. This application is now very close to general introduction into clinical practice.

Hyperpolarized gas imaging

MR imaging is versatile and has the capability to image other nuclei, including 3-helium and 129-xenon, provided the frequency of the system is adapted accordingly (for instance, for imaging 3-helium at a field strength of 1.5 Tesla, the radiofrequency amplifier and transmit/receive radiofrequency coils are tuned to 48 MHz, compared with 64 Mhz for proton imaging) [156].

Researchers discovered the potential of these noble, stable gas isotopes as a side-effect to nuclear physics experiments, which required hyperpolarization of 3-He to produce neutron mirrors. Hyperpolarization is a process in which the atoms are brought to a higher energy level by introduction of laser light at the appropriate bandwidth. When this is achieved within a low magnetic field, the normally random population of spins will change to have a relatively higher population of atoms with spins aligned along the magnetic field. When this gas is introduced in an MRI environment, the usual radio frequency (RF) and response will result in enhanced signal, and this application successfully obtained the first images in the early-mid 1990s [157–159].

Among the noble gases, the application of hyperpolarized 3-He has been used widely so far in clinical research studies, because the gas has better signal-to-noise ratio and remains in the airways without further interaction with the human body (in contrast to 129-Xe, which is lipid soluble and has anesthetic properties at higher concentrations) [156]. However, improvement in hyperpolarization systems has meant that 129-Xe MRI is making rapid strides forward, giving new insight in lung function [160–162]. One of the main features of hyperpolarized gas imaging is that the signal introduced in the system is so high that imaging is less dependent on field strength (which is not the case for proton imaging), and this has advantages as lower field-strength magnets may result in fewer artifacts [163–165]. A main disadvantage to this technique is that the contrast is exogenous and non-renewable. To maximize the use of the contrast, one must design special pulse sequences to minimize loss of polarization by RF pulses and the paramagnetic effects of oxygen.

Several such techniques have been developed for hyperpolarized 3-He MRI, and these techniques have found a broad range of applications that may be of interest for the future assessment of pathophysiology, normal lung function, and structure.

All hyperpolarized gas imaging techniques rely on the delivery of a single breath of gas mixture into the airways, with the hyperpolarization either performed on site or by a central distribution network [166]. This usually is achieved through the inhalation of the content of a plastic bag, followed by a breath-hold lasting up to 16 seconds. Several thousands of applications have now taken place worldwide, and no significant adverse events have been observed [167,168].

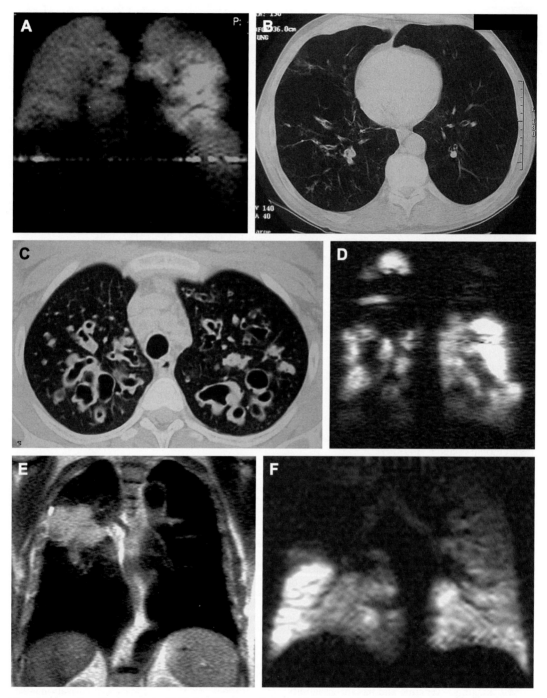

Fig. 10. Examples of hyperpolarized 3-He MRI and correlation with HRCT. (*A, B*) Patient who has alpha-1-antitrypsin deficiency. Notice basal ventilation defects on coronal MRI (*A*), with corresponding panlobular emphysema on axial CT (*B*). (*C, D*) Patient who has cystic fibrosis. Notice upper lobe cystic bronchiectasis on axial HRCT (*C*) with corresponding ventilation defects on coronal hyperpolarized 3-He MRI (*D*). (*E, F*) Patient who has lung cancer. On coronal proton image a large soft tissue mass is visualized in the right upper lung (*E*), which corresponds to upper lobe ventilation defect on hyperpolarized 3-He MRI (*F*).

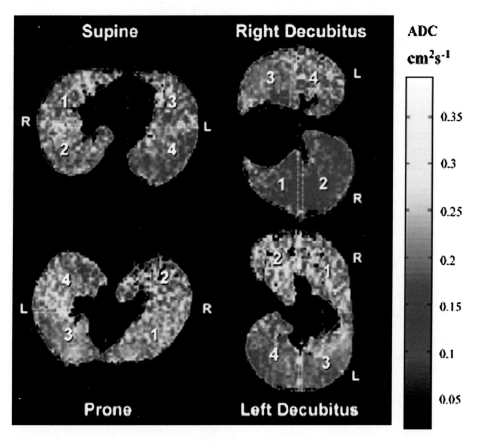

Fig. 11. ADC imaging in a normal volunteer in different positions, demonstrating gravity dependent changes with decreased ADC values in dependent lung portions. (*Reproduced from* Fichele S, Woodhouse N, Swift AJ, et al. MRI of helium-3 gas in healthy lungs: posture related variations of alveolar size. J Magn Reson Imaging 2004;20(2):333; with permission.)

Ventilation distribution is built on the notion that any area with signal is a reflection of the delivery of 3-He gas to this area. It is possible to obtain a 3-dimensional volumetric dataset of the lungs using this technique [169], and several authors have shown the use of this technique in normal volunteers and patients who have asthma, emphysema (including alpha-1-antitrypsin deficiency; Fig. 10A), cystic fibrosis (Fig. 10B), and lung cancer (Fig. 10C) [170–177]. There is homogeneous ventilation distribution in normal volunteers, although small ventilation defects are seen frequently [170,178–180]. In smoking subjects who have normal pulmonary function tests, ventilation defects usually are detectable [181]. In patients who have emphysema, ventilation defects tend to be worse than in normal smokers and correlate with pulmonary function tests [170,180]. In asthmatic subjects, ventilation defects can be provoked using methacholine; these defects are reversible using a bronchodilator and

correlate with pulmonary function tests, [171,182] but quantification can be slightly more problematic. One method, using a subtraction of the proton MR mask from the hyperpolarized 3-He images, has shown a very good repeatability with robust measurements and effectively yields "ventilated lung" as a percentage of overall chest cavity volume in a group of normal and smoking subjects [183].

A limited study has been performed in patients who have lung cancer, suggesting that it may be feasible to use hyperpolarized 3-He MRI as a tool for the planning of radiation fields, which offers the possibility of higher tumor dose and of sparing relatively healthy lung, and thereby the reduction of radiation pneumonitis [177]. Finally, limited studies in lung transplant recipients showed that 3-He MRI was capable of detecting abnormal ventilation [184] and was more sensitive than HRCT or spirometry for the detection of bronchiolitis obliterans and ventilation abnormalities [185,186].

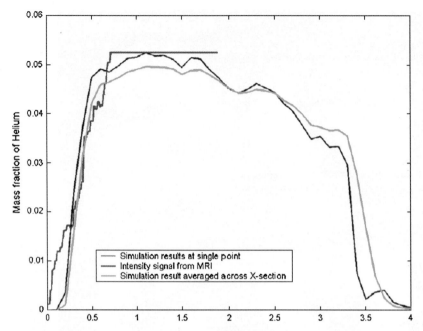

Fig. 12. Dynamic 3-He MRI reconstruction of signal change over time during single inspiration demonstrates the slope of the curve, which may be translated to forced inspiratory volume during 1 second. (*Data from* Koumellis P, van Beek EJ, Woodhouse N, et al. J Magn Reson Imaging 2005;22(3):420–6.)

Diffusion imaging is feasible, making use of the very high diffusivity of 3-He. When using several RF pulses separated by a pre-determined time interval, the MR system is capable of obtaining information on the distance traveled by the atoms. In a free open environment, this is compared further with a restricted environment that exists within the lung and airways. Thus, the lung structure actually reduces the effective diffusion distance caused by the Brownian motion of 3-He atoms and leads to what is known as apparent diffusion coefficient (ADC) measurements, which are a direct representation of small airway size and which correlate closely with histology [187]. Discussion has taken place as to whether these measurements represent terminal bronchioles, and different techniques are being developed to assess longer or shorter measurement times, thus allowing for assessment of collateral ventilation (longer time scales) or true alveolar measurements (shorter time scales) [188,189].

ADC works by application of gradient echo pulse sequences at two different intervals, resulting in changes of polarization loss between more or less confined atoms. The ratio of these polarization changes allow the spatial mapping of ADC, with higher values allocated to larger air

spaces (such as trachea and large bronchi) [190]. ADC is distributed homogeneously in normal subjects and becomes progressively more heterogeneous in normal smokers who have emphysema [191–194]. ADC has been shown to increase under the influence of aging [195,196] and emphysema [194,197,198] caused by gravity dependent compression of the lung [199]; Fig. 11). A significant issue is that ADC measurements can only take place in areas where 3-He signal is present. In disease states with airway obstruction, such as those seen in mucus plugging, this will affect the overall results.

Dynamic ventilation imaging enables the visualization of the 3-He signal as it flows into the main airways down to the peripheral airspaces and makes use of a combination of ultra-fast imaging sequences and image reconstruction techniques that effectively interpolate the changes that occur during the imaging process, resulting in frame rate in the order of 5–10 milliseconds [200,201]. Ventilation can be quantified by obtaining curves of signal change during the imaging time, and it appears that the resulting curves closely correlate with (overall) lung function tests, as demonstrated in Fig. 12 in a young patient who has cystic fibrosis [202,203]. In addition, by prolonging the duration of the imaging process or by starting the MR data acquisition later in the respiratory cycle, it is possible to assess for regional air trapping, which may be relevant in various types of airway outflow obstruction.

Oxygen sensitive imaging uses the paramagnetic effect of oxygen as a calculable decrease in the signal of 3-He caused by loss of polarization. Thus, in areas where oxygen is absorbed rapidly (eg, ventilation-perfusion matching), the signal of 3-He will remain, whereas in areas where oxygen remains in the airways, (eg, ventilation-perfusion mismatch) the 3-He signal will demonstrate a faster decay [204–206]. It is now feasible to obtain 3-dimensional maps of oxygen uptake ratios (or ventilation-perfusion maps) using a single breath-hold technique [207]. The method is still being developed, but it may be able to assist (among many other options) the assessment of pulmonary thromboembolic disease (in particular, chronic disease patients in the preoperative assessment of thromboendarterectomy), the planning of surgical or endobronchial interventions, and the preoperative assessment of patients who have borderline respectability of lung cancer. Several groups have demonstrated the feasibility of combining perfusion and ventilation studies in animal model settings [208,209].

References

[1] Ritman EL, Robb RA, Harris LD. Imaging physiological functions: experience with the DSR. Philadelphia: Praeger; 1985.

[2] Hoffman EA, Larsen RL. Regional pulmonary blood flow via X-ray CT and biodegradable radiopaque microspheres. Circulation 1990;4:111–24.

[3] Boyd DP, Lipton MJ. Cardiac computed tomography. Proceedings of the Institute of Electrical and Electronics Engineers 1983;71:298–307.

[4] Saito T, Misaki M, Shirato K, et al. Three-dimensional quantitative coronary angiography. IEEE Trans Biomed Eng 1990;37:768–77.

[5] Saito Y. Multislice X-ray CT scanner. Medical Review 1998;98:1–8.

[6] Wang G, Lin TH, Cheng PC, et al. A general cone-beam reconstruction algorithm. IEEE Trans Med Imaging 1993;12:486–96.

[7] McCollough CH, Primak AN, Saba O, et al. Dose performance of a 64-channel dual-source CT scanner. Radiology 2007;243:775–84.

[8] Flohr TG, McCollough CH, Bruder H, et al. First performance evaluation of a dual-source CT (DSCT) system. Eur Radiol 2006;16:256–68.

[9] Funabashi N, Mizuno N, Yoshida K, et al. Superiority of synchrony of 256-slice cone beam computed tomography for acquiring pulsating

[10] Mizuno N, Funabashi N, Imada M, et al. Utility of 256-slice cone beam tomography for real four-dimensional volumetric analysis without electrocardiogram gated acquisition. Int J Cardiol 2007; 120:262–7.

[11] Saba OI, Chon D, Beck K, et al. Static versus prospective gated non-breath hold volumetric MDCT imaging of the lungs. Acad Radiol 2005; 12:1371–84.

[12] Xu S, Taylor RH, Fichtinger G, et al. Lung deformation estimation and four-dimensional CT lung reconstruction. Acad Radiol 2006;13:1082–92.

[13] Sarrut D, Boldea V, Miguet S, et al. Simulation of four-dimensional CT images from deformable registration between inhale and exhale breath-hold CT scans. Med Phys 2006;33:605–17.

[14] Guerrero T, Sanders K, Castillo E, et al. Dynamic ventilation imaging from four-dimensional computed tomography. Phys Med Biol 2006;51: 777–91.

[15] Guerrero T, Sanders K, Noyola-Martinez J, et al. Quantification of regional ventilation from treatment planning CT. Int J Radiat Oncol Biol Phys 2005;62:630–4.

[16] Starkschall G, Desai N, Balter P, et al. Quantitative assessment of four-dimensional computed tomography image acquisition quality. J Appl Clin Med Phys 2007;8:2362.

[17] Rietzel E, Chen GT. Deformable registration of 4D computed tomography data. Med Phys 2006;33: 4423–30.

[18] Christensen GE, Song JH, Lu W, et al. Tracking lung tissue motion and expansion/compression with inverse consistent image registration and spirometry. Med Phys 2007;34:2155–63.

[19] Johnson TR, Nikolaou K, Fink C, et al. [Dual-source CT in chest pain diagnosis]. Radiologe 2007;47:301–9 [in German].

[20] Johnson TR, Krauss B, Sedlmair M, et al. Material differentiation by dual energy CT: initial experience. Eur Radiol 2007;17:1510–7.

[21] Saba OI, Fuld MK, Krauss B, et al. Dual energy MDCT for volumetric assessment of V/Q: initial experiences. American Thoracic Society Annual Meeting 2007;A938.

[22] Fuld M, Saba O, Krauss B, et al. Dual energy Xe-MDCT for automated assessment of the central airway tree: initial Experiences. American Thoracic Society Annual Meeting 2007;A250.

[23] Remy-Jardin M, Pistolesi M, Goodman LR, et al. Management of suspected acute pulmonary embolism in the era of CT angiography: a statement from the Fleischner Society. Radiology 2007;245: 315–29.

[24] Stillman AE, Oudkerk M, Ackerman M, et al. Use of multidetector computed tomography for the

objects. Comparison with conventional multislice computed tomography. Int J Cardiol 2007;118: 400–5.

assessment of acute chest pain: a consensus state-
ment of the North American Society of Cardiac
Imaging and the European Society of Cardiac
Radiology. Eur Radiol 2007;17:2196–207.

[25] Wildberger JE, Klotz E, Ditt H, et al. Multislice
computed tomography perfusion imaging for visualization of acute pulmonary embolism: animal
experience. Eur Radiol 2005;15:1378–86.

[26] Bayat S, Porra L, Suhonen H, et al. Differences in
the time course of proximal and distal airway
response to inhaled histamine studied by synchrotron radiation CT. J Appl Physiol 2006;100:
1964–73.

[27] Porra L, Monfraix S, Berruyer G, et al. Effect of
tidal volume on distribution of ventilation assessed
by synchrotron radiation CT in rabbit. J Appl
Physiol 2004;96:1899–908.

[28] Bayat S, Le Duc G, Porra L, et al. Quantitative
functional lung imaging with synchrotron radiation using inhaled xenon as contrast agent. Phys
Med Biol 2001;46:3287–99.

[29] Keller JM, Edwards FM, Rundle R. Automatic
outlining of regions on CT scans. J Comput Assist
Tomogr 1981;5:240–5.

[30] Kuhnigk H, Wunder C, Roewer N. Anaesthetic
considerations for a 2-month-old infant with
suspected complex I respiratory chain deficiency.
Paediatr Anaesth 2003;13:83–5.

[31] Brown RH, Herold CJ, Hirshman CA, et al. In vivo
measurements of airway reactivity using high-
resolution computed tomography. Am Rev Respir
Dis 1991;144:208–12.

[32] Amirav I, Kramer SS, Grunstein MM, et al. Assessment of methacholine-induced airway constriction
by ultrafast high-resolution computed tomography. J Appl Physiol 1993;75:2239–50.

[33] Brown RH, Herold CJ, Hirshman CA, et al. Individual airway constrictor response heterogeneity
to histamine assessed by high-resolution computed
tomography. J Appl Physiol 1993;74:2615–20.

[34] Brown RH, Mitzner W, Zerhouni E, et al. Direct in
vivo visualization of bronchodilation induced by
inhalational anesthesia using high-resolution
computed tomography. Anesthesiology 1993;78:
295–300.

[35] Zerhouni EA, Herold CJ, Brown RH, et al. High-
resolution computed tomography-physiologic
correlation. J Thorac Imaging 1993;8:265–72.

[36] Brown RH, Herold C, Zerhouni EA, et al. Spontaneous airways constrict during breath holding studied by high-resolution computed tomography.
Chest 1994;106:920–4.

[37] Palagyi K, Tschirren J, Hoffman EA, et al. Quantitative analysis of pulmonary airway tree structures.
Comput Biol Med 2006;36:974–96.

[38] Tschirren J, Hoffman EA, McLennan G, et al.
Intrathoracic airway trees: segmentation and
airway morphology analysis from low dose CT
scans. IEEE Trans Med Imaging 2005;24:1529–39.

[39] Tschirren J, McLennan G, Palagyi K, et al. Matching and anatomical labeling of human airway tree.
IEEE Trans Med Imaging 2005;24:1540–7.

[40] Saba OI, Hoffman EA, Reinhardt JM. Computed
tomographic-based estimation of airway size with
correction for scanned plane tilt angle. In: Chen
C-T, Clough AV, editors. SPIE Medical Imaging.
San Diego (CA); 2000. p. 58–66.

[41] Wood SA, Zerhouni EA, Hoford JD, et al.
Measurement of three-dimensional lung tree struc-
tures by using computed tomography. J Appl
Physiol 1995;79:1687–97.

[42] Hoffman EA, Clough AV, Christensen GE, et al.
The comprehensive imaging-based analysis of the
lung: a forum for team science. Acad Radiol
2004;11:1370–80.

[43] Hoffman EA, Reinhardt JM, Sonka M, et al. Characterization of the interstitial lung diseases via den-
sity-based and texture-based analysis of computed
tomography images of lung structure and function.
Acad Radiol 2003;10:1104–18.

[44] Nakano Y, Wong JC, de Jong PA, et al. The prediction of small airway dimensions using computed
tomography. Am J Respir Crit Care Med 2005;
171:142–6.

[45] Wananuki Y, Suzuki S, Nishikawa M, et al. Correlation of quantitative CT with selective alveolo-
bronchogram and pulmonary function tests in
emphysema. Chest 1994;106:806–13.

[46] Kinsella M, Muller NL, Abboud RT, et al. Quantitation of Emphysema by computed tomography
using a "density mask" program and correlation
with pulmonary function tests. Chest 1990;97:
315–21.

[47] Muller NL, Staples CA, Miller RR, et al. "Density
mask". An objective method to quantitate emphysema using computed tomography. Chest 1988;94:
782–7.

[48] Gould GA, Redpath AT, Ryan M, et al. Parenchymal emphysema measured by CT lung density
correlates with lung function in patients with
bullous disease. Eur Respir J 1993;6:698–704.

[49] Stern EJ, Webb WR, Gamsu G. Dynamic quantitative computed tomography: a predictor of pulmonary function in obstructive lung diseases. Invest
Radiol 1994;29:564–9.

[50] Newman KB, Lynch DA, Newman LS, et al. Quantitative computed tomography detects air trapping
due to asthma. Chest 1994;106:105–9.

[51] Millar AB, Fromson B, Strickland BA, et al.
Computed tomography based estimates of regional
gas and tissue volume of the lung in supine subjects
with chronic airflow limitation or fibrosing alveolitis. Thorax 1986;41:932–9.

[52] Rienmuller R, Behr J, Kalender WA. Standardized
quantitative high resolution CT in lung diseases.
J Comput Assisst Tomogr 1991;15:742–9.

[53] Biernacki W, Gould GA, Whyte KF, et al. Pulmonary hemodynamics, gas exchange, and the severity

of emphysema as assessed by quantitative CT scan in chronic bronchitis and emphysema. Am Rev Respir Dis 1989;139:1509–15.

[54] Gould KL. Coronary Artery Stenosis. New York: Elsevier; 1991.

[55] Gould GA, Macnee W, McLean A, et al. CT Measurements of Lung Density in Life can quantitate distal airspace enlargement-an essential defining feature of human emphysema. Am Rev Respir Dis 1988;137:380–92.

[56] Knudson RJ, Standen JR, Kaltenborn WT, et al. Expiratory computed tomography for assessmet of suspected pulmonary emphysema. Chest 1991; 99:1357–66.

[57] Hartley PG, Galvin JR, Hunninghake GW, et al. High-resolution CT-derived measures of lung density are valid indexes of interstitial lung disease. J Appl Physiol 1994;76:271–7.

[58] Hruban RH, Meziane MA, Zerhouni EA, et al. High resolution computed tomography of inflation fixed lungs: pathologic-radiologic correlation of centrilobular emphysema. Am Rev Respir Dis 1987;136:935–40.

[59] Miller RA, Muller NL, Vedal S, et al. Limitations of computed tomography in the assessment of emphysema. Am Rev Respir Dis 1989;139:980–3.

[60] Murata K, Itoh H, Senda M, et al. Stratified impairment of pulmonary ventilation in diffuse-panbronchiolitis. PET and CT studies. J Comput Assist Tomogr 1989;13:48–53.

[61] Webb WR. High-resolution computed tomography of the lung: normal and abnormal anatomy. Semin Roentgenol 1991;26:110–7.

[62] Sanders C. Imaging of emphysema. Seminars in Respiratory Medicine 1992;13:318–30.

[63] Sonka M, Hlavac V, Boyle R. Image Processing, analysis, and machine vision. London: Chapman and Hall; 1993.

[64] Schad LR, Bluml S, Zuna I. MR tissue characterization of intracranial tumors by means of texture analysis. Magn Reson Imaging 1993;11:889–96.

[65] Miller P, Astley S. Classification of breast tissue by texture analysis. Image and Vision Computing 1992;10:277–82.

[66] Wu C, Chen Y. Multi-threshold dimension vector for texture analysis and its application to liver tissue classification. Pattern Recognition 1993;1: 137–44.

[67] McPherson D, Aylward P, Knosp B, et al. Ultrasound chracterization of acute myocardial ischemia by quantitative texture analysis. Ultrason Imaging 1986;8:227–40.

[68] Skorton DJ, Collins SM, Nichols J, et al. Quantitative texture analysis in two-dimensional echocardiography: application to the diagnosis of experimental myocardial contusion. Circulation 1983;68:217–23.

[69] Chandrasekaran K, Aylward PE, Fleagle SR, et al. Feasibility of identifying amyloid and hypertrophic cardiomyopathy with the use of computerized

quantitative texture analysis of clinical echocardiographic data. J Am Coll Cardiol 1989;13:832–40.

[70] Uppaluri R, Mitsa T, Galvin JR. Fractal analysis of high-resolution CT images as a tool for quantification of lung diseases. Proceedings SPIE medical imaging, physiology and function from multidisciplinary images, San Diego, CA, 1995:133–42.

[71] Tully RJ, Conners RW, Harlow CA, et al. Towards computer analysis of pulmonary infiltration. Invest Radiol 1978;13:298–305.

[72] Katsuragawa S, Kunio D, MacMahon H. Image feature analysis and computer-aided diagnosis in digital radiography: classification of normal and abnormal lungs with interstitial disease in chest images. Med Phys 1989;16:38–44.

[73] Adams H, Bernard M, McConnochie K. An appraisal of CT pulmonary density mapping in normal subjects. Clin Radiol 1991;43:238–42.

[74] Fleagle S, Stanford W, Burns T, et al. Feasibility of quantitative texture analysis of cardiac magnetic resonance imagery: Preliminary results. SPIE Medical Imaging 1994;2168:23–32.

[75] Yuan R, Mayo JR, Hogg JC, et al. The effects of radiation dose and CT manufacturer on measurements of lung densitometry. Chest 2007;132: 617–23.

[76] Stolk J, Dirksen A, van der Lugt AA, et al. Repeatability of lung density measurements with low-dose computed tomography in subjects with alpha-1-antitrypsin deficiency-associated emphysema. Invest Radiol 2001;36:648–51.

[77] Shaker SB, Dirksen A, Laursen LC, et al. Volume adjustment of lung density by computed tomography scans in patients with emphysema. Acta Radiol 2004;45:417–23.

[78] Parr DG, Stoel BC, Stolk J, et al. Validation of computed tomographic lung densitometry for monitoring emphysema in alpha1-antitrypsin deficiency. Thorax 2006;61:485–90.

[79] Bakker ME, Stolk J, Putter H, et al. Variability in densitometric assessment of pulmonary emphysema with computed tomography. Invest Radiol 2005;40:777–83.

[80] Matsuoka S, Kurihara Y, Yagihashi K, et al. Quantitative assessment of peripheral airway obstruction on paired expiratory/inspiratory thinsection computed tomography in chronic obstructive pulmonary disease with emphysema. J Comput Assist Tomogr 2007;31:384–9.

[81] Goris ML, Zhu HJ, Blankenberg F, et al. An automated approach to quantitative air trapping measurements in mild cystic fibrosis. Chest 2003;123: 1655–63.

[82] Uppaluri R, Hoffman E, Schwartz D, et al. Quantitative analysis of the chest CT in asbestos-exposed subjects using an adaptive multiple feature method. Am J Respir Crit Care Med 1998;157:A276.

[83] Uppaluri R, Mitsa T, Sonka M, et al. Quantification of pulmonary emphysema from lung ct images

using texture analysis. Am J Respir Crit Care Med 1997;156:248–54.

[84] Uppaluri R, McLennan G, Enright P, et al. AMFM - A quantitative assessment of early parenchymal changes in smokers. Am J Respir Crit Care Med 1998;157:A788.

[85] Xu Y, Sonka M, McLennan G, et al. MDCT-based 3-D texture classification of emphysema and early smoking related lung pathologies. IEEE Trans Med Imaging 2006;25:464–75.

[86] Xu Y, van Beek EJ, Hwanjo Y, et al. Computer-aided classification of interstitial lung diseases via MDCT: 3D adaptive multiple feature method (3D AMFM). Acad Radiol 2006;13:969–78.

[87] Ball W, Stewart P, Newsham L, et al. Regional pulmonary function studied with Xenon133. J Clin Invest 1962;41:519–31.

[88] Jones R, Overton T, Sproule B. Frequency dependence of ventilation distribution in normal and obstructed lungs. J Appl Physiol 1977;42:548–53.

[89] Bunow B, Line B, Horton M, et al. Regional ventilatory clearance by xenon scintigraphy: a critical evaluation of two estimation procedures. J Nucl Med 1979;20:703–10.

[90] Hubmayr R, Walters B, Chevalier PA, et al. Topographical distribution of regional lung volume in anesthetized dogs. J Appl Physiol 1983;54:1048–56.

[91] Fredberg J, Keefe D, Glass G, et al. Alveolar pressure nonhomogeneity during small-amplitude high-frequency oscillation. J Appl Physiol 1984;57:788–800.

[92] van der Mark T, Rookmaker A, Kiers A, et al. Nitrogen-13 and xenon-133 ventilation studies. J Nucl Med 1984;25:1175–82.

[93] Berdine G, Lehr J, McKinley D, et al. Nonuniformity of canine lung washout by high-frequency ventilation. J Appl Physiol 1986;61:1388–94.

[94] Venegas J, Yamada Y, Custer J, et al. Effects of respiratory variables on regional gas transport during high-frequency ventilation. J Appl Physiol 1988;64:2108–18.

[95] Hubmayr R, Hill M, Wilson T. Nonuniform expansion of constricted dog lungs. J Appl Physiol 1996;80:522–30.

[96] Robertson H, Glenny R, Stanford D, et al. High-resolution maps of regional ventilation utilizing inhaled fluorescent microspheres. J Appl Physiol 1997;82:943–53.

[97] Gur D, Drayer BP, Borovetz HS, et al. Dynamic computed tomography of the lung: regional ventilation measurements. J Comput Assist Tomogr 1979;3:749–53.

[98] Gur D, Shabason L, Borovetz HS, et al. Regional pulmonary ventilation measurements by Xenon enhanced dynamic computed tomography: an update. J Appl Phys 1981;5:678–83.

[99] Snyder J, Pennock B, Herbert D, et al. Local lung ventilation in critically ill patients using nonradioactive

xenon-enhanced transmission computed tomography. Crit Care Med 1984;12:46–51.

[100] Murphy DMF, Nicewicz JT, Zabbatino SM, et al. Local pulmonary ventilation using nonradioactive xenon-enhanced ultrafast computed tomography. Chest 1989;96:799–804.

[101] Yonas H, Jungreis C. Xenon CT cerebral blood flow: past, present, and future. AJNR Am J Neuroradiol 1995;16:219–20.

[102] Marcucci C, Simon B. Distribution of regional pulmonary ventilation in prone and supine dogs using xenon-enhanced CT. Faseb Journal 1996;10:A363.

[103] Simon B, Marcucci C, Downie JM. CT measurement of regional specific compliance correlates with specific ventilation in intact dogs. Am J Resp Crit Care Med 1999;159:A480.

[104] Simon B, Chandler D. Regional differences in volume recruitment and ventilation in dogs after acute lung injury (ALI). Am J Respir Crit Care Med 1998;157:A214.

[105] Tajik JK, Tran BQ, Hoffman EA. Xenon enhanced CT imaging of local pulmonary ventilation. SPIE Medical Imaging Physiology and Function from Multidimensional Images 1996;2709:40–54.

[106] Simon B, Marcucci C, Fung M, et al. Parameter estimation and confidence intervals for Xe-CT ventilation studies: a Monte Carlo approach. J Appl Physiol 1998;84:709–16.

[107] Tajik JK, Chon D, Won C, et al. Subsecond multisection CT of regional pulmonary ventilation. Acad Radiol 2002;9:130–46.

[108] Suga K. Technical and analytical advances in pulmonary ventilation SPECT with xenon-133 gas and Tc-99m-Technegas. Ann Nucl Med 2002;16:303–10.

[109] Kreck TC, Krueger MA, Altemeier WA, et al. Determination of regional ventilation and perfusion in the lung using xenon and computed tomography. J Appl Physiol 2001;91:1741–9.

[110] Chon D, Simon BA, Beck KC, et al. Differences in regional wash-in and wash-out time constants for xenon-CT ventilation studies. Respir Physiol Neurobiol 2005;148:65–83.

[111] Chon D, Beck KC, Simon BA, et al. Effect of low-xenon and krypton supplementation on signal/noise of regional CT-based ventilation measurements. J Appl Physiol 2007;102:1535–44.

[112] Coselmon MM, Balter JM, McShan DL, et al. Mutual information based CT registration of the lung at exhale and inhale breathing states using thin-plate splines. Med Phys 2004;31:2942–8.

[113] Ayappa I, Brown LV, Wang PM, et al. Arterial, capillary, and venous transit times and dispersion measured in isolated rabbit lungs. J Appl Physiol 1995;79:261–9.

[114] Capen RL, Latham LP, Wagner WW Jr. Comparison of direct and indirect measurements of

pulmonary capillary transit times. J Appl Physiol 1987;62:1150–4.

[115] Clough AV, Linehan JH, Dawson C. Regional perfusion parameters from pulmonary microfocal angiograms. Am J Physiol 1997;272:H1537–48.

[116] Clough AV, Haworth ST, Hanger CC, et al. Transit time dispersion in the pulmonary arterial tree. J Appl Physiol 1998;85:565–74.

[117] Hoffman EA, Tajik JK. Dynamic and high resolution CT assessment of pulmonary blood flow distributions. Am Rev Respir Dis 1993;147:A201.

[118] Mintun MA, Ter-Pergossian MM, Green MA, et al. Quantitative measurement of regional pulmonary blood flow with positron emission tomography. J Appl Physiol 1986;60:317–26.

[119] Tajik JK, Tan BQ, Hoffman EA. CT-based assessment of regional pulmonary blood flow parameters: an update. In: Chen C-T, Clough AV, editors. Medical imaging 1999: physiology and function from multidimensional images. San Diego: SPIE; 1999. p. 181–7.

[120] Wolfkiel CJ, Rich S. Analysis of regional pulmonary enhancement in dogs by ultrafast computed tomography. Invest Radiol 1992;27:211–6.

[121] Bassingthwaighte JB, Raymond GR, Chan JIS. Principles of tracer kinetics. In: Zaret BL, Beller GA, editors. Nuclear cardiology: state of the art and future directions. St. Louis (MO); 1993. p. 3–23.

[122] Bentley MD, Lerman LO, Hoffman EA, et al. Measurement of renal perfusion and blood flow with fast computed tomography. Circ Res 1994;74: 945–51.

[123] Eigler NL, Schuhlen H, Whiting JS, et al. Digital angiographic impulse response analysis of regional myocardial perfusion. Estimation of coronary flow, flow reserve, and distribution volume by compartmental transit time measurement in a canine model. Circ Res 1991;68:870–80.

[124] Ritman EL. Temporospatial heterogeneity of myocardial perfusion and blood volume in the porcine heart wall. Ann Biomed Eng 1998;26: 519–25.

[125] Musch G, Layfield JD, Harris RS, et al. Topographical distribution of pulmonary perfusion and ventilation, assessed by PET in supine and prone humans. J Appl Physiol 2002;93:1841–51.

[126] Levin DL, Chen Q, Zhang M, et al. Evaluation of regional pulmonary perfusion using ultrafast magnetic resonance imaging. Magn Reson Med 2001; 46:166–71.

[127] Hatabu H, Tadamura E, Levin DL, et al. Quantitative assessment of pulmonary perfusion with dynamic contrast-enhanced MRI. Magn Reson Med 1999;42:1033–8.

[128] Johnson TR, Nikolaou K, Wintersperger BJ, et al. ECG-gated 64-MDCT angiography in the differential diagnosis of acute chest pain. AJR Am J Roentgenol 2007;188:76–82.

[129] Won C, Chon D, Tajik J, et al. CT-based assessment of regional pulmonary microvascular blood flow parameters. J Appl Physiol 2003;94:2483–93.

[130] Chon D, Beck KC, Larsen RL, et al. Regional pulmonary blood flow in dogs by 4D-X-ray CT. J Appl Physiol 2006;101:1451–65.

[131] Hoffman EA, Tajik JK, Kugelmass SD. Matching pulmonary structure and perfusion via combined dynamic multislice CT and thin-slice high-resolution CT. Comput Med Imaging Graph 1995;19: 101–12.

[132] Alford SK, Van Beek EJ, McLennan G, et al. Characterization of smoking related regional alterations in pulmonary perfusion via functional CT. Proceedings of the Annual Meeting of the American Thoracic Society, San Francisco, CA, 2007:A818.

[133] Fuld M, Chon D, Milchak R, et al. Global pulmonary hypoxia causes enhanced perfusion in regions of local inflammation. Proceedings of the Annual Meeting of the American Thoracic Society, San Diego, CA, 2006:A330.

[134] Easley RB, Fuld MK, Fernandez-Bustamante A, et al. Mechanism of hypoxemia in acute lung injury evaluated by multidetector-row CT. Acad Radiol 2006;13:916–21.

[135] Hoffman EA, Simon BA, McLennan G. State of the Art. A structural and functional assessment of the lung via multidetector-row computed tomography: phenotyping chronic obstructive pulmonary disease. Proc Am Thorac Soc 2006;3:519–32.

[136] Yeh EN, Stuber M, McKenzie CA, et al. Inherently self-calibrating non-Cartesian parallel imaging. Magn Reson Med 2005;54:1–8.

[137] Sodickson DK, Manning WJ. Simultaneous acquisition of spatial harmonics (SMASH): fast imaging with radiofrequency coil arrays. Magn Reson Med 1997;38:591–603.

[138] Pruessmann KP, Weiger M, Scheidegger MB, et al. SENSE: sensitivity encoding for fast MRI. Magn Reson Med 1999;42:952–62.

[139] Benamore RE, O'Doherty MJ, Entwisle JJ. Use of imaging in the management of malignant pleural mesothelioma. Clin Radiol 2005;60:1237–47.

[140] Erasmus JJ, Truong MT, Munden RF. CT, MR, and PET imaging in staging of non-small-cell lung cancer. Semin Roentgenol 2005;40:126–42.

[141] Puderbach M, Hintze C, Ley S, et al. MR imaging of the chest: a practical approach at 1.5T. Eur J Radiol 2007.

[142] Swift AJ, Woodhouse N, Fichele S, et al. Rapid lung volumetry using ultrafast dynamic magnetic resonance imaging during forced vital capacity maneuver: correlation with spirometry. Invest Radiol 2007;42:37–41.

[143] Eichinger M, Tetzlaff R, Puderbach M, et al. Proton magnetic resonance imaging for assessment of lung function and respiratory dynamics. Eur J Radiol 2007;64:329–34.

[144] Pedersen MR, Fisher MT, van Beek EJ. MR imaging of the pulmonary vasculature–an update. Eur Radiol 2006;16:1374–86.

[145] Kreitner KF, Kunz RP, Ley S, et al. Chronic thromboembolic pulmonary hypertension—assessment by magnetic resonance imaging. Eur Radiol 2007;17:11–21.

[146] Ley S, Zaporozhan J, Arnold R, et al. Preoperative assessment and follow-up of congenital abnormalities of the pulmonary arteries using CT and MRI. Eur Radiol 2007;17:151–62.

[147] Meaney JF, Weg JG, Chenevert TL, et al. Diagnosis of pulmonary embolism with magnetic resonance angiography. N Engl J Med 1997;336: 1422–7.

[148] Oudkerk M, van Beek EJ, Wielopolski P, et al. Comparison of contrast-enhanced magnetic resonance angiography and conventional pulmonary angiography for the diagnosis of pulmonary embolism: a prospective study. Lancet 2002;359:1643–7.

[149] Ohno Y, Higashino T, Takenaka D, et al. MR angiography with sensitivity encoding (SENSE) for suspected pulmonary embolism: comparison with MDCT and ventilation-perfusion scintigraphy. AJR Am J Roentgenol 2004;183:91–8.

[150] Iwasawa T, Saito K, Ogawa N, et al. Prediction of postoperative pulmonary function using perfusion magnetic resonance imaging of the lung. J Magn Reson Imaging 2002;15:685–92.

[151] Fink C, Puderbach M, Ley S, et al. Time-resolved echo-shared parallel MRA of the lung: observer preference study of image quality in comparison with non-echo-shared sequences. Eur Radiol 2005;15:2070–4.

[152] Ohno Y, Hatabu H, Murase K, et al. Primary pulmonary hypertension: 3D dynamic perfusion MRI for quantitative analysis of regional pulmonary perfusion. AJR Am J Roentgenol 2007;188: 48–56.

[153] Ley S, Mereles D, Risse F, et al. Quantitative 3D pulmonary MR-perfusion in patients with pulmonary arterial hypertension: correlation with invasive pressure measurements. Eur J Radiol 2007; 61:251–5.

[154] Hopkins SR, Garg J, Bolar DS, et al. Pulmonary blood flow heterogeneity during hypoxia and high-altitude pulmonary edema. Am J Respir Crit Care Med 2005;171:83–7.

[155] Roeleveld RJ, Marcus JT, Boonstra A, et al. A comparison of noninvasive MRI-based methods of estimating pulmonary artery pressure in pulmonary hypertension. J Magn Reson Imaging 2005; 22:67–72.

[156] Goodson BM. Nuclear magnetic resonance of laser-polarized noble gases in molecules, materials, and organisms. J Magn Reson 2002;155:157–216.

[157] Albert MS, Cates GD, Driehuys B, et al. Biological magnetic resonance imaging using laser-polarized 129Xe. Nature 1994;370:199–201.

[158] Middleton H, Black RD, Saam B, et al. MR imaging with hyperpolarized 3He gas. Magn Reson Med 1995;33:271–5.

[159] Black RD, Middleton HL, Cates GD, et al. In vivo He-3 MR images of guinea pig lungs. Radiology 1996;199:867–70.

[160] Ruset I, Hersman F. Novel low-pressure production method for hyperpolarized Xenon. Proceedings of the 11th Annual Scientific Meeting of the ISMRM, Toronto, Canada, 2003:514.

[161] Ruset IC, Ketel S, Hersman FW. Optical pumping system design for large production of hyperpolarized. Phys Rev Lett 2006;96:053002.

[162] Patz S, Hersman FW, Muradian I, et al. Hyperpolarized (129)Xe MRI: a viable functional lung imaging modality? Eur J Radiol 2007;64:335–44.

[163] Darasse L, Guillot G, Nacher P, et al. Low-field 3He nuclear magnetic resonance in human lungs. CR Acad Sci II B 1997;324:691–700.

[164] Durand E, Guillot G, Darrasse L, et al. CPMG measurements and ultrafast imaging in human lungs with hyperpolarized helium-3 at low field (0.1 T). Magn Reson Med 2002;47:75–81.

[165] Mair RW, Hrovat MI, Patz S, et al. 3He lung imaging in an open access, very-low-field human magnetic resonance imaging system. Magn Reson Med 2005;53:745–9.

[166] Wild JM, Schmiedeskamp J, Paley MN, et al. MR imaging of the lungs with hyperpolarized helium-3 gas transported by air. Phys Med Biol 2002;47: N185–90.

[167] de Lange E, Altes T, Wright C, et al. Hyperbolized gas MR imaging of the lung: safety assessment of inhaled helium-3. Proceedings of the 89th Scientific Assembly and Annual Meeting of the Radiological Society of North America, Chicago, IL, 2003: 525.

[168] Woodhouse N, Wild J, Mills G, et al. Comparision of hyperolarized 3 He adminstration methods in healthly and diseased subjects. Proceedings of the 14th Annual Scientific Meeting of the International Society of Magnetic Resonance in Medicine, Seattle, WA, 2006:1288.

[169] Wild JM, Woodhouse N, Paley MN, et al. Comparison between 2D and 3D gradient-echo sequences for MRI of human lung ventilation with hyperpolarized 3He. Magn Reson Med 2004;52:673–8.

[170] van Beek E, Wild J, Schreiber W, et al. Functional MRI of the lungs using hyperpolarized 3-helium gas. J Magn Reson Imaging 2004;20:540–54.

[171] de Lange EE, Altes TA, Patrie JT, et al. Evaluation of asthma with hyperpolarized helium-3 MRI: correlation with clinical severity and spirometry. Chest 2006;130:1055–62.

[172] de Lange EE, Altes TA, Patrie JT, et al. The variability of regional airflow obstruction within the lungs of patients with asthma: assessment with hyperpolarized helium-3 magnetic resonance imaging. J Allergy Clin Immunol 2007;119:1072–8.

[173] Donnelly LF, MacFall JR, McAdams HP, et al. Cystic fibrosis: combined hyperpolarized 3He-enhanced and conventional proton MR imaging in the lung–preliminary observations. Radiology 1999;212:885–9.

[174] van Beek EJ, Hill C, Woodhouse N, et al. Assessment of lung disease in children with cystic fibrosis using hyperpolarized 3-Helium MRI: comparison with Shwachman score, Chrispin-Norman score and spirometry. Eur Radiol 2007;17:1018–24.

[175] McMahon C, Dodd J, Hill C, et al. Hyperpolarized 3Helium magnetic resonance ventilation imaging in patients with cystic fibrosis: correlation with high resolution CT and spirometry. Eur Radiol 2006; 16:2483–90.

[176] Mentore K, Froh DK, de Lange EE, et al. Hyperpolarized HHe 3 MRI of the lung in cystic fibrosis: assessment at baseline and after bronchodilator and airway clearance treatment. Acad Radiol 2005;12:1423–9.

[177] Ireland RH, Bragg CM, McJury M, et al. Feasibility of image registration and intensity-modulated radiotherapy planning with hyperpolarized helium-3 magnetic resonance imaging for non-small-cell lung cancer. Int J Radiat Oncol Biol Phys 2007;68:273–81.

[178] MacFall JR, Charles HC, Black RD, et al. Human lung air spaces: potential for MR imaging with hyperpolarized He-3. Radiology 1996;200:553–8.

[179] Kauczor HU, Hofmann D, Kreitner KF, et al. Normal and abnormal pulmonary ventilation: visualization at hyperpolarized He-3 MR imaging. Radiology 1996;201:564–8.

[180] de Lange EE, Mugler JP 3rd, Brookeman JR, et al. Lung air spaces: MR imaging evaluation with hyperpolarized 3He gas. Radiology 1999;210:851–7.

[181] Guenther D, Eberle B, Hast J, et al. (3)He MRI in healthy volunteers: preliminary correlation with smoking history and lung volumes. NMR Biomed 2000;13:182–9.

[182] Samee S, Altes T, Powers P, et al. Imaging the lungs in asthmatic patients by using hyperpolarized helium-3 magnetic resonance: assessment of response to methacholine and exercise challenge. J Allergy Clin Immunol 2003;111:1205–11.

[183] Woodhouse N, Wild JM, Paley MN, et al. Combined helium-3/proton magnetic resonance imaging measurement of ventilated lung volumes in smokers compared to never-smokers. J Magn Reson Imaging 2005;21:365–9.

[184] McAdams HP, Palmer SM, Donnelly LF, et al. Hyperpolarized 3He-enhanced MR imaging of lung transplant recipients: preliminary results. AJR Am J Roentgenol 1999;173:955–9.

[185] Zaporozhan J, Ley S, Gast KK, et al. Functional analysis in single-lung transplant recipients: a comparative study of high-resolution CT, 3He-MRI, and pulmonary function tests. Chest 2004;125:173–81.

[186] Gast KK, Zaporozhan J, Ley S, et al. (3)He-MRI in follow-up of lung transplant recipients. Eur Radiol 2004;14:78–85.

[187] Woods JC, Choong CK, Yablonskiy DA, et al. Hyperpolarized 3He diffusion MRI and histology in pulmonary emphysema. Magn Reson Med 2006;56:1293–300.

[188] Woods JC, Yablonskiy DA, Choong CK, et al. Long-range diffusion of hyperpolarized 3He in explanted normal and emphysematous human lungs via magnetization tagging. J Appl Physiol 2005;99:1992–7.

[189] Wang C, Miller GW, Altes TA, et al. Time dependence of 3He diffusion in the human lung: measurement in the long-time regime using stimulated echoes. Magn Reson Med 2006;56:296–309.

[190] Morbach AE, Gast KK, Schmiedeskamp J, et al. Diffusion-weighted MRI of the lung with hyperpolarized helium-3: a study of reproducibility. J Magn Reson Imaging 2005;21:765–74.

[191] Saam BT, Yablonskiy DA, Kodibagkar VD, et al. MR imaging of diffusion of (3)He gas in healthy and diseased lungs. Magn Reson Med 2000;44: 174–9.

[192] Owers-Bradley JR, Fichele S, Bennattayalah A, et al. MR tagging of human lungs using hyperpolarized 3He gas. J Magn Reson Imaging 2003;17: 142–6.

[193] Schreiber WG, Morbach AE, Stavngaard T, et al. Assessment of lung microstructure with magnetic resonance imaging of hyperpolarized Helium-3. Respir Physiol Neurobiol 2005;148:23–42.

[194] Swift AJ, Wild JM, Fichele S, et al. Emphysematous changes and normal variation in smokers and COPD patients using diffusion 3He MRI. Eur J Radiol 2005;54:352–8.

[195] Fain SB, Altes TA, Panth SR, et al. Detection of age-dependent changes in healthy adult lungs with diffusion-weighted 3He MRI. Acad Radiol 2005;12:1385–93.

[196] Altes TA, Mata J, de Lange EE, et al. Assessment of lung development using hyperpolarized helium-3 diffusion MR imaging. J Magn Reson Imaging 2006;24:1277–83.

[197] Salerno M, de Lange EE, Altes TA, et al. Emphysema: hyperpolarized helium 3 diffusion MR imaging of the lungs compared with spirometric indexes–initial experience. Radiology 2002;222: 252–60.

[198] Fain SB, Panth SR, Evans MD, et al. Early emphysematous changes in asymptomatic smokers: detection with 3He MR imaging. Radiology 2006;239: 875–83.

[199] Fichele S, Woodhouse N, Said Z, et al. MRI of Helium-3 Gas in Healthy Lungs: posture related variations of alveolar size. J Magn Reson Imaging 2004;20:331–5.

[200] Salerno M, Altes TA, Brookeman JR, et al. Dynamic spiral MRI of pulmonary gas flow using hyperpolarized (3)He: preliminary studies in healthy and diseased lungs. Magn Reson Med 2001;46:667–77.

[201] Wild JM, Paley MN, Kasuboski L, et al. Dynamic radial projection MRI of inhaled hyperpolarized 3He gas. Magn Reson Med 2003;49:991–7.

[202] Dupuich D, Berthezene Y, Clouet PL, et al. Dynamic 3He imaging for quantification of regional lung ventilation parameters. Magn Reson Med 2003;50:777–83.

[203] Koumellis P, van Beek EJ, Woodhouse N, et al. Quantitative analysis of regional airways obstruction using dynamic hyperpolarized 3He MRI - preliminary results in children with cystic fibrosis. J Magn Reson Imaging 2005;22(3):420–6.

[204] Eberle B, Weiler N, Markstaller K, et al. Analysis of intrapulmonary O(2) concentration by MR imaging of inhaled hyperpolarized helium-3. J Appl Physiol 1999;87:2043–52.

[205] Deninger AJ, Eberle B, Ebert M, et al. (3)he-MRI-based measurements of intrapulmonary p(O2) and its time course during apnea in healthy volunteers: first results, reproducibility, and technical limitations. NMR Biomed 2000;13:194–201.

[206] Deninger AJ, Eberle B, Bermuth J, et al. Assessment of a single-acquisition imaging sequence for oxygen-sensitive (3)He-MRI. Magn Reson Med 2002;47:105–14.

[207] Wild JM, Fichele S, Woodhouse N, et al. 3D volume-localized pO2 measurement in the human lung with 3He MRI. Magn Reson Med 2005;53:1055–64.

[208] Cremillieux Y, Berthezene Y, Humblot H, et al. A combined 1H perfusion/3He ventilation NMR study in rat lungs. Magn Reson Med 1999;41:645–8.

[209] Hong C, Leawoods JC, Yablonskiy DA, et al. Feasibility of combining MR perfusion, angiography, and 3He ventilation imaging for evaluation of lung function in a porcine model. Acad Radiol 2005;12:202–9.

Clin Chest Med 29 (2008) 217–223

Index

Note: Page numbers of article titles are in **boldface** type.

A

Acquired immunodeficiency syndrome (AIDS). See *AIDS.*

ACR. See *American College of Radiology (ACR).*

Acute interstitial pneumonia, imaging of, 133–135

AIDS, patients with, infections in
 detection of, 93–94
 imaging of, 93–101
  bacterial infections, 95
  fungal infections, 98–101
  mycobacterial infections, 96–99
  Pneumocystis jiroveci pneumonia, 95–96
  radiologic patterns, 94–95
  viral infections, 101

Air bronchiolograms, CT of, 23

Air bronchograms, CT of, 23

Airway(s)
 large
  anatomy of, 181–183
  imaging of, **181–193**
   CT in, 183–184. See also
    Multidetector-row CT (MDCT);
    specific disorder and Computed
    tomography (CT).
 small
  anatomy of, 165–166
  normal, CT findings in, 165–166

Airways disease
 intrinsic, in connective tissue disease,
  histopathological aspects of, 150
 radiologic detection of, HRCT in, 153
 small, inflammatory, imaging of, 169–172

AJCC. See *American Joint Committee on Cancer (AJCC).*

Aluminum pneumoconiosis, imaging of, 125–126

American Cancer Society, 39

American College of Radiology (ACR), 59

American Joint Committee on Cancer (AJCC), 39

American Society of Clinical Oncology (ASCO), 39

Anatomy, of large airways, 181–183

Angiography, magnetic resonance, in pulmonary thromboembolism, 113

Arteriography, pulmonary, imaging of, 108

Arthritis, rheumatoid, pulmonary complications of, 154

Asbestos-related disorders, imaging of, 120–124

ASCO. See *American Society of Clinical Oncology (ASCO).*

Aspiration, imaging of, in ICU, 70

Atelectasis, imaging of, in ICU, 66–69

B

Bacterial infections
 in AIDS patients, imaging of, 95
 in non-AIDS immune compromised hosts,
  imaging of, CT in, 92

Berylliosis, 124

Biomarker(s), molecular, in lung cancer screening, 10–12

Biopsy(ies), transthoracic needle, in SPN evaluation, 34–36

Bronchiolitis
 cellular, imaging of, 169–170
 classification of, image-based, 167
 constrictive, imaging of, 172–174
 CT signs of, 168
 follicular, imaging of, 171
 respiratory, imaging of, 172

Bronchus(i), tracheal, imaging of, CT in, 190

"Bubbly" lucencies, CT of, 23

0272-5231/08/$ - see front matter © 2008 Elsevier Inc. All rights reserved.
doi:10.1016/S0272-5231(08)00016-6